ADVANCES IN NEUROLOGY

Volume 99

ADVANCES IN NEUROLOGY

Volume 99

Tourette Syndrome

Editors

John T. Walkup, MD
Associate Professor
Division of Child and Adolescent Psychiatry
Department of Psychiatry and Behavioral Sciences
The Johns Hopkins Medical Institutions
Baltimore, Maryland

Jonathan W. Mink, MD, PhD
Associate Professor
Departments of Neurology, Neurobiology & Anatomy, and Pediatrics
Chief
University of Rochester
Division of Child Neurology
Golisano Children's Hospital at Strong Memorial
Rochester, New York

Peter J. Hollenbeck, PhD
Professor and Associate Head
Department of Biological Sciences
Purdue University
West Lafayette, Indiana

Lippincott Williams & Wilkins
a Wolters Kluwer business
Philadelphia · Baltimore · New York · London
Buenos Aires · Hong Kong · Sydney · Tokyo

Aquisitions Editor: Frances DeStefano
Managing Editor: Scott Scheidt
Project Manager: Fran Gunning
Marketing Manager: Kathy Neely
Manufacturing Manager: Ben Rivera
Design Coordinator: Doug Smock
Production Services: Nesbitt Graphics, Inc.
Printer: Edwards Brothers

© 2006 by Lippincott Williams & Wilkins
530 Walnut Street
Philadelphia, PA 19106 USA
www.LWW.com

Library of Congress Cataloging-in-Publication Data

ISBN : 0781799708
ISSN : 0091-3952

Care has been taken to confirm the accuracy of the information presented and to describe generally accepted practices. However, the authors, editors, and publisher are not responsible for errors or omissions or for any consequences from application of the information in this book and make no warranty, expressed or implied, with respect to the currency, completeness, or accuracy of the contents of the publication. Application of this information in a particular situation remains the professional responsibility of the practitioner.

The authors, editors, and publisher have exerted every effort to ensure that drug selection and dosage set forth in this text are in accordance with current recommendations and practice at the time of publication. However, in view of ongoing research, changes in government regulations, and the constant flow of information relating to drug therapy and drug reactions, the reader is urged to check the package insert for each drug for any change in indications and dosage and for added warnings and precautions. This is particularly important when the recommended agent is a new or infrequently employed drug.

Some drugs and medical devices presented in this publication have Food and Drug Administration (FDA) clearance for limited use in restricted research settings. It is the responsibility of the health care provider to ascertain the FDA status of each drug or device planned for use in their clinical practice.

To purchase additional copies of this book, call our customer service department at (800) 638-3030 or fax orders to (301) 223-2320. International customers should call (301) 223-2300.

Visit Lippincott Williams & Wilkins on the Internet: at http://www.LWW.com. Lippincott Williams & Wilkins customer service representatives are available from 8:30 am to 6 pm, EST.

10 9 8 7 6 5 4 3 2 1

Advances in Neurology Series

Contents

Section 5: Genetics and Molecular Biology of TS

Section 6: Immunology and TS

Section 7: Epidemiology and Defining the Phenotype

Section 8: Advances in Treatment

Contributing Authors

Roger L. Albin, MD
Professor
Department of Neurology
University of Michigan
Ann Arbor, Michigan

Chief, Neuroscience Research
GREXX
Ann Arbor VAMC
Ann Arbor, Michigan

Judy Applegate
Yale University School of Nursing
New Haven, Connecticut

Juliana Belo Diniz, MD
Resident
Institute of Psychiatry
University of São Paulo Medical School
São Paulo, Brazil

Cathy L. Budman, MD
Associate Professor
Department of Psychiatry and Neurology
New York University
New York, New York

Director, Movement Disorders in Psychiatry
Department of Psychiatry and Neurology
North Shore Hospital-LIJ Health System
Manhasset, New York

Geraldo F. Busatto, MD, PhD
Associate Professor
Department of Psychiatry
University of São Paulo
São Paulo, Brazil

Tracy Butler, MD
Assistant Professor of Neurology
  in Psychiatry
Department of Psychiatry, Functional
  Neuroimaging Laboratory
Weill Medical College of Cornell University
New York, New York

Assistant Attending Neurologist
Departments of Psychiatry and Neurology
Division of Neuropsychiatry
New York Presbyterian Hospital
White Plains, New York

Susanna W. Chang, PhD
Psychologist
Department of Psychiatry and Biobehavioral Sciences
University of California, Los Angeles
Medical Psychology Program
UCLA Neuropsychiatric Hospital
Los Angeles, California

Barbara J. Coffey, MD, MS
Associate Professor
Department of Psychiatry
New York University School of Medicine
New York, New York

Director
Institute for Tourette's and Movement Disorders
NYU Child Study Center
NYU School of Medicine
New York, New York

Christine A. Conelea, BA
Graduate Student
Department of Psychology
University of Wisconsin-Milwaukee
Milwaukee, Wisconsin

Martha Bridge Denckla, MD
Batza Family Endowed Chair
Director, Developmental Cognitive Neurology
Kennedy Krieger Institute

Professor, Neurology, Pediatrics, Psychiatry
John Hopkins University School of Medicine
Baltimore, Maryland

Jennifer DeWolfe, DO
Epilepsy Fellow
Department of Neurology
Division of Clinical Neurophysiology
The University of Alabama at Birmingham
Birmingham, Alabama

Leon S. Dure IV, MD
Bew White Professor of Pediatrics
Department of Pedicatrics and Neurology
The University of Alabama at Birmingham

Director, Division of Pediatric Neurology
Department of Pediatrics
The Children's Hospital of Alabama
Birmingham, Alabama

Paula J. Edge, AA
Senior Behavior Program Specialist
Division of Child & Adolescent Psychiatry
Department of Psychiatry
University of Florida
Gainesville, Florida

Ygor A. Ferrão, MD, PhD
Professor, Department of Anatomy
Centro Universit rio Metodista IPA
Porto Alegre, Rio Grande do Sul, Brazil

Director, Department of Psychiatry
Hospital São Pedro
Porto Alegre, Rio Grande do Sul, Brazil

Kenneth D. Gadow, PhD
Professor, Department of Psychiatry
State University of New York
Stony Brook, New York

Roseli Gendaki Shavitt, MD, PhD
Pos Doctoral Student
Institute of Psychiatry
University of São Paulo Medical School
São Paulo, Brazil

Donald L. Gilbert, MD, MS
Associate Professor of Pediatrics and Neurology
Department of Neurology
Cincinnati Children's Hospital Medical Center
Cincinnati, Ohio

Gavin Giovannoni, MD
Reader in Neuroimmunology
Department of Neuroinflammation
Institute of Neurology, UCL

Honorary Consultant Neurologist
Department of Clinical Neurology
National Hospital for Neurology and Neurosurgery,
  UCLH
London, United Kingdom

Ana Gabriela Hounie, MD, PhD
Pos-Doctorate Fellow
Department of Psychiatry
Faculty of Medicina
University of São Paulo
São Paulo, Brazil

Michael B. Himle, MS
Graduate Student
Department of Psychology
University of Wisconsin-Milwaukee
Milwaukee, Wisconsin

Peter J. Hollenbeck, PhD
Professor and Associate Head
Department of Biological Sciences
Purdue University
West Lafayette, Indiana

David S. Husted, MD
Fourth Year Resident
Division of Child & Adolescent Psychiatry
Department of Psychiatry
University of Florida
Gainesville, Florida

Cornelia L. Illmann, PhD
Instructor, Department of Psychiatry
Harvard Medical School

Research Assistant
Center for Human Genetic Research
Massachusetts General Hospital
Boston, Massachusetts

Joseph Jankovic, MD
Professor of Neurology
Director, Parkinson's Disease Center
  and Movement Disorders Clinic
Department of Neurology
Baylor College of Medicine
Houston, Texas

Nancy M. P. King, JD
Professor, Department of Medicine
School of Medicine
University of North Carolina-Chapel Hill
Chapel Hill, North Carolina

Robert A. King, MD
Professor of Child Psychiatry, Medical Director,
Tourette's Disorder/OCD Clinic
Yale Child Study Center
Yale University School of Medicine
New Haven, Connecticut

Attending Physician
Yale-New Haven Hospital
New Haven, Connecticut

Roger Kurlan, MD
Professor, Department of Neurology
University of Rochester
Rochester, New York

Attending Neurologist
Department of Neurology
Strong Memorial Hospital
Rochester, New York

James F. Leckman
Yale University Child Study Center
New Haven, Connecticut

Antonio Carlos Lopes, MD
Research Psychiatrist
Department of Psychiatry
Faculty of Medicine, University of São Paulo
São Paulo, Brazil

Donald A. Malone Jr., MD
Staff Psychiatrist
Section Head, Adult Psychiatric Services
Department of Psychiatry
Cleveland Clinic Foundation
Cleveland, Ohio

Meghan M. McGinn, BA
Research Assistant
Center for Human Genetic Research
Massachusetts General Hospital
Boston, Massachusetts

William M. McMahon
Tourette Research Program
University of Utah
Division of Child and Adolescent Psychiatry
Salt Lake City, Utah

Nicte Mejia, MD
Research Assistant, Department of Neurology
Baylor College of Medicine
Houston, Texas

Marcos T. Mercadante, MD, PhD
Associate Professor, PDD Program
Mackenzie Presbyterian University
São Paulo, Brazil

Euripedes Constantino Miguel, MD, PhD
Associate Professor
Department of Psychiatry
Faculty of Medicine
University of São Paulo
São Paulo, Brazil

Jonathan W. Mink, MD, PhD
Associate Professor
Department of Neurology, Neurobiology
* and Anatomy, Pediatrics*
University of Rochester
Rochester, New York

Chief, Department of Child Neurology
Golisano Children's Hospital at Strong Memorial
Rochester, New York

Tanya K. Murphy, MD
Associate Professor and Chief
Division of Child & Adolescent Psychiatry
Department of Psychiatry
University of Florida
Gainesville, Florida

Michael Orth, MD, PhD
Department of Neurology
Universitatsklinikum Eppendorf
Hamburg, Germany

Mayur Pandya, DO
Resident, Department of Psychiatry
Cleveland Clinic Foundation
Cleveland, Ohio

David L. Pauls, MD
Professor, Department of Psychiatry
Harvard Medical School

Psychiatry/Center for Human Genetic Research
Massachusetts General Hospital
Boston, Massachusetts

John C. Piacentini, PhD, ABPP
Professor, Department of Psychiatry and
* Biobehavioral Sciences*
University of California, Los Angeles

Chief Child Psychologist
Medical Psychology Program
UCLA Neurospychiatric Hospital
Los Angels, California

Mary Robertson
Emeritus Professor
Department of Mental Health Sciences
University College London
London, United Kingdom

Consultant, Department of Neurology
St. George's Hospital
London, United Kingdom

Maria Conceição do Rosario-Campos, MD, PhD
Researcher, OCD Spectrum Disorder Project
University of São Paulo
São Paulo, Brazil

Lawrence Scahill
Associate Professor of Nursing
* and Child Psychiatry*
Yale Child Study Center
New Haven, Connecticut

Mary Schwab-Stone
Yale University Child Study Center
New Haven, Connecticut

Rachel L. Shechter, BA
Project Associate
Institute for Tourette's and Movement Disorders
NYU Child Study Center, NYU School of Medicine
New York, New York

Harvey S. Singer, MD
Haller Professor of Pediatric Neurology
Department of Neurology and Pediatrics
Johns Hopkins University School of Medicine
Baltimore, Maryland

Director, Child Neurology
Department of Neurology and Pediatrics
Johns Hopkins Hospital
Baltimore, Maryland

David Silbersweig, MD
Associate Professor
Department of Psychiatry, Neurology
Weill Medical College of Cornell University

Associate Attending Physician
Department of Psychiatry, Neurology
New York Presbyterian Hospital
New York, New York

Emily Stern, MD
Assistant Professor
Department of Psychiatry
Weill Medical College of Cornell University
New York, New York

Ashley N. Sutherland, BS
Graduate Student
Department of Psychology

San Diego State University
San Diego, California

Jeffrey Sverd, MD
Associate Professor of Clinical Psychiatry
Department of Psychiatry and Behavioral Science
State University of New York at Stony Brook
Health Sciences Center
Stony Brook, New York

Medical Director, Children's Psychiatric Inpatient
Department of Psychiatry and Behavioral Science
University Hospital
State University of New York at Stony Brook
Stony Brook, New York

Neal R. Swerdlow, MD, PhD
Professor
Department of Psychiatry
UCSD School of Medicine
La Jolla, California

Phillip N. Williams
Departments of Neurology and Pediatrics
Johns Hopkins University School of Medicine
Baltimore, Maryland

Susan Williams
Yale University, Child Study Center
New Haven, Connecticut

Douglas W. Woods, PhD
Associate Professor
Department of Psychology
University of Wisconsin-Milwaukee
Milwaukee, Wisconsin

Preface

Tourette Syndrome (TS) is a neurobehavioral disorder characterized by a persistent pattern of motor and vocal tics. Motor tics can be expressed as brief, rapid and darting movements of the face, shoulders, and extremities, or manifest as more complex and purposeful movements. Vocal tics may be simple sounds such as sniffing, grunting, and throat clearing or more complex vocalizations such as repeated words and phrases. Tics have a waxing and waning course with a peak severity in early teenage years; many individuals experience improvement in adulthood. Despite the overall positive prognosis, a minority of those affected have more severe symptoms and a persistent course into adulthood. The exact cause of TS is unknown; however, genetic and environmental factors both play a role. Dysfunction of cortical and subcortical regions, circuitry involving the thalamus, basal ganglia, and the frontal cortex, in addition to the neurotransmitters on which these regions and circuits depend have all been implicated in the etiology of TS.

In addition to tics, people with TS often experience an array of concomitant problems that for some patients can be more disabling than tics themselves and are often the reason for seeking medical help. The range of these difficulties is broad and includes problems with attention and learning, impulse control, obsessive-compulsive behaviors, other anxiety and mood disorders, as well as difficulties with living and adaptation. Treatments for the myriad of problems faced by some people with TS are available and often effective, but much more needs to be done to identify improved treatments and pinpoint the underlying mechanisms of their efficacy.

Founded in 1972, the Tourette Syndrome Association (TSA) has been the major driving force in scientific and clinical progress relevant to TS. For more than 30 years, this small family/patient-based organization has been highly effective in using its modest resources to steadfastly encourage interest in TS research and directly support talented investigators and promising scientific initiatives in the field. Many of the new research findings presented at the Fourth International Scientific and Clinical Symposium and included in this volume are the direct result of past and current TSA-funding as well as TSA's active facilitation of large collaborative research consortia in genetics, neuroimaging, clinical trials, and the behavioral sciences.

The TSA is equally effective in broadly disseminating research findings among the professional community. The Fourth International Scientific and Clinical Symposium is part of the TSA's concerted effort to identify current research advances, disseminate them among the scientific and clinical communities, and establish networks of basic and clinical scientists from all over the world. As with the published proceedings of the First, Second, and Third International Scientific Symposia (*Advances in Neurology* volumes 35, 58, and 85), it is anticipated that this volume of *Advances in Neurology* will once again serve as an important reference book for the field.

The Fourth Symposium was convened at a time of an unprecedented increase in TS-related publications, grant activity, and heightened public awareness of TS. This confluence of factors provided an excellent opportunity for a summary review of all recently published and ongoing research activities. TS research advances have emanated from studies across many relevant disciplines, including phenomenology, epidemiology, genetics, neuroimaging, neurophysiology, neuroimmunology neuropathology, and clinical trials (medication and non-medication). Because TS research in each field is informed and thereby influenced by findings from the other fields, the symposium program emphasized information flow and communication across disciplines, as clearly reflected in this volume. Indeed, such cross fertilization is vital for the effective study of this disorder into the future.

A Medline search of the term *Tourette* completed prior to the symposium listed 517 newly published reports since the Third International Scientific Symposium in 1999. This high level of productivity reflects the rapid advances in TS science, which is accelerating at an exponential rate (figure below). Even these publication data underestimate the true rate of advances, as several National Institutes of Health-funded efforts in TS science are underway and on the verge of reporting new findings in important areas of investigation. A brief summary of progress discussed at the Fourth International Scientific Symposium and reviewed in this volume is provided here.

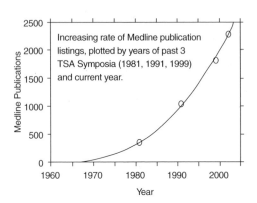

Increasing rate of Medline publication listings, plotted by years of past 3 TSA Symposia (1981, 1991, 1999) and current year.

PHENOMENOLOGY AND EPIDEMIOLOGY

New findings reported since the Third International Scientific Symposium in 1999 greatly alter the way clinicians view several clinical features of TS. Careful epidemiologic studies now estimate the prevalence of TS to be substantially higher than previously thought (1—6). Furthermore, new studies highlight important findings regarding the longitudinal outcome of TS (7), suggesting that symptoms may extend longer into adulthood than was previously believed to occur in most TS patients (8). New, important descriptive information regarding the clinical phenomenology of TS is now available. This information relates to issues such as sensory tics (9,10), anger and explosive outbursts (11), and co-morbid attention deficit hyperactivity disorder (12), obsessive compulsive disorder (7,13—18) and other psychiatric (19) and neurologic disorders.

GENETICS

Progress in TS genetics has occurred in four important areas. Perhaps most importantly, technological advances have made possible approaches to the identification of susceptibility genes that were unheard of even 10 years ago. In addition, several key developments have occurred. First, the TSA has supported the creation of a clinical database that facilitates the identification of empirically derived phenotypes for TS that will be critical for identifying susceptibility gene(s) for TS. Second, the TSA International Genetic Consortium has collected a very large number of sib-pairs and trios as part of its National Institutes of Mental Health-funded sib-pair study. Data from this grant plus existing data on large extended families comprise a large and detailed data set that will allow for varied and complex approaches to identifying the susceptibility genes for TS. Third, individuals with TS and their families who have chromosomal rearrangements affecting regions previously linked to TS, and/or genes for brain substrates implicated in the pathophysiology of this disorder have been identified (20—22). These rare families also provide an important and highly informative approach to finding chromosomal regions with susceptibility genes for TS. Lastly, work in other areas have identified or supported (via association and mutation screening studies) potential candidate genes of interest to TS (23,24).

NEUROIMAGING

The past 4 years have seen an acceleration in the number of studies of volumetric and neurochemical neuroimaging in TS patients (25–35). Studies have employed novel, semi-automated and automated segmentation and voxel classification approaches to identify cortical and subcortical volumetric differences and differential hemispheric asymmetries between TS and control subjects. Moreover, positron emission tomography has been used to identify increased [18F] fluorodopa accumulation in the left caudate and right midbrain as well as increased binding of vesicular monoamine transporter type-2 (VMAT2) positron emission tomography ligand in the ventral striatum of individuals with TS. Advances in neurochemical imaging have applied on-line activation strategies to identify regional neurochemical and blood oxygen-level dependent patterns associated both with tic expression, and with functional/cognitive deficits in TS patients. On the "cutting edge" of this field, sib-pairs from genetic studies described above have undergone detailed MRI-based morphometric analyses as part of a novel strategy to identify heritable neuroanatomical abnormalities that will serve as endophenotypic markers for identifying TS genes.

NEUROPHYSIOLOGY AND NEUROPATHOLOGY

Attempts to characterize the functional deficits in TS and link them to specific brain mechanisms are enhanced by studies of TS neurophysiology and neuropathology. Since 1999, a number of important findings have linked TS to quantifiable deficits in laboratory measures of automatic and volitional response inhibition (36–41). Ultimately, these new physiological markers may have utility across a number of research domains, ranging from genetics (via their potential use as endophenotypes) to drug development.

New TS neuropathology studies have taken advantage of the recent acquisitions to the TSA sponsored brain bank (42–44). Although these are small studies, they represent a significant addition to the six TS cases that previously constituted the entire TS neuropathology literature. These new reports identify regional cortical and subcortical differences in cell counts and neurochemistry that may impact the design and interpretation of TS studies at several levels, from neuroimaging to animal models.

CLINICAL TRIALS

Since the 1999 symposium, several new, controlled clinical trials for TS therapeutics have been reported. These have included trials that focus specifically on tic suppression (45), common co-occurring conditions such as attention deficit hyperactivity disorder (46) and obsessive compulsive disorder (47–49) as well as novel strategies for the treatment of tics that deviate substantially from past approaches to pharmacotherapy of tics, including the use of delta 9-tetrahydrocannabinol (50), direct and indirect dopamine agonists (51,52) and botulinum toxin (53). Very well-designed studies have also yielded negative findings that are equally important to disseminate to the TS community (54–56). Highly promising applications of targeted behavioral therapies have now been validated in controlled studies (57,58) and novel clinical uses of these therapies are being explored (59–61). In response to this important work the TSA developed a Behavioral Sciences Consortium. Members of this group have recently received National Institutes of Health funding for both a child and adolescent, and an adult multisite clinical trial. Finally, although controversial, reports on behavioral neurosurgical approaches to TS, (62,63) including deep brain stimulation T (63,64), may be the precursor to safer and more effective procedures in the future. In this regard, the TSA Medical and Scientific Advisory Boards have just recently completed a manuscript with recommendations for the evaluation of patients with TS prior to deep brain stimulation (Mink et al., under review).

TOURETTE SYNDROME AND AUTOIMMUNITY

One of the most important and controversial areas of TS science involves the relationship between TS and brain injury associated with group A beta-hemolytic streptococcal infections, or other infectious processes. In August 2000, the TSA and National Institutes of Health co-sponsored a Round-table Forum on Pediatric Autoimmune Disorders Associated with Streptococcus (PANDAS), and a detailed report from this meeting was published on the internet. This report distilled information from multiple sources to identify critical gaps in knowledge about PANDAS and its relationship to TS and also to establish critical research questions designed to bridge these gaps. In addition, during the past 5 years, a number of important theoretical and empirical reports were published that bear directly on this critical topic, including findings of: A) elevated antineuronal antibodies in TS sera directed specifically against striatal neurons (65–69); B) increased antistreptococcal M12 and M19 proteins in TS sera (70), and C) the development of a potential animal model based on behavioral and neuropathological changes after intrastriatal infusion of TS sera into rat striatum (71) that was not replicated in a similar study [Loiselle et al., 2004].

This volume reflects the significant advances and breadth of TS science, yet much more research needs to be done. Clinicians now know more about the phenomenology of TS than ever before, including some basic understanding of TS subtypes. But there is still controversy regarding how best to classify TS. The specific issue in question involves how closely TS is linked to other movement disorders or other psychiatric disorders characterized by repetitive behaviors. Although there is a much better understanding of the prevalence of tics and TS, researchers still lack the kind of epidemiologic data that facilitates powerful advocacy for the specific needs of people with TS across the life span. Years of research into the genetics of TS has taught researchers how difficult it is to identify genes for complex traits. However, new technologies and increasingly large and detailed data sets give hope that this important first discovery isn't far away. In many respects, understanding TS will require a clearer understanding of how the brain works in people with and without TS. Although the tools lack the current power to answer all of the researchers' questions, today's basic neuroscience research clearly sets the stage for future efforts. Although treatments for tics and comorbid conditions are generally effective and safe, they are not risk free and often not well tolerated. New treatments that offer improved efficacy and safety are needed to address the multiple problems faced by people with TS. Just like the early success of dopamine blocking agents in TS launched research into the role of dopamine in TS, so future treatment advances may also provide clues about the neurologic underpinnings of this often complex and fascinating disorder.

John Walkup
Johns Hopkins University, Baltimore, Maryland

Peter Hollenbeck
Purdue University, West Lafayette, Indiana

Jonathan Mink
University of Rochester, Rochester, New York

Neal Swerdlow
University of California, San Diego, California

REFERENCES

1. Hornse H, Banerjee S, Zeitlin H, et al. The prevalence of Tourette syndrome in 13-14-year-olds in mainstream schools. *J Child Psychol Psychiatry* 2001;42:1035–1039.

2. Jin R, Zheng RY, Huang WW, et al. [Study on the prevalence of Tourette syndrome in children and juveniles aged 7-16 years in Wenzhou area]. *Zhonghua Liu Xing Bing Xue Za Zhi.* 2004;25:131–133.

3. Khalifa N, von Knorring AL. Prevalence of tic disorders and Tourette syndrome in a Swedish school population. *Dev Med Child Neurol.* 2003;45:315–319.

4. Robertson MM. Diagnosing Tourette syndrome: is it a common disorder? *J Psychosom Res.* 2003;55:3–6.

5. Stefanoff P, Mazurek J. [Epidemiological methods used in studies in the prevalence of Tourette syndrome]. *Psychiatr Pol.* 2003;37:97–107.

6. Wang HS, Kuo MF. Tourette's syndrome in Taiwan: an epidemiological study of tic disorders in an elementary school at Taipei County. *Brain Dev.* 2003;25: S29–S31.

7. Leckman JF, Peterson BS, King RA, et al. Phenomenology of tics and natural history of tic disorders. *Adv Neurol.* 2001;85:1–14.

8. Pappert EJ, Goetz CG, Louis ED, et al. Objective assessments of longitudinal outcome in Gilles de la Tourette's syndrome. *Neurology* 2003;61:936–940.

9. Banaschewski T, Siniatchkin M, Uebel H, et al. [Compulsive phenomena in children with tic disorder and attention deficit-hyperactive disorder]. *Z Kinder Jugendpsychiatr Psychother.* 2003;31:203–211.

10. Miguel EC, do Rosario-Campos MC, Prado HS, et al. Sensory phenomena in obsessive-compulsive disorder and Tourette's disorder. *J Clin Psychiatry.* 2000;61: 150–156.

11. Budman CL, Rockmore L, Stokes J, et al. Clinical phenomenology of episodic rage in children with Tourette syndrome. *J Psychosom Res.* 2003;55:59–65.

12. Spencer TJ, Biederman J, Faraone S, et al. Impact of tic disorders on ADHD outcome across the life cycle: findings from a large group of adults with and without ADHD. *Am J Psychiatry.* 2001;158:611–617.

13. Banaschewski T, Woerner W, Rothenberger A. Premonitory sensory phenomena and suppressibility of tics in Tourette syndrome: developmental aspects in children and adolescents. *Dev Med Child Neurol.* 2003; 45:700–703.

14. Cath DC, Spinhoven P, van Woerkom TC, et al. Gilles de la Tourette's syndrome with and without obsessive-compulsive disorder compared with obsessive-compulsive disorder without tics: which symptoms discriminate? *J Nerv Ment Dis.* 2001;189:219–228.

15. Gilbert DL, Bansal AS, Sethuraman G, et al. Association of cortical disinhibition with tic, ADHD, and OCD severity in Tourette syndrome. *Mov Disord.* 2004;19:416–425.

16. Grados MA, Riddle MA, Samuels JF, et al. The familial phenotype of obsessive-compulsive disorder in relation to tic disorders: the Hopkins OCD family study. *Biol Psychiatry.* 2001;50:559–565.

17. Kano Y, Ohta M, Nagai Y, et al. Obsessive-compulsive symptoms in parents of Tourette syndrome probands and autism spectrum disorder probands. *Psychiatry Clin Neurosci.* 2004;58:348–352.

18. Leckman JF, Pauls DL, Zhang H, et al. Obsessive-compulsive symptom dimensions in affected sibling pairs diagnosed with Gilles de la Tourette syndrome. *Am J Med Genet B Neuropsychiatr Genet.* 2003;116:60–68.

19. Coffey BJ, Biederman J, Smoller JW, et al. Anxiety disorders and tic severity in juveniles with Tourette's disorder. *J Am Acad Child Adolesc Psychiatry.* 2000;39: 562–568.

20. Crawford FC, Ait-Ghezala G, Morris M, et al. Translocation breakpoint in two unrelated Tourette syndrome cases, within a region previously linked to the disorder. *Hum Genet.* 2003;13:154–161.

21. State MW, Greally JM, Cuker A, et al. Epigenetic abnormalities associated with a chromosome 18(q21-q22) inversion and a Gilles de la Tourette syndrome phenotype. *Proc Natl Acad Sci USA.* 2003;100:4684–4689.

22. Verkerk AJ, Mathews CA, Joosse M, et al. CNTNAP2 is disrupted in a family with Gilles de la Tourette syndrome and obsessive compulsive disorder. *Genomics* 2003;82:1–9.

23. Diaz-Anzaldua A, Joober R, Riviere JB, et al. Tourette syndrome and dopaminergic genes: a family-based association study in the French Canadian founder population. *Mol Psychiatry.* 2004;9:272–277.

24. Stober G, Hebebrand J, Cichon S, et al. Tourette syndrome and the norepinephrine transporter gene: results of a systematic mutation screening. *Am J Med Genet.* 1999;88:158–163.

25. Albin RL, Koeppe RA, Bohnen NI, et al. Increased ventral striatal monoaminergic innervation in Tourette syndrome. *Neurology* 2003;61:310–315.

26. Black KJ, Carl JL, Hartlein JM, et al. Rapid intravenous loading of levodopa for human research: clinical results. *J Neurosci Methods.* 2003;127:19–29.

27. Kates WR, Frederikse M, Mostofsky SH, et al. MRI parcellation of the frontal lobe in boys with attention deficit hyperactivity disorder or Tourette syndrome. *Psychiatry Res.* 2002;116:63–81.

28. Kim KJ, Peterson BS. Cavum septi pellucidi in Tourette syndrome. *Biol Psychiatry.* 2003;54:76–85.

29. Peterson BS, Thomas P, Kane MJ, et al. Basal ganglia volumes in patients with Gilles de la Tourette syndrome. *Arch Gen Psychiatry.* 2003;60:415–424.

30. Ernst M, Zametkin AJ, Jons PH, et al. High presynaptic dopaminergic activity in children with Tourette's disorder. *J Am Acad Child Adolesc Psychiatry.* 1999;38:86–94.

31. Jeffries KJ, Schooler C, Schoenbach C, et al. The functional neuroanatomy of Tourette's syndrome: an FDG PET study III: functional coupling of regional cerebral metabolic rates. *Neuropsychopharmacology* 2002;27: 92–104.

32. Meyer P, Bohnen NI, Minoshima S, et al. Striatal presynaptic monoaminergic vesicles are not increased in Tourette's syndrome. *Neurology* 1999;53:371–374.

33. Muller-Vahl KR. Cannabinoids reduce symptoms of Tourette's syndrome. *Expert Opin Pharmacother.* 2003;4:1717–1725.

34. Singer HS, Szymanski S, Giuliano J, et al. Elevated intrasynaptic dopamine release in Tourette's syndrome measured by PET. *Am J Psychiatry.* 2002;159:1329–1336.

35. Stern E, Silbersweig DA, Chee KY, et al. A functional neuroanatomy of tics in Tourette syndrome. *Arch Gen Psychiatry.* 2000;57:741–748.

36. Farber RH, Swerdlow NR, Clementz BA. Saccadic performance characteristics and the behavioural neurology of Tourette's syndrome. *J Neurol Neurosurg Psychiatry.* 1999;66:305–312.

37. Johannes S, Wieringa BM, Nager W, et al. Tourette syndrome and obsessive-compulsive disorder: event-related brain potentials show similar [mechanisms] of frontal inhibition but dissimilar target evaluation processes. *Behav Neurol.* 2003;14:9–17.

38. LeVasseur AL, Flanagan JR, Riopelle RJ, et al. Control of volitional and reflexive saccades in Tourette's syndrome. *Brain* 2001;124:2045–2058.

39. Mei Yoke Goh A, Bradshaw JL, Bradshaw JA, et al. Inhibition of expected movements in Tourette's Syndrome. *J Clin Exp Neuropsychol.* 2002;24:1017–1031.

40. Mostofsky SH, Lasker AG, Singer HS, et al. Oculomotor abnormalities in boys with Tourette syndrome with and without ADHD. *J Am Acad Child Adolesc Psychiatry.* 2001;40:1464–1472.

41. Swerdlow NR, Karban B, Ploum Y, et al. Tactile prepuff inhibition of startle in children with Tourette's syndrome: in search of an "fMRI-friendly" startle paradigm. *Biol Psychiatry.* 2001;50:578–585.

42. Hong JJ, Loiselle CR, Yoon DY, et al. Microarray analysis in Tourette syndrome postmortem putamen. *J Neurol Sci.* 2004225:57–64.

43. Kalanithi PS, Zheng W, Kataoka Y, et al. Altered parvalbumin-positive neuron distribution in basal ganglia of individuals with Tourette syndrome. *Proc Natl Acad Sci U S A.* 2005;102:13307–13312.

44. Minzer K, Lee O, Hong JJ, et al. Increased prefrontal D2 protein in Tourette syndrome: a postmortem analysis of frontal cortex and striatum. *J Neurol Sci.* 2004;219:55–61.

45. Scahill L, Leckman JF, Schultz RT, et al. A placebo-controlled trial of risperidone in Tourette syndrome. *Neurology* 2003;60:1130–1135.

46. TSA Study Group. Treatment of ADHD in children with tics: a randomized controlled trial. *Neurology* 2002;4:527.

47. Geller DA, Hoog SL, Heiligenstein JH, et al. Fluoxetine treatment for obsessive-compulsive disorder in children and adolescents: a placebo-controlled clinical trial. *J Am Acad Child Adolesc Psychiatry* 2001;40:773–779.

48. POTS. Cognitive-behavior therapy, sertraline, and their combination for children and adolescents with obsessive-compulsive disorder: the Pediatric OCD Treatment Study (POTS) randomized controlled trial. *JAMA* 2004; 292:1969–1976.

49. Riddle MA, Reeve EA, Yaryura-Tobias JA, et al. Fluvoxamine for children and adolescents with obsessive-compulsive disorder: a randomized, controlled, multicenter trial. *J Am Acad Child Adolesc Psychiatry.* 2001; 40:222–229.

50. Muller-Vahl KR, Berding G, Kolbe H, et al. Dopamine D2 receptor imaging in Gilles de la Tourette syndrome. *Acta Neurol Scand.* 2000;101:165–171.

51. Black KJ, Mink JW. Response to levodopa challenge in Tourette syndrome. *Mov Disord.* 2000;15:1194–1198.

52. Gilbert DL, Dure L, Sethuraman G, et al. Tic reduction with pergolide in a randomized controlled trial in children. *Neurology* 2003;60:606–611.

53. Marras C, Andrews D, Sime E, et al. Botulinum toxin for simple motor tics: a randomized, double-blind, controlled clinical trial. *Neurology* 2001;56:605–610.

54. Munchau A, Bloem BR, Thilo KV, et al. Repetitive transcranial magnetic stimulation for Tourette syndrome. *Neurology* 2002;59:1789–1791.

55. Silver AA, Shytle RD, Philipp MK, et al. Transdermal nicotine and haloperidol in Tourette's disorder: a double-blind placebo-controlled study. *J Clin Psychiatry.* 2001;62:707–714.

56. Silver AA, Shytle RD, Sheehan KH, et al. Multicenter, double-blind, placebo-controlled study of mecamylamine monotherapy for Tourette's disorder. *J Am Acad Child Adolesc Psychiatry.* 2001;40:1103–1110.

57. Piacentini J, Chang S. Behavioral treatments for Tourette syndrome and tic disorders: state of the art. *Adv Neurol.* 2001;85:319–331.

58. Wilhelm S, Deckersbach T, Coffey BJ, et al. Habit reversal versus supportive psychotherapy for Tourette's disorder: a randomized controlled trial. *Am J Psychiatry.* 2003;160:1175–1177.

59. Woods DW, Himle MB. Creating tic suppression: comparing the effects of verbal instruction to differential reinforcement. *J Appl Behav Anal.* 2004;37:417–420.

60. Woods DW, Hook SS, Spellman DF, et al. Case study: Exposure and response prevention for an adolescent with Tourette's syndrome and OCD. *J Am Acad Child Adolesc Psychiatry.* 2000;39:904–907.

61. Woods DW, Twohig MP, Flessner CA, et al. Treatment of vocal tics in children with Tourette syndrome: investigating the efficacy of habit reversal. *J Appl Behav Anal.* 2003;36:109–112.

62. Anandan S, Wigg CL, Thomas CR, et al. Psychosurgery for self-injurious behavior in Tourette's disorder. *J Child Adolesc Psychopharmacol.* 2004;14: 531–538.

63. Temel Y, Visser-Vandewalle V. Surgery in Tourette syndrome. *Mov Disord.* 2004;19:1:3–14.

64. Visser-Vandewalle V, Temel Y, Boon P, et al. Chronic bilateral thalamic stimulation: a new therapeutic approach in intractable Tourette syndrome. Report of three cases. *J Neurosurg.* 2003;99:1094–1100.

65. Hallett JJ, Harling-Berg CJ, Knopf PM, et al. Anti-striatal antibodies in Tourette syndrome cause neuronal dysfunction. *J Neuroimmunol.* 2000;111:195–202.

66. Loiselle CR, Wendlandt JT, Rohde CA, et al. Antistreptococcal, neuronal, and nuclear antibodies in Tourette syndrome. *Pediatr Neurol.* 2003;28:119–125.

67. Morshed SA, Parveen S, Leckman JF, et al. Antibodies against neural, nuclear, cytoskeletal, and streptococcal epitopes in children and adults with Tourette's syndrome, Sydenham's chorea, and autoimmune disorders. *Biol Psychiatry.* 2001;8:566–577.

68. Muller N, Riedel M, Straube A, et al. Increased anti-streptococcal antibodies in patients with Tourette's syndrome. *Psychiatry Res.* 2000;94:43–49.

69. Wendlandt JT, Grus FH, Hansen BH, et al. Striatal antibodies in children with Tourette's syndrome: multivariate discriminant analysis of IgG repertoires. *J Neuroimmunol.* 2001;1:106–113.

70. Muller N, Kroll B, Schwarz MJ, et al. Increased titers of antibodies against streptococcal M12 and M19 proteins in patients with Tourette's syndrome. *Psychiatry Res.* 2001;101:2:187–193.

71. Loiselle CR, Lee O, Moran TH, et al. Striatal microinfusion of Tourette syndrome and PANDAS sera: failure to induce behavioral changes. *Mov Disord.* 2004;19: 390–396.

1

Phenomenology of Tics and Natural History of Tic Disorders

James F. Leckman,[1] Michael H. Bloch,[2] Robert A. King,[3]
and Lawrence Scahill[4]

[1]*Child Study Center, Sterling Hall of Medicine, Yale University School of Medicine, New Haven,
Connecticut;* [2,3]*Tourette's/OCD Clinic, Yale Child Study Center, New Haven;*
[4]*Yale Child Study Center.*

"There is really no adequate description of the sensations that signal the onset of the actions. The first one seems irresistible, calling for an almost inevitable response... Intense concentration on the site can, itself, precipitate the action... Tourette syndrome movements are intentional body movements... The end of the Tourette syndrome action is the 'feel' that is frequently accompanied by a fleeting and incomplete sense of relief." —Joseph Bliss (1)

"Tics are rapid, coordinated caricatures of normal motor acts." —A. J. Lees (2)

"Tourette's syndrome illuminates the need to see the child as a growing, differentiating whole person, a psychosomatic entity, living in the complex environment of home and family, not just the bearer of symptoms in need of elimination." —D. J. Cohen et al. (3)

THE PHENOMENOLOGY OF TICS

Tics are a curious assemblage of abrupt repetitive movements and sounds. In 1791, James Boswell (4) characterized Samuel Johnson's tics as "convulsive starts and odd gesticulations, which tended to excite at once surprise and ridicule." His description remains apt today. During the past several decades, clinical investigators have focused their attention on tics—cataloging both their overt features and the mental states that accompany them. Insights gained have led to the development of valid and reliable clinical rating instruments and have shed some light on the timing of tics and their usual waxing and waning course, as well as other features of their natural history and underlying neurobiology.

Definition

Tics are sudden, repetitive, stereotyped motor movements or phonic productions that involve discrete muscle groups. Tics may be usefully seen as fragments of normal motor action or vocal productions that are misplaced in context and that can be easily mimicked and at times confused with goal-directed behavior. Clinicians characterize tics by their anatomical location, number, frequency, and duration. The intensity or "forcefulness" of the tic can also be an important characteristic because some tics are noteworthy simply by virtue of the exaggerated fashion in which they are performed or uttered. Finally, tics vary in terms of their complexity. The term *complexity* in this context usually refers to how simple or involved a movement or sound is, ranging from brief, meaningless, abrupt fragments (simple tics) to ones that are longer, more involved, and seemingly more goal-directed in character (complex tics). Each of these elements has been incorporated into clinician rating scales that have proven to be useful in monitoring tic severity (5–7).

Another feature of tics is their suppressibility because almost always patients can willfully withhold their tics for brief periods of time. So, if they are told to "stop making those funny movements," they can. Unfortunately, voluntary tic suppression can be associated with a build-up of inner tension so that when the tics are expressed they can be more forceful than they would otherwise be.

The suggestibility of tics is another typical trait such that when a person with Tourette syndrome (TS) is systematically interviewed about their repertoire of tic symptoms, old tics that have been absent for some time may transiently reappear.

Clinical descriptions from the 19th century onward, including those of JMG Itard (8) and Georges de la Tourette (9), have focused on cataloguing and classifying tics as viewed objectively. Following their lead, this chapter will first review the external character of tics before considering the subjective states that accompany tics.

Motor Tics

The observed range of motor tics is extraordinary, so that virtually any voluntary motor movement can emerge as a motor tic (10). Table 1-1 presents a brief compendium of some of the more common motor tics.

Motor tics may be described as simple or complex. Simple motor tics are sudden, brief (usually less than 1 second in duration), meaningless movements. Common examples include eye blinking, facial grimacing, mouth movements, head jerks, shoulder shrugs, and arm and leg jerks. Younger patients often are totally unaware of their simple motor tics.

Over time, many patients develop complex motor tics, which are sudden, more purposive appearing, stereotyped movements of longer duration. Examples are myriad and include facial gestures and movements such as brushing hair back, possibly in combination with head jerk, and body shrugs. Gyrating, bending, and more dystonic appearing movements of the head or torso are also seen. These complex motor tics rarely are seen in the absence of simple motor tics. Paroxysms, or continuous orchestrated displays of simple and complex motor tics, can occur in more severe cases. Lewd and absence gestures with hands or tongue (copropraxia) and self-abusive acts (hitting the face, biting a hand or wrist) are observed in a small number of patients. At times, it may be difficult to distinguish complex tics from motor dyskinesias and other choreas and hyperkinetic movement disorders (11). The dividing line between complex tics and compulsions can be even more difficult to establish reliably (12).

TABLE 1-1. *Examples of simple and complex motor and vocal tics*

Tic symptom dimensions	Examples
Simple motor tics: *Sudden, brief, meaningless movements*	Eye blinking, eye movements, grimacing, nose twitching, mouth movements, lip pouting, head jerks, shoulder shrugs, abdominal tensing, kicks, finger movements, jaw snaps, rapid jerking of any part of the body
Complex motor tics: *Slower, longer, more "purposeful" movements*	Sustained "looks," facial gestures, biting, touching objects or self, thrusting arms, throwing, banging, gestures with hands, gyrating and bending, dystonic postures, copropraxia (obscene gestures)
Simple phonic tics: *Sudden, meaningless sounds or noises*	Throat clearing, coughing, sniffling, spitting, screeching, barking, grunting, gurgling, clacking, hissing, sucking, animal noises, and innumerable other sounds
Complex phonic tics: *Sudden, more "meaningful" utterances*	Syllables, words, phrases, statements such as "shut up," "stop that," "oh, okay," "I've got to," "honey," "what makes me do this?" "how about it," or "now you've seen it," speech atypicalities (usually rhythms, tone, accents, intensity of speech); echo phenomenon (immediate repetition of one's own [palillalia] or another's words or phrases [echolalia]); and coprolalia (obscene, inappropriate, and aggressive words and statements)

[From Leckman JF, King RA, Cohen DJ. Tics and tic disorders. In: Leckman JF, Cohen DJ with Colleagues from the Yale Child Study Center. *Tourette's Syndrome—Tics, Obsessions, Compulsions: Developmental Psychopathology and Clinical Care.* New York: John Wiley and Sons; 1998:23–42.]

The degree of impairment and disruption associated with particular motor tics is variable and a salient clinical feature. Partly dependent on frequency, intensity, complexity, and duration of specific tics, estimates of impairment also need to include the impact on the individual's self-esteem, family life, social acceptance, school or job functioning, and physical well-being. For example, a very frequent simple motor wrist tic may be less impairing than an infrequently occurring, forceful copropraxic gesture. Patients are often aware of their complex motor tics and their impact on other people, setting the stage for detrimental intrapsychic consequences. The mental elaborations associated with the behaviors may also have a detrimental effect on self-esteem and affect socialization. Physical injuries (e.g., blindness from retinal detachment) can occur in a small minority of adolescent and adult cases secondary to severe self-abusive tics.

Vocal Tics

The range of possible vocal or phonic symptoms is extraordinary with any noise or sound having the potential to be enlisted as a tic (Table 1-1). As with motor tics, phonic symptoms are characterized by their number, frequency, duration, intensity (volume), and complexity (noises versus syllables or words).

Simple vocal tics are fast, meaningless sounds or noises that can be characterized by their frequency, duration, volume intensity, and potential for disrupting speech. Sniffing, throat clearing, grunting, barks, and high-pitched squeaks are common simple phonic symptoms. Complex vocal tics are quite diverse and can include syllables, words or phrases, as well as odd patterns of speech in which there are sudden changes in the rate, volume, and/or rhythm. Immediate echo phenomena such as repeating words and phrases occur in some patients (echolalia and palilalia). In a small minority of patients, coprolalia is present in which obscene or socially inappropriate syllables, words, or phrases are expressed, at times in a loud explosive manner. Complex vocal tics are rarely, if ever, present in the absence of simple motor and vocal tics of one sort or another. Provocative and insulting vocal symptoms have a high potential

for stigmatizing the patient and his or her family and can indirectly lead to physical injury.

In more severely affected patients multiple motor tics and one or more vocal tic can occur simultaneously or in a set sequence. Similarly, a few very severely affected patients will report the occurrence of several of these orchestrated tic sequences.

In summary, tics present as fragments of innate behavioral routines that are expressed inappropriately. This viewpoint leads naturally to questions about the neurobiological substrates of TS and related conditions. Although this topic is discussed in greater depth later in this volume, it is worth pointing out that many human behavioral programs are selected and integrated within the circuitry of the basal ganglia and its connections with the thalamus and cortex and that the circuitry contained in these structures are somatotopically organized (13). That is to say that these neuroanatomical structures have "body plans" or maps built in to their structure. It is also true that there is a convergence of both motor and sensory inputs onto the same neurons located within these circuits (14,15). This is a fact that may account for the role that bodily sensations play in tic disorders.

Premonitory Sensory Urges and Momentary Relief

Many patients report a variety of sensory and mental states associated with their tics. Detailed descriptions of these phenomena have appeared in first-person and biographical accounts of celebrated ticquers (1). These phenomena are more frequently reported by adolescents and adults than by younger children. The presence of premonitory sensory urges are reported to prompt the tics, as well as complex states of inner conflict over if and when to yield to these urges. A sensation of relief frequently accompanies the successful performance of a tic (16–20).

Joseph Bliss, a lifelong TS patient, drew the attention of the medical community to these urges in an article published in 1980 (1). In that paper, he set down the knowledge he had gained from his lifelong effort to understand the sequence of events that lead to tics. To quote Mr. Bliss:

"There is really no adequate description of the sensations that signal the onset of the actions. The first one seems irresistible, calling for an almost inevitable response… Intense concentration on the site can, in itself, precipitate the action…. Tourette syndrome movements are intentional body movements…. The end of a Tourette syndrome action is the 'feel' at the terminal site of the movement, a feel that is frequently accompanied by a fleeting and incomplete sense of relief."

This description is wholly congruent with those of other patients with TS (16): "A need to tic is an intense feeling that unless I tic or twitch I feel as if I am going to burst. Unless I can physically tic, all of my mental thoughts center on ticcing until I am able to let it out. It's a terrible urge that needs to be satisfied…"; "A feeling of pressure—a need that's very hard to describe, like something itches deep inside you—but no place you can describe; and the only way you can relieve this need is by ticcing. It's like your brain itches, or your insides are being tickled…"; "I guess it's sort of an aching feeling, in a limb or a body area, or else in my throat if it precedes a vocalization. If I don't relieve it, it either drives me crazy or begins to hurt (or both)—in that way it's both mental and physical." Much of what investigators have learned since 1980 is a footnote to Mr. Bliss' lucid description.

Children younger than age 10 years with simple tics—a forceful eye blink or a quick head jerk—usually do not have or are not aware of these sensory urges. For them, TS is truly an involuntary movement disorder. The urges typically show up later, on average more than 3 years after the onset of the tics. In contrast, precocious children as young as age 7 years have spontaneously offered compelling descriptions of this phenomenon. One 7-year-old boy described his "Tourette" going to his lips and making him grimace. In the largest study to date, Banaschewski et al. (19) gathered data using a questionnaire from 254 outpatients (212 males, 42 females) with TS, age 8 to 19 years and found increasing rates of premonitory urges when the total group was stratified into three age groups (8 to 10, 11 to 14, and 15 to 19 years). They also found no evidence that tic duration and age at tic onset influenced the onset of the premonitory urges.

A second point is that, just because an individual may have some premonitory urges, not every tic is preceded by such an urge. More than 90% of all of the 134 TS patients that participated in a study of these premonitory urges reported having experienced such urges during the past week, but often tics involving more automatic behaviors, like eye blinking, do not have urges that precede them (16).

Third, the shoulder girdle, throat, hands, the midline of the stomach, the front of the thighs and the feet are "hot spots" for such urges (16) (Fig. 1-1). The urges are often located in a small discrete area that can be readily identified. For others, these urges are more generalized and are best captured by a sense of inner tension. Many individuals report having both types of sensations.

Fourth, these urges are sometimes more troublesome than the tics. This finding is true particularly for some adults who are able partially to resist the tics but are left with these distracting urges. Indeed, it seems likely that these premonitory urges contribute to a greater or lesser extent to the attentional problems that so frequently accompany TS. Usually when the tics get better so do the urges. During the waxing and waning of symptoms or improvement with treatment, as the tics improve so do the urges.

Finally, a full consideration of these premonitory urges reveals another troublesome aspect of TS in that the tics themselves are at least partially voluntary acts, or as Bliss said "intentional" capitulations to these virtually irresistible sensory invitations. Indeed, in one study of premonitory urges, investigators found that 92% of the subjects reported that they experienced their tics to be partly or wholly "voluntary" in character (16). Taken out of context, this forced intentionality can be misunderstood and become a source of anguish and guilt ("Why can't I resist, what's wrong with me?").

This debate concerning the partially "voluntary" nature of tics has also been addressed without a clear resolution by clinical neurophysiologists. Using back-averaging techniques, Obeso et al. (21) initially observed normal *Bereitschaftspotential* in six subjects who voluntarily simulated tic-like movements, but no such pre-movement potential was noted in

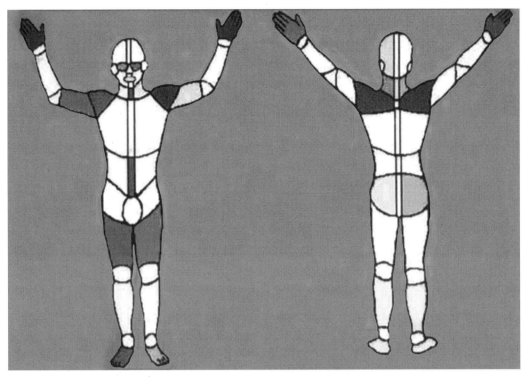

FIG. 1-1. Density of premonitory urges. The densities of premonitory urges for each of 89 anatomical regions are depicted. The highest density on the scale represents 0.40 total premonitory urges per region per person, the lowest represents 0 urges per region per person, and the midpoint represents 0.20 urges per region per person. These data are based on premonitory urges "ever" experienced as assessed in a self-report questionnaire. See Leckman et al. (16) for details.

association with tics. Karp et al. (22), however, documented premotor negativity in two of five patients with simple motor tics, suggesting that even some simple motor tics have a voluntary component (unvoluntary) and may be a response to some internal or external cue.

Speculations concerning the origins of these urges often begin with an acknowledgement that these pre-tic signals are likely to arise within the inner body space. In some form, everyone may be capable of experiencing something like premonitory urges, but those without TS may need to sit in a quiet room without distractions to notice them. They are normal signals from the body that are ordinarily screened out of conscious awareness. Viewed from this perspective, TS is a sensorimotor disorder characterized by a heightened, but selective, sensitivity to internal as well as external stimuli (as discussed later in text). Alternatively, it is possible these urges are secondary to the experience

of incessant tics because these habitual actions claim a disproportionate share of sensorimotor space within the brain. The truth is likely in between these theories.

Advances in the neurosciences have also helped clinicians realize how "plastic" the brain is, that is, how one set of neurons originally programmed to monitor one function can during the course of days be reprogrammed to attend to another related function. Whether these urges arise due to a heightened sensitivity of matrisomal medium spiny neurons in the direct pathway that receive convergent somatosensory and motor cortical inputs as well as projections from the midline thalamic nuclei and crucially important signals from fast-spiking gamma-aminobutyric acid striatal interneurons acting in concert with the tonically active neurons in the striatum or through some other mechanism (14,15, 23–26), it is likely that a more complete understanding of these phenomena will lead to novel therapeutic interventions. For example, one component of habit reversal training involves awareness training in which patients are assisted in developing awareness of premonitory urges in an effort to interrupt the urge-tic sequence (27–29). There is also evidence that successful anti-tic treatments, including botulinum toxin injections and intrathalamic deep brain stimulation, also diminish the premonitory urges (30–32).

Heightened Sensitivity to Selective Set of External Phenomena

In a comparable fashion, many patients with TS are remarkably sensitive to and at times their attention is too easily captured by phenomena in the external world (33). As first noted by Gilles de la Tourette, patients may unconsciously mirror the behavior (echopraxia) and speech (echolalia) of others as well as of themselves (palilalia): they do and say what they have just seen or heard.

Other instances include "site sensitization": being unusually aware, distracted, and distressed by a particular sensory stimuli. The classic example is tags in new clothing that in some remarkable way serve as a distracting focus of attention. Unless they are removed, it proves difficult for the child to attend to other things. Other related phenomena are "triggering perceptions." One example of this was reported by a man who goes into a bout of severe vocal tics if he hears a particular woman's cough who rides the same bus with him in the morning. Other disinhibited behaviors seen in a minority of TS patients also appear to be perceptually mediated. Specifically some rare patients report the emergence of urges to perform more complex acts that are dangerous, forbidden, or simply senseless and bizarre in response to proscriptive injunctions. An extreme example was told by an electrician who had to give up his job because whenever he saw the sign "Danger—High Voltage" he had the urge to touch the apparatus. Related phenomena may include the urge to touch a hot iron, to put the car in reverse gear while driving down a highway, touch the breast of an unknown woman in an adjacent seat, or to shout out in a quiet church service. In these cases the proscription against these behaviors is more internal. Finally, it may be that some of the "just right" phenomena (e.g., the need for things to be arranged repetitively until they look just right), which are usually described as obsessions or compulsions, also belong in this category (34,35). Those patients with stimulus-bound tics may also report the distress and frustration over the unwitting acts of others that may provoke their tic symptoms; for example, a person's cough or gesture may set off a bout of tics in response. Complex permutations of these mental events are also frequently encountered. They include needing to perform the tic a certain number of times or in a particular way to satisfy the internal urge.

This stimulus-dependent property of tics provides intriguing parallels with animal studies in which investigators have documented plasticity of neural firing in monkey striatum during a sensorimotor-conditioning task and well as other reward-conditioned stimuli (23). Perhaps most germane is the observation by Fried et al. (36) that electrical stimulation in the supplementary motor area can lead to the urge to perform a movement or utter some sound or phrase.

DIAGNOSIS AND CLASSIFICATION OF TIC DISORDERS

There is no sensitive and specific diagnostic test for TS or other tic disorders at present. Consequently, the current diagnostic classifications of tic disorders are based on the clinical criteria that focus on the individual's history and clinical presentation.

Diagnostic categories can be useful to families, educators, and other professionals. They provide a common basis for discussion and are an essential tool in epidemiological and clinical research. Several widely used diagnostic classifications systems currently include tic disorders including the *Diagnostic and Statistical Manual—Fourth Edition—Text Revision* (*DSM-IV-TR*) classification system offered by the American Psychiatric Association (37) (Table 1-2), the *International Classification of Disease and*

TABLE 1-2. *Diagnostic and Statistical Manual of Mental Disorders, Fourth Edition, Text Revision (DSM-IV-TR) Tic Disorder Classification*

I. Diagnostic criteria for Tourette syndrome (307.23):

A. Both multiple motor and one or more vocal tics have been present at some time during the illness, although not necessarily concurrently.
B. The tics occur many times a day (usually in bouts), nearly every day or intermittently throughout a period of more than a year; and during this period, there was never a tic-free period of more than 3 consecutive months.
C. Onset before age 18 years.
D. The disturbance is not due to the direct physiological effects of a substance (e.g., stimulants) or a general medical condition (e.g., Huntington's chorea or postviral encephalitis).

II. Diagnostic criteria for chronic motor or vocal tic disorder (307.22):

A. Single or multiple motor or vocal tics, but not both, have been present at some time during the illness.
B. The tics occur many times a day, nearly every day, or intermittently throughout a period of more than 1 year; during this period, there was never a tic-free interval of more than 3 months.
C. Onset before age 18 years.
D. The disturbance is not due to the direct physiological effects of a substance (e.g., stimulants) or a general medical condition (e.g., Huntington's chorea or postviral encephalitis).
E. Criteria have never been met for Tourette disorder.

III. Diagnostic criteria for transient tic disorder (307.21):

A. Single or multiple motor and/or vocal tics.
B. The tics may occur many times a day, nearly every day for at least 4 weeks, but for no longer than 12 consecutive months.
C. Onset before age 18 years.
D. Disturbance is not due to the direct physiological effects of a substance (e.g., stimulants) or a general medical condition (e.g., Huntington's chorea or postviral encephalitis).
E. Criteria have never been met for Tourette's disorder or chronic motor or vocal disorder.

IV. Diagnostic criteria for tic disorder not otherwise specified (307.20):

This category is for a tic disorder that does not meet criteria for a specific tic disorder. Examples include tics lasting less than 4 weeks or tics with an onset after age 18 years.

From American Psychiatric Association. *Diagnostic and Statistical Manual of Mental Disorders, Fourth Edition, Text Revision.* Washington, DC: American Psychiatric Association; 2000:108–116.

Related Health Problems—10th Revision (ICD-10) criteria by the World Health Organization (38), and the *Classification of Tic Disorders (CTD)* by the Tourette Syndrome Classification Group (39) (Table 1-3). Although clear differences exist comparing these classification schemes, they are broadly congruent with each containing three major well-specified categories: TS or its equivalent; chronic motor or vocal tic disorder or its equivalent; and transient tic disorder or its equivalent (Tables 1-2 and 1-3).

Transient Tic Disorder

Almost invariably a disorder of childhood, transient tic disorder is usually characterized by one or more simple motor tics that wax and wane in severity during a period of weeks to months. The anatomical distribution of these tics is usually confined to the head, neck, or upper extremities. Transient phonic tics, in the absence of motor tics, can also occur, though more rarely (40). Although sound epidemiological studies have not focused on this category, this is a common condition affecting a sizable percentage of all children. The age of onset is typically 3 to 10 years (41–43). Boys are at greater risk, and there may be a family history of tics or TS. The initial presentation may be unnoticed. If medical consultation is sought, family practitioners, pediatricians, allergists, and ophthalmologists are typically the first to see the child. Missed diagnoses are common, particularly as the symptoms may have completely disappeared by the time of the consultation. As prescribed by the prevailing diagnostic criteria, the subsequent natural history of this condition is limited to fewer than 12 consecutive months of active symptomatology. As such, this is often a retrospective

TABLE 1-3. *Classification of tic syndromes (The Tourette Syndrome Classification Study Group)*

I. Diagnostic criteria for Tourette syndrome (A-1 and A-2)

A. Both multiple motor and one or more vocal tics have been present at some time during the illness, although not necessarily concurrently.
B. The tics occur many times a day, nearly every day, or intermittently throughout a period of more than 1 year.
C. The anatomic location, number, frequency complexity, type, severity of tics changes over time.
D. Onset before age 21 years.
E. Involuntary movements and noises cannot be explained by other medical conditions.
F. Motor and/or vocal tics must be witnessed by a reliable examiner directly at some point in the illness or be recorded by videotape or cinematography (for definite Tourette syndrome, A-1) or tics not witnessed by a reliable examiner, but tics were witnessed by a reliable family member or close friend and description of tics as demonstrated is accepted by reliable examiner (for Tourette syndrome by history, A-2).

II. Diagnostic criteria for chronic multiple motor tic or phonic tic disorder (B-1 and B-2)

A. Either multiple motor or vocal tics, but not both, have been present at some time during the illness.
B. The tics occur many times a day, nearly every day, or intermittently throughout a period of more than 1 year.
C. The anatomic location, number, frequency, complexity, or severity of tics changes over time.
D. Onset before age 21 years.
E. Involuntary movements and noises cannot be explained by other medical conditions.
F. Motor and/or vocal tics must be witnessed by a reliable examiner directly at some point in the illness or by videotape or cinematography (definite chronic multiple motor tic or phonic tic disorder, B-1) or tics were not witnessed by a reliable examiner, but tics were witnessed by a reliable family member or close friend, and description of tics as demonstrated is accepted by a reliable examiner (chronic multiple motor tic or phonic tic disorder by history, B-2).

III. Diagnostic criteria for chronic single tic disorder (C-1 and C-2)

A. Same as in II (B-1 and B-2), but with single motor or vocal tic.

IV. Diagnostic criteria for transient tic disorder (D-1 and D-2)

A. Single or multiple motor and/or vocal tics.
B. The tics occur many times a day nearly every days for at least 2 weeks, but for no longer than 12 consecutive months, although the disorder began more than 1 year ago.
C. The anatomic location, number, frequency, complexity, or severity of tics changes over time.
D. No history of Tourette syndrome or chronic motor or vocal tic disorders.
E. Onset before age 21 years.
F. Motor and/or vocal tics must be witnessed by a reliable examiner directly at some point in the illness or by videotape or cinematography (definite transient tic disorder, D-1) or tics were not witnessed by a reliable examiner, but tics were witnessed by a reliable family member or close friend, and description of tics as demonstrated is accepted by a reliable examiner (transient tic disorder by history, D-2).

V. Diagnostic criteria for nonspecific tic disorder (E-1 and E-2)

A. Tics that do not meet the criteria for a specific tic disorder; an example would be a tic disorder with the tics lasting less than 1 year, and without any change over that period of time.
B. Motor and/or vocal tics must be witnessed by a reliable examiner directly at some point in the illness or by videotape or cinematography (definite nonspecific tic disorder, E-1) or tics were not witnessed by a reliable examiner, but tics were witnessed by a reliable family member or close friend, and description of tics as demonstrated is accepted by a reliable examiner (nonspecific tic disorder by history, E-1).

VI. Diagnostic criteria for definite tic disorder, diagnosis deferred (F)

A. Meets all criteria of definite Tourette syndrome (first definition), but duration of illness has not yet extended to 1 year.

VII. Diagnostic criteria for probable Tourette syndrome (G)

A. Type 1: Fulfills all criteria for definite Tourette syndrome (first definition) completely, but excludes the third and fourth criteria; or:
B. Type 2: Fulfills all criteria for definite Tourette syndrome (first syndrome) except for the first criterion; this type can be either a single motor tic with vocal tics or multiple motor tics with possible vocal tic(s).

VIII. Diagnostic criteria for probable multiple tic disorder—motor and/or vocal (H)

A. Fulfills all criteria for definite multiple tic disorder (second definition) completely, except for the third and/or fourth criteria.

[From Tourette Syndrome Classification Study Group. Definitions and classification of tic disorders. *Arch Neurol.* 1993;50:1013–1016.]

diagnosis as the clinician is unable to know with certainty which children will show progression of their symptoms and which children will display a self-limiting course. This uncertainty points to the value of deferring the diagnosis as codified in the Tourette Syndrome Classification Study Group Criteria-F (28) (Table 1-3).

Chronic Motor or Vocal Tic Disorder

Chronic motor or vocal tic disorder can be observed among children and adults. The prevalence of this disorder among school-age children may be as high as 6% (42). As with other tic disorders, boys are at greater risk and there may be a family history of tics or TS. Occasionally tic disorders are found on both sides of the family tree (44). This disorder is characterized by a waxing and waning course and a broad range of clinical severity. Chronic simple and complex motor tics are the most common manifestations. Most tics involve the head, neck, and upper extremities. Although some children may display other developmental difficulties, such as attention deficit hyperactivity disorder (ADHD), the disorder is not incompatible with an otherwise normal course of development. This condition can also appear as a residual state, particularly in adulthood. In such instances, a predictable repertoire of tic symptoms may only be seen during periods of heightened stress or fatigue. Chronic vocal tic disorder by all accounts is a rare condition. Some authors exclude "chronic cough of adolescence" from this category (45).

Tourette Syndrome: Chronic Motor and Phonic (Vocal) Tic Disorder

The eponym *Gilles de la Tourette syndrome* describes the best known, if not the most prototypic tic disorder. Typically this condition begins in early childhood with transient bouts of simple motor tics such as eye blinking or head jerks. These tics may initially come and go, but eventually they become persistent and begin to have adverse effects on the child and his or her family. As noted previously, the repertoire of motor tics can be vast, incorporating virtually any voluntary movement by any portion of the body. Although some authors have drawn attention to a "rostral-caudal" progression of motor tics (head, neck, shoulders, arms, torso), this course is not predictable. As the syndrome develops, complex motor tics may appear. Often they have a camouflaged appearance (e.g., brushing hair away from the face with an arm) and can only be distinguished as tics by their repetitive character. Rarely, complex motor tics can result in self-injury and further complicate management (e.g., punching one side of the face or biting a wrist).

On average, vocal tics begin 1 to 2 years after the onset of motor symptoms and are usually simple in character (e.g., throat clearing, grunting, squeaks). More complex vocal symptoms such as echolalia, palilalia, and coprolalia occur in a minority of cases. Other complex vocal symptoms include dramatic and abrupt changes in rhythm, rate, and volume.

The forcefulness of motor tics and the volume of vocal tics can also vary tremendously, from behaviors that are not noticeable (a slight shrug or a hushed guttural noise) to strenuous displays (arm thrusts or loud barking) that are frightening and exhausting.

Because the clinical characteristics of TS present challenges for the systematic determination of whether individuals are affected, Robertson et al. (46) developed a diagnostic confidence index (DCI) to estimate the lifetime likelihood of having had this disorder. The DCI generates a score from 0 to 100 that is a measure of the likelihood of having or ever having had TS. The DCI was administered to 280 consecutive patients with TS attending a TS clinic. This initial report indicates that the DCI is a useful, practicable instrument in the clinic or research practice allowing an assessment of lifetime likelihood of TS. However, further work is needed to test the psychometric properties of the DCI, such as its validity and reliability in populations of interest.

In addition to the tic behaviors, associated behavioral and emotional problems frequently complicate TS or other chronic tic disorders. These difficulties range from impulsive, "disinhibited," and immature behavior to compulsive touching or sniffing. There is no clear dividing line between these abrupt and disruptive behaviors and complex tics from co-morbid conditions of ADHD and obsessive-compulsive disorder.

Other Tic Disorder Diagnoses

These classification systems also include one or more additional diagnostic categories. The *CTD* includes five additional categories, including: definite single tic disorder, nonspecific tic disorder, definite tic disorder—diagnosis deferred, probable TS, and probable multiple tic disorder (Table 1-3). The major virtue of these additional categories is that they provide a more precise system for classifying cases that do not neatly fit into one of the principal categories. The *DSM-IV-TR* and *ICD-10* classifications employ fewer diagnostic options and tend to group the remaining cases into "not otherwise specified," "other," or "unspecified" categories.

Nosological Controversies

With the publication of *DSM-IV* in 1994 a notable difference between the *CTD* and *DSM-IV* classification schemes emerged, namely the *DSM-IV* requirement that the tic symptoms need to "cause marked distress of significant impairment in social, occupational or other important areas of functioning" (47). This criterion is based on a conceptualization of mental disorder articulated by the framers of the *DSM-IV* and was intended to distinguish between normality and pathology. In the case of tic disorders, this criterion is vague and open to widely varying interpretation. For example, it is unclear who needs to be distressed or for how long. The frequent presence of co-morbid diagnoses that, in combination with the tic symptoms cause distress or impairment, may result in further difficulties in applying the "distress" criterion of *DSM-IV*. Finally, problems arise in research settings where all of the *DSM-IV* may be satisfied except the "distress" criterion, leaving open how such cases should be classified.

Fortunately, the section on TS and other tic disorders in text revision of *DSM-IV* dropped the controversial distress criterion (37). With this change there should be less controversy about who has TS so that individuals who have adjusted well to the presence of tics can still be considered to have the diagnosis even if the syndrome is not a major source of distress.

Another minor but substantive difference between the *DSM-IV* and the Tourette Syndrome Classification Group criteria is a differing age of onset criterion (tic onset prior to age 18 years in *DSM-IV* and prior to 21 years in the Tourette Syndrome Classification Group). Until a more objective diagnostic test is developed this point is likely to remain unresolved. However, as the most individuals report the onset of their tic symptoms in the first decade of life, this 3-year difference is unlikely to have much practical import.

Caveats on the Topic of Diagnostic Categories

Before leaving the discussion of diagnostic categories, a few caveats are in order. First, it is important to recognize that diagnostic categories, despite their value, change and can be misapplied to suit the fashion of the day (33).

Second, even if TS is the correct diagnosis, it will be important for families, educators, and clinicians to focus on the whole person with TS rather than the relevant diagnostic category. Overly focusing on the disorder can potentially have a number of adverse consequences, not the least of which is the implicit message to the patient concerning his or her identity. To place TS at the center of one's identity is to invite distortion and a negative expectancy rather than a more adaptive outcome. For example, it is common for families to arrive at an initial consultation with the firmly held belief that their child, who today has a few troublesome tics, is destined to become someone whose life has been devastated by TS. Active clinical intervention is required to adjust and correct these potentially harmful expectancies.

Third, the potential explanatory power of diagnostic categories, at times, can lure families

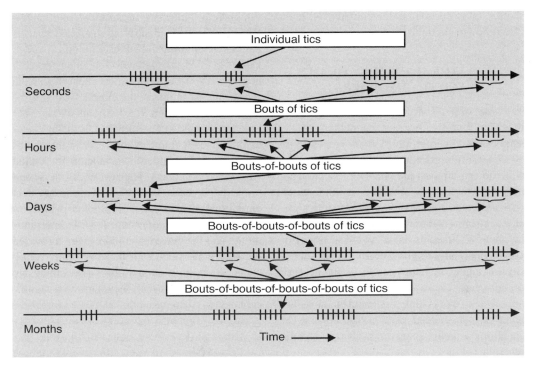

FIG. 1-2. Fractal character of the temporal occurrence of tics. Progressively longer time dimensions (seconds to months) are heuristically depicted in this figure. Over the course of seconds tics occur in bouts. Over the course of minutes bouts of tics occur in bouts. If this description is accurate, in each time scale, the bout-like appearance of tics (or higher order combinations of bouts and bouts of bouts of tics) will be observed. This fractal quality may well underlie the waxing and waning of tics observed over weeks to months as well as other features of the natural history of Tourette syndrome. See Leckman (24) for details.

and professionals into attributing more to the disorder than is reasonable. In the experience of these authors, this attribution is particularly true when a child's development has been encumbered with other difficulties such as pervasive developmental disorders, dyslexia, or disruptive behavior problems.

THE OCCURRENCE OF TICS IN BOUTS: A CLUE TO THE WAXING AND WANING COURSE

Individual tics tend to occur in bouts with brief inter-tic intervals that can be measured in seconds. These bouts themselves occur in bouts and may account for transient periods of tic exacerbation that occur during the course of a typical day. Empirical studies of this phenomenon are just getting underway (34).

Speculation has focused on the "fractal" occurrence of tics. This fractal quality means that regardless of the time increments studied, seconds, minutes, hours, days, weeks, or years, the nonlinear temporal patterning of tics or bouts of tics or bouts-of-bouts of tics or bouts-of-bouts-of-bouts of tics or bouts-of-bouts-of-bouts-of-bouts of tics remains basically the same (Fig. 1-2). This quality, if confirmed, may elucidate a fundamental property of tics and tic disorders. For example, the well known waxing and waning course of tics may simply be another way to refer to bouts-of-bouts-of-bouts-of-bouts of tics and the time interval between them. At the other end of the time scale, it is possible that an examination of the neural mechanisms underlying this fractal phenomenon may identify related events that can be measured in milliseconds or even shorter intervals that are associated with the generation of tic phenomena.

THE NATURAL HISTORY OF TICS AND TIC DISORDERS

The onset of tics is usually in the first decade of life. Most investigators report a median onset of simple motor tics at age 5 or 6 years (16,45, 49–55). Of interest, this time interval coincides with the very highest prevalence of isolated and persistent motor tics observed in kindergarten and first-grade classrooms (42). Motor tics usually begin first with brief bouts of transient tics involving the face or head. A typical report involves bouts of eye blinking of variable intensity beginning in kindergarten or in the early school years. These symptoms often disappear after a few weeks only to reappear at a later point in time. Indeed, the "classic" history includes a wax and waning course and a changing repertoire of tics.

Phonic or vocal tics usually appear several years after the onset of motor tics. In most cases the onset is between ages 8 to 15 years. Less than 5% of patients have isolated phonic tics in the absence of motor symptoms. Phonic tics often show a similar progression from transient episodes to more sustained period of phonic symptoms.

Typically, in cases of TS, the symptoms multiply and worsen by early adolescence and so that even during the waning phases the tics are troublesome. Current research is focused on prospective longitudinal studies of children either at increased risk of TS (56) or who have been diagnosed with the disorder (57–62). This work has largely been driven by efforts to determine whether or not stressful life events and newly acquired streptococcal infections regularly antedate periods of tic symptom exacerbation. While both of these topics remain a source of controversy (59–62), it does appear that daily life stressors are more likely to be important determinants of future tic outcome than are major life events (59,61). There is also a hint that antecedent mood and anxiety symptoms may be important mediators of future tic severity.

These studies have emphasized the waxing and waning course of TS and the need to establish an objective, prospective, and quantitative method for identifying symptom exacerbations in children and adults with this disorder. Lin et al (53) prospectively obtained monthly consecutive Yale Global Tic Severity Scale scores in 64 children diagnosed with TS for periods ranging from 3 to 39 months. Exacerbation thresholds were estimated by using state-of-the-art bootstrap methods. These thresholds were then independently evaluated by asking two expert clinicians. The severity of tic symptoms displayed a high degree of intrasubject variability. Exacerbation thresholds, which incorporated the change score from the previous month and the current symptom score, provided the best agreement with those of expert clinicians. When both tic and obsessive-compulsive symptoms were present, they showed a significant degree of co-variation.

In most patients, the worst-ever tic severity is also age-dependent and usually falls between ages 7 and 15 years after which there is a steady decline in tic severity (51–55) (Fig. 1-3). This peak in tic severity coincides with a second peak in tic prevalence observed in community-based studies (42,43). The decrease in tic symptoms over the course of adolescence is consistent with available epidemiologic data that indicate a lower prevalence of TS among adults compared with children. It is also consistent with follow-up studies of clinically referred TS patients (49–55). In many instances, the vocal symptoms become increasingly rare or may disappear altogether, and the motor tics may be reduced in number and frequency. Estimates of the degree of improvement appear to depend on the assessment tools used. "Objective" ratings that incorporate videotaped ratings indicate that tics improve over time, but not to the same degree as more subjective estimates (53). All studies point to the persistence of some tics into adulthood in most individuals often in association with less subjective distress. The physiological basis for these age-dependent changes remains in doubt. Candidates include normal age-dependent alterations in the number and nature of dopaminergic receptors and dopamine transporter sites in the striatum (63,64).

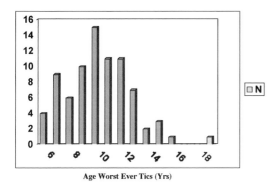

FIG. 1-3. Age distribution of when tic symptoms are at their worst. This histogram presents the age, in years, of worst-ever tics as reported at follow-up. This figure combines data from the studies of Leckman et al (American Psychiatric Association. *Diagnostic and Statistical Manual of Mental Disorders*, Fourth ed., Text Revision. Washington, DC: American Psychiatric Association; 2000) ($N = 36$) and Bloch et al; Bloch MH, Peterson BS, Scahill L, et al. Clinical predictors of future tic and OCD severity in children with Tourette syndrome, submitted. **nd** ($N = 46$) using similar methodologies.

Volumetric differences in the caudate nucleus and subgenual cortical regions also appear to have predictive value in estimating future tic severity (65,66). Although the developmental and/or intramorbid events responsible for these findings are unknown, speculation has focused on epigenetic factors such as transient perinatal hypoxia and/or as yet to be determined autoimmune phenomena.

In adulthood, a patient's repertoire of tics usually stabilizes, meaning fewer varieties of tics appearing just during periods of fatigue and heightened emotionality. Complete remission of both motor and phonic symptoms has also been reported, but estimates vary considerably with some studies reporting rates of remission as high as 50% (49–55). In such cases, the legacy of TS in adult life is most closely associated with the significance of having severe tics as a child. For example, the individual who was misunderstood and punished at home and at school for tics or who was teased mercilessly by peers and stigmatized by communities will fare worse than a child whose interpersonal environment was more understanding and supportive.

Even with the available interventions, the average overall quality of life of patients with TS is significantly worse than the general population (67). Indeed, persistently severe tics in adulthood can be associated with marked impairment. However, global outcome and social and educational functional capacities in adulthood are not synonymous with tic outcomes. Indeed, the presence of chronic motor and vocal tics alone in the absence of other difficulties often heralds a positive outcome—especially in the presence of other strengths. Unfortunately, tics alone are the exception rather than the rule. Psychiatric co-morbidities—ADHD, other disruptive behavior problems, obsessive-compulsive disorder, mood and anxiety disorders, as well as social difficulties and/or learning problems—are often important determinates of global outcome. In one recent follow-up study of 31 adults with TS, 52% of patients had some social or educational dysfunction during adolescence or adulthood (53). All patients completed high school, 52% had finished at least 2 years of college, and 71% were currently employed or pursuing higher education full time.

In another recent study (55), global outcome was assessed near the beginning of the third decade of life (Fig. 1-4). Approximately 20% of individuals diagnosed with TS in childhood were rated as being moderately impaired or worse. Global outcome was associated not only with the level of severity of tics ($P <.03$) and obsessive-compulsive disorder, ($P <.004$) in early adulthood, but also with the level of tic severity in childhood ($P <.006$) and a childhood diagnosis of ADHD ($P <.03$). Subsequent chapters address the range of co-morbid conditions seen in patients with TS. The frequency and prognostic significance of these co-morbid conditions challenge "tic-only" formulations of TS and reinvigorate the debate over what constitutes the essential nature of this complex and multifaceted disorder.

CONCLUSIONS

Tic symptoms—the hallmark of TS may simply be fragments of innate behavioral programs that are normally assembled collaboratively by the basal ganglia acting in concert with cortical and

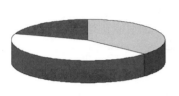

□ >90 Superior
Functioning
(37%)

□ 70-90 Slight
Impairment
(43%)

■ <70 Moderate
Impairment or
Worse (20%)

FIG. 1-4. Global functioning at age 19 years. Overall psychosocial functioning was rated using the Global Assessment Scale (GAS, 0-100) at the age of 19 years. The average GAS score was fairly high at 84.4 ± 14.7 (median = 86, range: 35–100) at time 2. Seventeen subjects (37%) received GAS ratings at follow-up of greater than 90, indicating that the examiner judged their psychiatric disorder(s) had minimal impact on overall functioning. Twenty subjects (43%) received GAS scores (>70 but ≤90), suggesting that their illness had only a mild impact on global functioning. Nine subjects (20%) had GAS ratings (≤70), indicating that their disorder had at least a moderate impact on their overall functioning. For further details see Bloch et al. (55).

thalamic sites. The sensory urges that precede many of the motor and phonic tics may further illuminate the normal internal cues that typically aid in the assembly of these behavioral programs. Diagnostic schemata for tic disorders are clinically useful, but evolving, conventions. The occurrence of tics in time appears to have fractal characteristics that may help to the waxing and waning course of chronic tic disorders and surprisingly may point the way to the identification of neurons with the same burst-pause pattern of reactivity that play a crucial role as tic-generators. The natural history of tics usually shows a marked decline during the course of adolescence. A consideration of what regularly makes tics better or worse may provide clues concerning the underlying neurobiology of this condition. Specifically, future studies examining the timing and nature of depressive symptoms (as well as other co-morbid conditions) in children with TS—combined with prospective collection of stress, immunologic and neuroendocrine markers as well as longitudinal measurements of brain structure and function may provide deeper insights into the factors that influence tic outcomes.

Finally, in the search for understanding the nature and course of TS, the clinician must not lose sight of the whole person. The long-term goal of research on phenomenology and natural history is to anticipate potential problems, optimize adaptation, and keep development on track. In addition to scientific knowledge, the capacity for health care providers to build on an individual's strengths and interests and to encourage an optimistic attitude and so prevent tics and related problems form getting the best of individuals with TS. A complete review of the phenomenology and natural history of TS would include an assessment of the impact of these aptitudes and attitudes.

ACKNOWLEDGMENTS

This review is dedicated to the memory of Donald J. Cohen—a unique individual who dedicated a significant portion of his professional life to the care and understanding of individuals with Tourette syndrome and their families. This research was supported by grants from the Tourette Syndrome Association; NIH: P01 MH49351, P01 HD03008, T32 MH18268, M01 RR0125, P30 MH30929, and R01 MH061940. Portions of this chapter are adapted from Leckman et al. (69) and Leckman JF, Cohen DJ: *Tourette's Syndrome—Tics, Obsessions, Compulsions: Developmental Psychopathology and Clinical Care.* New York: John Wiley and Sons, 1998.

REFERENCES

1. Bliss J. Sensory experiences in Gilles de la Tourette syndrome. *Arch Gen Psychiatry.* 1980;37:1343–1347.
2. Lees AJ. *Tics and Related Disorders.* New York: Churchill Livingstone; 1985.
3. Cohen DJ, Detlor J, Shaywitz BA, Leckman JF. Interaction of biological and psychological factors in the natural history of Tourette's syndrome: A model of childhood neuropsychiatric disorders. *Adv Neurology.* 1982;35:31–40.
4. Murray TJ. Doctor Samuel Johnson's abnormal movements. In: Friedhoff AJ, Chase TN, eds. *Advances in Neurology: Volume 35. Gilles de la Tourette syndrome.* New York: Raven Press; 1982:25–30.
5. Leckman JF, Cohen DJ. *Tourette's Syndrome—Tics, Obsessions, Compulsions: Developmental Psychopathology and Clinical Care.* New York: John Wiley and Sons; 1998.

6. Leckman JF, Riddle MA, Hardin MT, et al. The Yale Global Tic Severity Scale (YGTSS): Initial testing of a clinician-rated scale of tic severity. *J Am Acad Child Adol Psychiatry*. 1989;28:566–573.

7. Robertson MM, Banerjee S, Kurlan R, et al. The Gilles de la Tourette Syndrome Diagnostic Confidence Index: Development, acceptability and association with clinical factors, *Neurology* 2005. In press.

8. Itard JMG. Mémoire sur quelques functions involontaires des appareils de la locomotion, de la préhension et de la voix. *Arch Gen Med*. 1825;8:385–407.

9. Gilles de la Tourette G, Goetz CG, Klawans HL, trans. Étude sur une affection nerveuse caractérisée par de l'incoordination mortice accompagnee d'echolaliae et de coprolalie. In: Friedhoff AJ, Chase TN, eds. *Advances in Neurology: Volume 35. Gilles de la Tourette syndrome*. New York: Raven Press; 1982:1–16.

10. Leckman JF, King RA, Cohen DJ. Tics and tic disorders. In: Leckman JF, Cohen DJ with Colleagues from the Yale Child Study Center. *Tourette's Syndrome—Tics, Obsessions, Compulsions: Developmental Psychopathology and Clinical Care*. New York: John Wiley and Sons; 1998:23–42.

11. Jankovic J. Differential diagnosis and etiology of tics. *Adv Neurol*. 2001;85:15–29.

12. Towbin KE, Peterson BS, Cohen DJ, Leckman JF. Differential diagnosis. In: Leckman JF, Cohen DJ with Colleagues from the Yale Child Study Center. *Tourette's Syndrome—Tics, Obsessions, Compulsions: Developmental Psychopathology and Clinical Care*. New York: John Wiley and Sons; 1998:118–139.

13. Alexander GE, Crutcher MD, DeLong MR. Basal ganglia-thalamocortical circuits: parallel substrates for motor, oculomotor, "prefrontal" and "limbic" functions. *Prog Brain Res*. 1990;85:119–146.

14. Wilson CJ. The contribution of cortical neurons to the firing pattern of medium spiny neurons. In: Houk JC, Davis JL, Beiser DG, eds. *Models of Information Processing in the Basal Ganglia*. Cambridge, MA: MIT Press; 1995:29–50.

15. Flaherty AW, Graybiel AM. Motor and somatosensory corticostriatal projection magnifications in the squirrel monkey. *J Neurophysiol*. 1995;74:2638–2648.

16. Leckman JF, Walker DE, Cohen DJ. Premonitory urges in Tourette's syndrome. *Am J Psychiatry*. 1993;150:98–102.

17. Kurlan R, Lichter D, Hewitt D. Sensory tics in Tourette's syndrome. *Neurology* 1989;39:731–734.

18. Lang A. Patient perception of tics and other movement disorders. *Neurology* 1991;41:223–228.

19. Banaschewski T, Woerner W, Rothenberger A. Premonitory sensory phenomena and suppressibility of tics in Tourette syndrome: developmental aspects in children and adolescents. *Dev Med Child Neurol*. 2003;45:700–703.

20. Kwak C, Dat Vuong K, Jankovic J. Premonitory sensory phenomenon in Tourette's syndrome. *Mov Disord*. 2003;18:1530–1533.

21. Obeso JA, Rothwell JC, Marsden CD. Simple tics in Gilles de la Tourette's syndrome are not prefaced by a normal premovement EEG potential. *J Neurol Neurosurg Psychiatry*. 1981;44:735–738.

22. Karp BI, Porter S, Toro C, Hallett M. Simple motor tics may be preceded by a premotor potential. *J Neurol Neurosurg Psychiatry.* 1996;61:103–106.

23. Graybiel AM, Aosaki T, Flaherty AW, Kimura M. The basal ganglia and adaptive motor control. *Science* 1994;265:1826–1831.

24. Leckman JF. Gilles de la Tourette syndrome. *Lancet* 2002;360:1577–1586.

25. Graybiel AM, Canales JJ. The neurobiology of repetitive behaviors: clues to the neurobiology of Tourette syndrome. *Adv Neurol*. 2001;85:123–131.

26. Mink JW. Neurobiology of basal ganglia circuits in Tourette syndrome: Faulty inhibition of unwanted motor patterns. *Adv Neurol*. 2001;85:113–122.

27. Azrin NH, Nunn RG. Habit reversal: a method of eliminating nervous habits and tics. *Behav Res Ther*. 1973;11:619–628.

28. Wilhelm S, Deckersbach T, Coffey BJ, et al. Habit reversal versus supportive psychotherapy for Tourette's disorder: a randomized, double-blind controlled trial. *Am J Psychiatry*. 2003;160:1175–1177.

29. Piacentini J. Behavioral therapy: Habit reversal. *Adv Neurol*, 2005. In press.

30. Kwak C, Hanna P, Jankovic J. Botulinum toxin in the treatment of tics. *Arch Neurol*. 2000;57:1190–1193.

31. Marras C, Andrews D, Sime E, Lang A. Botulinum toxin for simple motor tics: a randomized, double-blind, controlled clinical trial. *Neurology* 2001;56:605–610.

32. Visser-Vandewalle V, Temel Y, van der Linden Ch, Ackermans L, Beuls E. Deep brain stimulation in movement disorders. The applications reconsidered. *Acta Neurol Belg*. 2004;104:33–36.

33. Cohen AJ, Leckman JF. Sensory phenomena associated with Gilles de la Tourette syndrome. *J Clin Psychiatry*. 1992;53:319–323.

34. Leckman JF, Walker WK, Goodman WK, Pauls DL, Cohen DJ. "Just right" perceptions associated with compulsive behaviors in Tourette's syndrome. *Am J Psychiatry*. 1994;151:675–680.

35. Miguel EC, Rosário-Campos MC, da Silva Prado H, et al. Sensory phenomena in patients with obsessive-compulsive disorder and Gilles de la Tourette syndrome. *J Clin Psychiatry*. 2000;61:150–156

36. Fried I, Katz A, McCarthy G, et al. Functional organization of human supplementary motor cortex studied by electrical stimulation. *J Neurosci*. 1991;11:3656–3666.

37. American Psychiatric Association. *Diagnostic and Statistical Manual of Mental Disorders,* Fourth ed., Text Revision. Washington, DC: American Psychiatric Association; 2000.

38. World Health Organization. *International Classification of Diseases*, Tenth ed. Geneva: World Health Organization; 1992.

39. Tourette Syndrome Classification Study Group. Definitions and classification of tic disorders. *Arch Neurol*. 1993;50:1013–1016.

40. Kurlan R, Behr J, Medved L, Como P. Transient tic disorder and the spectrum of Tourette's syndrome. *Arch Neurol*. 1988;45:1200–1201.

41. Costello EJ, Angold A, Burns BJ, et al. The Great Smoky Mountains Study of Youth. Goals, design, methods, and the prevalence of DSM-III-R disorders. *Arch Gen Psychiatry*. 1996;53:1129–1136.

42. Snider LA, Seligman LD, Ketchen BR, et al. Tics and problem behaviors in schoolchildren: prevalence, characterization, and associations. *Pediatrics* 2002;110:331–336.

43. Gadow KD, Nolan EE, Sprafkin J, Schwartz J. Tics and psychiatric comorbidity in children and adolescents. *Dev Med Child Neurol.* 2002;44:330–338.

44. Hanna PA, Janjua FN, Contant CF, Jankovic J. Bilineal transmission in Tourette syndrome. *Neurology* 1999; 53:813–818.

45. Shapiro AK, Shapiro ES, Young JG, Feinberg T. *Gilles de la Tourette syndrome*, Second ed. New York: Raven Press; 1988.

46. Robertson MM, Banerjee S, Kurlan R, et al. The Tourette syndrome diagnostic confidence index: development and clinical associations. *Neurology* 1999; 53:2108–2112.

47. Kushner HI. *A Cursing Brain? The Histories of Tourette Syndrome.* Cambridge, MA: Harvard University Press; 1999.

48. Peterson BS, Leckman JF. Temporal characterization of tics in Gilles de la Tourettes syndrome. *Biol Psychiatry.* 1998;44:1337–1348.

49. Erenberg G, Cruse RP, Rothner AD. The natural history of Tourette syndrome: a follow-up study. *Ann Neurol.* 1987;22:383–385.

50. Sandor P, Musisi S, Moldofsky H. Lang A. Tourette syndrome: a follow-up study. *J Clin Psychopharmacol.* 1990;10:197–199.

51. Goetz CG, Tanner CM, Stebbins GT, Leipiz G, Carr WC. Adult tics in Gilles de la Tourette's syndrome: description and risk factors. *Neurology.* 1992; 42:784–788.

52. Leckman JF, Zhang H, Vitale A, et al. Course of tic severity in Tourette's syndrome: the first two decades. *Pediatrics* 1998;102:14–19.

53. Pappert EJ, Goetz CG, Louis ED, Blasucci L, Leurgans S. Objective assessments of longitudinal outcome in Gilles de la Tourette's syndrome. *Neurology* 2003; 61:936–940.

54. Coffey BJ, Biederman J, Geller D, et al. Re-examining tic persistence and tic-associated impairment in Tourette's disorder: findings from a naturalistic follow-up study. *J Nerv Mental Dis*, 2005. In press.

55. Bloch MH, Peterson BS, Scahill L, et al. Clinical predictors of future tic and OCD severity in children with Tourette syndrome, submitted.

56. McMahon WM, Carter AS, Fredine N, Pauls DL. Children at familial risk for Tourette's disorder: child and parent diagnoses. *Am J Med Genet.* 2003; 121B: 105–111.

57. Peterson BS, Pine DS, Cohen P, Brook JS. Prospective, longitudinal study of tic, obsessive-compulsive, and attention-deficit/hyperactivity disorders in an epidemiological sample. *J Am Acad Child Adolesc Psychiatry.* 2001;40:685–695.

58. Lin H, Yeh CB, Peterson BS, et al. Assessment of symptom exacerbations in a longitudinal study of children with Tourette's syndrome or obsessive-compulsive disorder. *J Am Acad Child Adolesc Psychiatry.* 2002; 41:1070–1077.

59. Findley DB, Leckman JF, Katsovich L, et al. Development of the Yale Children's Global Stress Index (YCGSI) and its application in children and adolescents with Tourette's syndrome and obsessive-compulsive disorder. *J Am Acad Child Adolesc Psychiatry.* 2003;42:450–457.

60. Murphy TK, Sajid M, Soto O, et al. Detecting pediatric autoimmune neuropsychiatric disorders associated with streptococcus in children with obsessive-compulsive disorder and tics. *Biol Psychiatry.* 2004;55:61–68.

61. Hoekstra PJ, Steenhuis MP, Kallenberg CG, Minderaa RB. Association of small life events with self reports of tic severity in pediatric and adult tic disorder patients: a prospective longitudinal study. *J Clin Psychiatry.* 2004;65:426–431.

62. Luo F, Leckman JF, Katsovich L, et al. Prospective longitudinal study of children with tic disorders and/or obsessive-compulsive disorder: relationship of symptom exacerbations to newly acquired streptococcal infections. *Pediatrics* 2004;113:e578–585.

63. Seeman P, Bzowej NH, Guan HC, et al. Human brain dopamine receptors in children and aging adults. *Synapse* 1987;1:399–404.

64. Meng SZ, Ozawa Y, Itoh M, Takashima S. Developmental and age-related changes of dopamine transporter, and dopamine D1 and D2 receptors in human basal ganglia. *Brain Res.* 1999;843:136–144.

65. Bloch MH, Leckman JF, Peterson BS: Basal ganglia volumes and future tic severity in children with Tourette syndrome, submitted.

66. Bloch MH, Leckman JF, Bansal R, et al. Regional brain volumes and future tic and OCD severity in children with Tourette syndrome, submitted.

67. Elstner K, Selai CE, Trimble MR, Robertson MM. Quality of Life (QOL) of patients with Gilles de la Tourette's syndrome. *Acta Psychiatr Scand.* 2001; 103:52–59.

68. Endicott J, Spitzer RL, Fleiss JL, Cohen J. The Global Assessment Scale. *Arch Gen Psychiatry.* 1976;33: 766–771.

69. Leckman JF, Peterson BS, King RA, Scahill L, Cohen DJ. Phenomenology of tics and natural history of tic disorders. *Adv Neurol.* 2001;85:1–14.

2

Attention Deficit Hyperactivity Disorder

The Childhood Co-Morbidity That Most Influences the Disability Burden in Tourette Syndrome

Martha Bridge Denckla

Kennedy Krieger Institute, Baltimore, Maryland

Considerable evidence supports the view that attention deficit hyperactivity disorder (ADHD) represents a group of related neurobiological disorders characterized by inattention, overactivity and/or impulsivity. The heterogeneity of ADHD as well as its co-occurrence with multiple other conditions remains a major focus for future research. Although identification of "endophenotypes" would do much to sort out these complexities (1), it is equally important to determine whether the ADHD that occurs in conditions such as Tourette syndrome (TS) is distinctive from or similar to one of the endophenotypes or indeed any of the heterogeneous disorders subsumed under the name ADHD (2). The results of a decade of research suggests two important findings: 1) the ADHD in TS has many similarities to ADHD alone, and 2) children with TS alone do not appear to have the pattern of motor or executive control deficits seen in children with ADHD.

INTRODUCTION

The diagnosis of ADHD is made by historical report of the parents or others involved with the child (e.g., teachers). Historical information can be collected via clinical interview or may include semi-quantitative rating scales or questionnaires such as the Child Behavior Checklist and the Teacher Report Form (5). No clinical examinations or laboratory tests are currently accepted as either relevant to "ruling in" or "ruling out" the diagnosis of ADHD.

Although it is not uncommon for symptoms of ADHD to be considered simply immature levels of activity, attention, and impulsivity (i.e., "had the child been younger, the findings would be normal"), one should not therefore infer that there is evidence for "outgrowing" the disorder or that ADHD is trivial in its ultimate impact on academic, vocational, social, and emotional functioning.

The diagnosis of ADHD is often challenging because of the between-setting variability in symptoms and the variable standards of those performing the ratings. In this sense ADHD "is in the eye of the beholder." The various "beholders" in the life of the child often provide information that is setting specific and may reflect a different degree of appropriate/inappropriate handling of the child, further complicating the diagnostic process.

The sex of the child also complicates the diagnosis of ADHD. Girls are more likely to present to the clinic with the predominantly inattentive type and often at an older age (although, retrospectively, they may at a very early age have passed through a hyperactive-impulsive stage). The late age for diagnosis is particularly critical because the consequences of ADHD in women who have lived with the disorder are grave, ranging from chronic low self-esteem/dysphoric state to a greater vulnerability to major depression and drug abuse. Generally, even the most attenuated and subtle aspects of ADHD, those commonly regarded as "disorganization," are less well tolerated by society in girls and women than in boys and even men (4).

A comprehensive review of the neurobiology of ADHD is beyond the scope of this chapter, which discusses ADHD as a co-morbidity with TS. To date, ADHD research implicates the parallel circuits that run between the frontal lobe and the basal ganglia and another set of parallel circuits that run between the frontal lobes and the cerebellum. The thalamus represents a relay station and a convergence zone for both of these sets of circuits. Although compelling, neurobiological inferences drawn from treatment effects of stimulants should be considered independently from biomedical research findings of ADHD; it is neither necessary nor sufficient for a neurobiological view of ADHD for one to connect the response to stimulant medication with the particulars of this neuroanatomy (3).

The pattern of co-morbidity in TS may also provide clues to the underlying neurobiology of ADHD. It is well known how common ADHD is in child psychiatry clinics, so that the co-morbidity seen with TS is not distinctive; co-morbidity in the range of 50% is reported many times in literature for almost any clinical syndrome presenting in child psychiatry practice. The conditions most frequently associated with ADHD include mood/anxiety disorders (>20%) and the other "disruptive" disorders, including oppositional defiant and conduct disorders (>30%). In neurology clinics, developmental motor coordination disorder is commonly observed in all subtypes of ADHD.

Although the link between the co-morbid conditions observed in TS and the dysfunction at the various levels of the nervous system is unclear, the range of co-morbidity observed by psychiatrists and neurologists suggest that there may be three control circuits: 1) motor control, 2) executive control cognitively, and 3) executive control socially/emotionally. In addition to this threefold organization, there are three important levels potentially to be co-localized: the frontal lobe, basal ganglia, and cerebellum (3).

The neuropsychological study of ADHD has had a significant impact on the entire field of academic skills deficits; however executive function, also known as *executive control*, is the domain of direct interest to ADHD. There are many publications on executive function deficits in ADHD and a burgeoning literature on what is within the domain of executive function/control specific to ADHD (6). Many studies have indicated that within the domain of executive function, it is the set of functions described as response inhibitions that are most specific to the group with ADHD; whereas domains such as working memory, planning, cognitive flexibility, and various kinds of fluency may be equally or even more impaired in other developmental disorders, most specifically in high functioning autism (6). Abnormalities in executive function have always implicated "frontal" circuits; however, one must be cautious not to assign executive function only to the top or frontal level.

Problems with motor control and executive function observed in ADHD have implication for the assessment of children with ADHD. The clinician is advised to look for the signs of inhibitory insufficiency on the motor examination because these are completely "unconscious" signs that can be observed as excess-for-age extraneous overflow movements, either in the form of feet-to-hands overflow with gaits or the better-known mirror movements with fine motor coordination. Development of these inhibitory skills (announced by the absence of extraneous movement) presents as an orderly developmental "milestone" record. Poor visual-motor organization, usually judged by copying of designs, and a lack of strategies or plans of visual search is also readily observed during a clinical assessment. (The experienced neurologist also finds that the degree of childish unreliability in meeting the "entry requirement" of sensory testing is particularly prominent with ADHD.)

Lastly, there is increasing enthusiasm for, but unfortunately not increasing utilization of, behavioral treatments for the symptoms of ADHD. Although stimulant treatment has a powerful effect on ADHD symptoms as noted in the Multimodal Treatment of ADHD study (MTA) behavioral treatments were also helpful for enhancing response and addressing the needs of children with ADHD and co-morbid conditions. Clinically, the use of a well-formulated and supervised behavior modification plan has many benefits, yet skilled clinicians who are trained in applied behavior analysis, including the "ABC" sequence (antecedent–behavior–consequence) are uncommon in many communities. In fact, the behavioral treatment of ADHD both at home and in school is at the present time woefully underappreciated and underutilized (personal observations of the author in clinical practice).

In summary, there is considerable evidence for the concept of ADHD representing a heterogeneous group of related neurobiological-developmental disorders involving a "three-by-three" matrix of parallel control circuits with "nodal" points in frontal lobe, basal ganglia, and cerebellum; cross-talk between these circuits seems at the very least to be most likely at the level of the thalamus.

ATTENTION DEFICIT HYPERACTIVITY DISORDER CO-MORBID WITH TOURETTE SYNDROME

The relationships between ADHD and TS have been well summarized in several review articles by prominent clinicians/clinical investigators. The comprehensive review by Dr. Mary Robertson (see elsewhere this volume) will certainly bring out the important relationship (7). Pauls has suggested that there are possibly two genetic types of ADHD, one that is independent of TS and the other in which ADHD is "embedded" as an endophenotype in TS. Others, such as Towbin and Riddle, have postulated a threshold effect in which the entire group of persons with TS have some degree of the symptom/sign constellation of ADHD, subthreshold in some cases and above threshold for diagnosis in other cases. The question remains to be resolved whether the ADHD in TS is clearly different from ADHD alone (8).

More than a decade of research in this author's laboratory, conducted in collaboration with Dr. Harvey Singer and involving Kennedy Krieger Institute and Johns Hopkins University School of Medicine, has addressed the issue of ADHD and TS in neurobehavioral and anatomical terms. It is always very tempting to look at the syndrome of multiple tics as one of a particular kind of inhibitory insufficiency, so that the affiliation of tics with ADHD appears quite compelling and directs attention to the level of the basal ganglia. Behaviorally, however, ratings on the Behavior Rating Inventory of Executive Function (BRIEF) provide some evidence of difference and similarities between TS alone, TS plus ADHD, and ADHD alone. Both ADHD groups and TS plus ADHD groups are impaired on the five primary indices of the BRIEF. The BRIEF indices for the TS alone group are almost identical to those of the control group, with the subtle exception of a borderline elevation on the index labeled *working memory* (9). Further, on a computerized go/no-go continuous performance test, the test of variables of attention (TOVA), all three groups studied (TS alone, TS plus ADHD, ADHD alone) showed no error types of any excess but all were slow in reaction time and variable (10). It was very difficult to demonstrate any other executive dysfunctions in the pure TS group. In fact, two samples within this author's laboratory yielded opposite results on the only task previously found to be impaired in the TS sample, which was letter-word fluency (11,12). In the second sample, in which greater care was taken to completely remove significant elevations on obsessive-compulsive symptoms (not even reaching threshold of disorder) the letter-word fluency score was normal (12). This approach allowed a 10-year overview to the effect that pure TS, constituting perhaps only a 40% minority within the total picture of presenting with TS, is not associated with any significant executive dysfunction. In other words, the dysexecutive characteristics, the deficits in executive control, are associated with the ADHD co-morbidity and do not in this respect differ from what is seen with ADHD alone.

In addition to the "clean bill of health" given to the executive function in children with pure TS, this author also found incidentally a rather remarkable "advantage" to this group (11). When tested for full-scale intelligence quotient (IQ) and compared with the mean or mid-parental IQ, children with pure TS deviated upward from expectation; that is, their IQ scores were higher than that predicted by the usual model of regression to the mean, in which the mean is that taken from maternal and paternal IQ. In contrast, children with TS plus ADHD showed IQ scores that deviated to the lower side of the mid-parental regression line (11). Thus in the 40% of children with TS alone, there is reason to give some credence to common clinical lore, namely, that these children are unusually intellectually gifted youngsters who show no cognitive deficits. What remains unresolved and is still a major limitation to these studies is the impact of obsessive-compulsive symptomatology, even at a subthreshold level, on executive function.

The theme of "clean bill of health" for pure TS continues when one looks at all the data on motor testing. As has been found in many previous studies using the physical and neurological examination for soft signs (PANESS) for developmental neuromotor integrity, children with ADHD and TS plus ADHD showed slow-for-age timed movements, whereas most children with TS alone performed all movements with normal speed and half of all movements faster than average (13). It can be stated that 76% of children who have TS alone are faster than average on timed motor coordination. With respect to the eye movement experiments, the data is somewhat more complicated but equally demonstrative of a divergence of findings between pure TS and the ADHD groups. All the ADHD subjects, including those with TS, showed signs of deficient inhibition and excessive variability in their eye movements. The deficient inhibition was indicated by failure-for-age on the antisaccade (look away) task. The only problem found with the pure TS group was a prolonged latency of prosaccade initiation. Interestingly, this finding was an overlap because it was also found in the group with TS plus ADHD. Thus oculomotor function in the group with TS plus ADHD demonstrated a combination of the deficits of both the pure TS and the pure ADHD group (14).

This author's research team was able to perform anatomical (volumetric) magnetic resonance imaging measurements of the basal ganglia and the frontal lobes in the study groups. It should be noted that the research team took a very different approach from that of other groups who use ADHD status as a covariate. Because of behavioral evidence, the research team chose instead to analyze the small anatomical magnetic resonance imaging data by groups, pure TS, pure ADHD, and the co-morbid group.

The study of basal ganglia volumes found that both boys with TS plus ADHD and ADHD alone had smaller left globus pallidus volumes (15,16). TS alone was associated only with some subtle anomalies of lateral asymmetry of the basal ganglia. The research team also examined the midsaggital section to look at the corpus callosum as a body of white matter connections reflective of hemispheric relationships and found that there was a peculiar "cancellation of pathology" phenomenon. The boys with TS alone showed increased areas of four of five subdivisions of the corpus callosum, including the rostral body of the corpus callosum; in contrast, children with ADHD alone showed decreased area of the rostral body of the corpus callosum. Strangely, children with TS plus ADHD showed no difference in area of any region of the corpus callosum from what was found in the control group. It appeared from the data on the corpus callosum that there were independent effects in the direction of enlargement with TS and decrement with ADHD, such that those with TS plus ADHD were "pseudonormal" in size of corpus callosum rostrally (17).

Several studies carried out with a variety of novel volumetric programs compared the frontal lobes in TS alone, TS plus ADHD, and ADHD alone. In one study, it was found that there was increased right frontal white matter associated with TS alone, whereas ADHD alone was associated with smaller total frontal lobes bilaterally (18). Another study showed that there was some decrease in deep left white matter in TS alone, a finding not shared with other groups. Children with ADHD alone again demonstrated volumetric reductions in both gray and white matter bilaterally (19).

SUMMARY AND CONCLUSIONS

ADHD is a complex co-morbidity, as it is heterogeneous in terms of the clinical subtypes, but also in terms of the circuits involved and the level of involvement within those circuits. Specifically focusing on the relationship of ADHD to TS, this author's studies have added some neurobehavioral and some anatomical magnetic resonance imaging evidence suggesting the ADHD occurring with TS, appears like "garden-variety" ADHD, at least in the matched research sample. The similarities of neuro-anatomical findings in the TS plus ADHD and ADHD groups and their distinctness from neuro-anatomical findings in children with "pure" TS provide some parallels to the observed similarity of functional deficit in TS plus ADHD and ADHD alone groups and the relative lack of functional deficits in children with TS only. More specifically, the results of a decade of this author's research with the approximately 40% of children with TS who are free of ADHD indicate that they are entirely free of the motor control and executive control deficits of children with ADHD alone or TS plus ADHD, but they do have oculomotor control deficits in the initiation of prosaccades, regardless of their ADHD status. The neuroanatomical data in TS only is also of interest because it reflects increased white matter, particularly in the right frontal lobe and four out of five regions of the corpus callosum, including the rostral portion most affiliated with the frontal lobes. It should be emphasized that almost everything summarized above is true for boys, whereas samples of girls grouped similarly have not yielded the same results.

ACKNOWLEDGMENTS

Research cited in references 9 through 19 was supported by research grants P50 NS 35359, HD 25806 and P30 HD 024061. Grateful acknowledgments to Pamula Yerby-Hammack for preparation of this manuscript.

REFERENCES

1. Castellanos FX, Tannock R. Neuroscience of attention deficit hyperactivity disorder: The search for endophenotypes. *Nat Rev.* 2002;3:617–628.
2. American Psychiatric Association. *Diagnostic and Statistical Manual of Mental Disorders, 4th edition.* Washington, DC: American Psychiatric Association, 1994.
3. Denckla MB. ADHD: Topic update. *Brain Dev.* 2003;25:383–389.
4. Biederman J, Faraone SV, Mick E, et al. Clinical correlates of ADHD in females: findings from a large group of girls ascertained from pediatric and psychiatric referral sources. *J Am Acad Child Adolesc Psychiatry.* 1999;38:966–975.
5. McConaughey SH, Achenbach TM. Test Observation Form (TOF). Itasca, IL: Riverside Publishing, 2004.
6. Geurts HM, Verté S, Oosterlaan J, et al. How specific are executive functioning deficits in attention deficit hyperactivity disorder and autism. *J Child Psychol Psychiatry.* 2004;45:836–854.
7. Robertson MM. Behavioral and affective disorders in Tourette syndrome. In: Advances in neurology: Tourette syndrome. Philadelphia: Lippincott Williams & Wilkins, 2005:39–60.
8. Robertson MM. Invited review: Tourette syndrome, associated conditions and the complexities of treatment. *Brain* 2000;123:425–462.
9. Mahone EM, Cirino PT, Cutting LE, et al. Validity of the behavior rating inventory of executive function in children with ADHD and/or Tourette syndrome. *Arch Clin Neuropsychol.* 2002;17:643–662.
10. Harris EL, Schuerholz LJ, Singer HS et al. Executive function in children with Tourette syndrome and/or attention deficit hyperactivity disorder. *J Int Neuropsychol Soc.* 1995;1:511–516.
11. Schuerholz LJ, Baumgardner TL, Singer HS, et al. Neuropsychological status of children with Tourette's syndrome with and without attention deficit hyperactivity disorder. *Neurology* 1996;46:958–965.
12. Mahone EM, Koth CW, Cutting LE, et al. Executive function in fluency and recall measures among children with Tourette syndrome or ADHD. *J Int Neuropsychol Soc.* 2001;7:102–111.
13. Schuerholz LJ, Cutting LE, Mazzocco MM, et al. Neuromotor functioning in children with Tourette syndrome with and without attention deficit hyperactivity disorder. *J Child Neurol.* 1997;12:438–442.
14. Mostofsky SH, Lasker AG, Singer HS, et al. Oculomotor abnormalities in boys with Tourette syndrome with and without ADHD. *J Am Acad Child Adolesc Psychiatry.* 2001;40:1464–1472.
15. Singer HS, Reiss AL, Brown JE, et al. Volumetric MRI changes in basal ganglia of children with Tourette syndrome. *Neurology* 1993;43:950–956.
16. Aylward EH, Reiss AL, Reader MJ, et al. Basal ganglia volumes in children with attention deficit hyperactivity disorder. *J Child Neurol.* 119;11:112–115.
17. Baumgardner TL, Singer HS, Denckla MB, et al. Corpus callosum morphology in children with Tourette syndrome and attention deficit hyperactivity disorder. *Neurology* 1996;47:1–6.
18. Fredericksen KA, Cutting LE, Kates WR, et al. Disproportionate increases of white matter in right frontal lobe in Tourette syndrome. *Neurology* 2002;58:85–89.
19. Kates WR, Frederikse M, Mostofsky SH, et al. MRI parcellation of the frontal lobe in boys with attention deficit hyperactivity disorder or Tourette syndrome. *Psychiatry Res Neuroimaging.* 2002;116:63–81.

3

Obsessive-Compulsive Disorder in Tourette Syndrome

Ana Gabriela Hounie,[1] Maria Conceição do Rosario-Campos,[1] Juliana Belo Diniz,[3] Roseli Gendaki Shavitt,[1] Ygor A. Ferrão, Antonio Carlos Lopes,[1] Marcos T. Mercadante,[2] Geraldo F. Busatto,[1] and Euripedes Constantino Miguel[1]

[1]*Department of Psychiatry, University of São Paulo Medical School, São Paulo, Brazil;*
[2]*Pervasive Development Disorder Program, Mackenzie Presbyterian University, São Paulo, Brazil;*
[3]*OCD Spectrum Disorder Project, University of São Paulo, São Paulo, Brazil*

Obsessive compulsive disorder (OCD) is a chronic disorder that affects approximately 2% of the world population and is characterized by intrusive unwanted thoughts, fears or images (obsessions), and/or ritualized behaviors or mental acts (compulsions), generally performed to relieve the anxiety and/or distress caused by the obsessions (1).

Even though the *Diagnostic and Statistical Manual–Fourth Edition–Text Revision* (DSM-IV-TR), and *International Classification of Disease and Related Health Problems–10th Revision* (ICD-10) criteria define OCD as a unitary disorder, obsessive-compulsive (OC) symptoms are in fact remarkably diverse, and the clinical presentation varies among patients and even within the same patient across time (2,3). This variability in the phenotypic expression has led to the hypothesis that OCD is in fact a heterogeneous disorder with several different subgroups. One of the putative subgroups is the tic-related OCD.

The clinical association between vocal and motor tics and OC symptoms has been observed since the first descriptions of Tourette syndrome (TS) by Itard (4), and subsequently by Gilles de La Tourette (5). More recent clinical studies have shown that approximately one third of TS patients also have OCD and at least 50% would present OC symptoms (6). Likewise,

approximately 30% of OCD patients also have chronic tics and 10% fulfill criteria for TS (7–9).

This review article focuses on recent OCD studies that emphasize the relationship between OCD and TS. Different areas of research have provided scientific support to this association, investigating aspects of psychopathology, molecular and epidemiologic genetics, neuroanatomy, and neuroimaging. This review also explores the role of common environmental factors such as a streptococcal infection in the expression of OCD and TS and presents some of the treatment implications for this subgroup of patients. Finally, the article concludes with the proposal of an additive polygenic genetic model for OCD and TS, in which different sets of genes predispose to overlapping phenotypes that are in part both quantitative and qualitative distinct.

PHENOMENOLOGIC STUDIES

Many different approaches developed to describe the clinical features that characterize the tic-related OCD phenotype are reviewed.

Categorical Approach

Many studies have characterized the tic-related OCD phenotype based on the comparison of

TABLE 3-1. *The tic-related obsessive-compulsive disorder (OCD) phenotype: Phenotypic features found more frequently in patients with OCD and tic disorders compared with OCD patients without tics*

Study	Phenotypic features
Miguel et al. (3,21)	Presence of sensory phenomena
Miguel et al. (3); Pitman (11); George et al. (12); Holzer et al. (13); Petter et al. (14); Rasmussen et al. (10); Swerdlow et al. (15)	Intrusive violent and sexual images or thoughts, hoarding, and counting rituals
Miguel et al. (3); Leckman et al. (16); George et al. (12); Holzer et al. (13); Leckman et al. (15); Petter et al. (14); Leckman et al. (24); Eapen et al. (19); Rosario-Campos et al. (8)	"Tic-like" compulsions
Baer (23); Mataix-Cols et al. (27)	High scores on symmetry/hoarding factor
Leckman et al. (24)	High scores on harmful, sexual, somatic, and religious obsessions and related compulsions and symmetry/ordering factors
Miguel et al. (3)	Higher number and variety of obsessive-compulsive symptoms
Coffey et al. (37)	Higher comorbidity with trichotillomania, body dysmorphic disorder, bipolar disorder, attention deficit/hyperactivity disorder, social phobia, substance abuse

Adapted from Miguel EC, Leckman JF, Rauch S, et al. The obsessive-compulsive disorder phenotypes: Implications for genetic studies. Submitted.

patients with OCD and tics or TS and OCD without tics as mutually exclusive categorical subgroups. Tic-related and non-tic-related OCD differ with respect to the content of obsessions and compulsions and the number and nature of OCS. Tic-related OCD patients are more likely to present with intrusive violent and sexual images or thoughts, hoarding, and counting rituals (3,10–15).

"Tic-like" compulsions have also been reported as more frequent in OCD patients with tics and may be defined as behaviors similar to complex tics but performed to relieve the distress caused by physical sensations, such as the need to touch, tap or rub items, or blinking and staring compulsions (3,8,12,13,16–18) (Table 3-1).

Some of these phenotypic differences have also been reported in genetic studies. For instance, Eapen et al. (19) compared the OC symptom profile of patients with OCD with the profile of patients with TS and OC symptoms. They found that OCD patients with the tic-related OC symptom profile (i.e., aggressive, violent, and sexual obsessions and symmetry; "just right" perceptions; and tic-like compulsions) had also family history of OCD. Accordingly, OCD patients without family history of OCD reported the non-tic profile more frequently, including obsessions of contamination, cleaning and washing compulsions, and fear of things going wrong (Table 3-1). Furthermore, TS patients with parents who have OCD had a later age of onset of tic symptoms and more complex tics, suggesting that the presence of OCD in the family may also affect the TS phenotype in the proband (20).

OCD patients with and without tics also differ in terms of the subjective experiences that precede or accompany their repetitive behaviors. Although these experiences have been reported with different names, the authors of this chapter proposed to group these various descriptions of sensory phenomena into *bodily sensations* (i.e., focal or generalized body sensations occurring before the patient performed the repetitive behaviors) and *mental sensations* (i.e., general, uncomfortable feelings or perceptions occurring before or while the patient performs the repetitive behaviors) (21). Sometimes these sensory phenomena are responsible for significant psychosocial distress (21). To assess the different kinds of sensory phenomena, the authors developed an instrument in which patients are asked to identify which phenomena precede or accompany each of their repetitive behaviors (22). To study patients with both OCD and TS, the authors suggested the term *intentional repetitive behavior* (from the DSM-III-R) to include overlapping symptoms with distinct definitions such as complex tics (characteristic of TS) and compulsions (characteristic of OCD). The sensory phenomena associated with repetitive behaviors in patients with TS alone, TS plus OCD and pure OCD were compared. As expected, the OCD plus TS group reported significantly more intentional repetitive behaviors preceded by sensory phenomena than the OCD alone or the TS alone groups (3,21) (Table 3-1).

In a recent article, the authors of this chapter attempted to measure the impact of the presence of chronic motor tics and TS in the OC symptom profile by comparing three groups of OCD patients from a total sample of 162 patients (22a). Of these patients, 97 (61%) had OCD without tics; 34 (21%) had OCD plus chronic motor/vocal tics (CMVT), and 30 (18%) had OCD plus TS. OCD plus CMVT patients were similar to OCD plus TS patients compared with patients without tics in terms of higher frequency of intrusive sounds, repeating behaviors, counting compulsions, and tic-like compulsions. Regarding somatic obsessions, bodily sensations, just-right perceptions, presence of sensory phenomena, number of psychiatric co-morbidities, age at interview, and age at OC symptom onset, the OCD plus CMVT patients tended to be intermediate compared to the other two groups. In contrast, OCD plus CMVT patients were differentiated from patients with TS or no tics in regard to religious obsessions and depressive mood disorders, which were specifically high in OCD plus CMVT patients. In conclusion, these data suggest that the OCD phenotype may vary according to the presence of chronic tics or TS. In most of these measures, the OCD plus CMVT group resembles the OCD plus TS group. However, the results of these variables in the OCD plus CMVT were also intermediate in magnitude compared with patients with OCD without tics and OCD with TS. This finding may reflect different numbers or types of genes underlying each phenotype.

Dimensional Approach

Most studies describing the clinical, genetic, and neuroimaging features that characterize the tic-related OCD phenotype have focused on the comparison of OCD patients with or without tic disorders, thus considering these subgroups as mutually exclusive categories. Despite the usefulness of this approach, there is a consistent overlap between those potential subgroups, and it is difficult clinically to identify "pure" patients representing each group. Some more recent studies have used a dimensional approach. This strategy regards OCD as composed of sets of OC symptom dimensions, with each dimension corresponding to a distinctive set of biobehavioral mechanisms and allowing quantitative measures of phenotypic traits. The main difference between mutually exclusive categories and the dimensional approach is that in the latter approach each patient can score on one or more symptom dimensions at one time.

Baer (23) was the first to try to correlate these OC symptom factors with biological variables. He identified three OC symptom factors: contamination/cleaning; pure obsessions; and symmetry and hoarding. The third factor was found more frequently in OCD patients with tics.

Following Baer's work, Leckman et al. (24) proposed a four-factor model, comprising the following factors: aggressive, sexual, and religious obsessions and checking compulsions (factor one); symmetry and ordering obsessions and compulsions (factor two); contamination obsessions and cleaning/washing compulsions (factor three); hoarding obsessions and compulsions (factor four).

These factors or dimensions have been replicated by 10 other studies, with more than 2,000 patients. The most consistent models using this approach are composed of four or five OC symptoms factors (or dimensions) that can explain more than 60% of the total group variance (25–32). These dimensions have been shown to be temporally stable (31) and with meaningful biological correlates. For example, some studies have associated high scores on factors one and two with co-morbid tic disorders (23,24,27). Interestingly, Alsobrook et al. (33) have found an association between high scores on factors one and two and greater familial risk for OCD. In a recent study, Leckman et al. (32) found that factors one and two significantly correlated in sib-pairs concordant for TS and also noted that mother-child correlations were significant for these two factors.

Zhang et al. (34) completed a genome scan using the data from the same TS sib-pair study and assessed the hoarding dimension. Significant allele sharing was observed for markers at 4q34-35, 5q35.2-35.3 and 17q25. The 4q site is in proximity to D4S1625, the marker that was identified by the same dataset as being in a genomic region with suggestive linkage to the TS phenotype. The 17q site has also been implicated in some TS families (34a). Thus, the 4q and 17q results could simply be coming from linkage to the TS phenotype and not represent a separate locus for hoarding. Another possibility is that the same gene in each of these regions predisposes to both TS and the hoarding OCD phenotype. Finally, the chromosome 5 site, which has not been implicated in any other study of TS, might suggest a separate locus for hoarding.

Broadening the Phenotype

Another possible approach suggests broadening the investigation of possible phenotypes including other disorders related to OCD. The disorders included in this spectrum share some phenomenologic similarities with OCD, such as co-morbidity, family history, and treatment response patterns. In addition to tic disorders, other putative OCD spectrum disorders include body dysmorphic disorder (BDD), hypochondriasis, anorexia nervosa, and grooming behaviors (e.g., trichotillomania [TTM], skin picking) (35,36). Both BDD and TTM have been associated with TS in previous studies (22a,37) (Table 3-1). These findings suggest that OCD may be better conceptualized from a genetic standpoint as a quantitative trait. In such a model, the same genes would predispose to a variety of phenotypes. Although the OC spectrum concept theoretically increases the chances of finding genes associated to OCD, it is still unclear which disorders should be included in this spectrum.

In a recent study, Nestadt et al. (38) have used latent cluster analyses as a way of identifying subgroups from the subjects assessed in the Johns Hopkins OCD Family Study Group. Subsequently, the authors of this chapter have elaborated on the conclusions raised by Nestadt et al. (38) and proposed the existence of two OCD subgroups (39). One of the OCD subgroups would be represented by OC spectrum disorders (including tic disorders, BDD, TTM, and grooming behaviors), recurrent major depression, and generalized anxiety disorder. This subgroup would be associated with an early OCD age of onset and higher genetic susceptibility. Another OCD subgroup with different etiologic factors would be characterized by separation anxiety and panic disorder/agoraphobia, with lower genetic risk and later age of onset. Although this hypothesis must be tested in future studies, Fig. 3-1 attempts to represent these different possibilities in terms of the OCD phenotypic expression (40). Based on additional evidence, we have also added co-morbid diagnoses such as hypochondriasis (41), attention deficit/hyperactivity disorder (37), and eating disorders (42).

GENETIC FACTORS

Genetic Epidemiologic Studies

Genetic epidemiologic studies provide the most compelling evidence for the association between OCD and TS. Whether the probands are ascertained based on the diagnosis of TS (43–48) or of OCD (49–51), the first-degree relatives have higher frequency of both OCD or tic disorders compared with control relatives. Studies with OCD families have also reported that the earlier the age at onset of the OC symptoms in the proband, the higher the genetic loading in the family (36,49,50) (Table 3-2). A twin study of TS reported higher concordance of OC symptoms (52). Price et al. (52) reported that, among 43 twin pairs in which one member had TS, 83% of the TS patients had OC symptoms.

The importance of the age at onset of OC symptoms was also investigated in studies using OCD probands of children and adolescents (53–56). The small sample sizes and varied methodologies adopted in these studies yielded divergent findings.

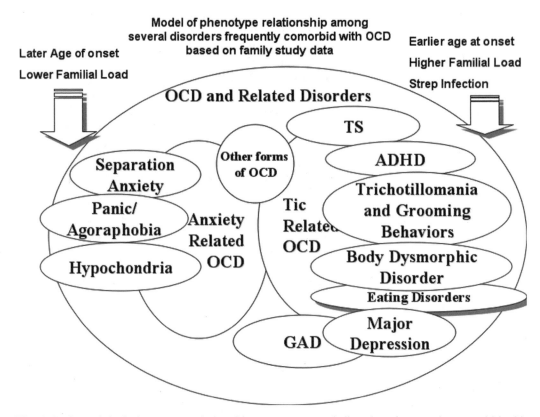

Fig. 3-1. A model of phenotype relationship among several disorders frequently comorbid with obsessive-compulsive disorder based on family study data.

TABLE 3-2. *Comparison of prevalence rates of obsessive-compulsive disorder (OCD), sub-clinical OCD, and tic disorders in family studies ascertained from adult probands and from children and adolescents*

	OCD	OCD + Sub-clinical OCD	Tic disorders	Total OCD + Sub-clinical OCD
Pauls et al. (49)	10.3 ± 1.4	7.9 ± 1.3	4.6	18.2 ± 1.8
Nestadt et al. (50)*	11.7 ± 1.8	4.6 ± 1.3	4.6**	16.3 ± 2.0*
Grados et al. (51)**				
Rosario-Campos et al. (68)	22.7 ± 2.6	6.5 ± 1.6	11.6	29.2 ± 2.8

OCD, obsessive-compulsive disorder.
*Findings of the first study on the familial aggregation pattern of obsessive-compulsive disorder
**Findings of the second study on the familial relationship between obsessive-compulsive disorder

The authors of this chapter recently conducted a study to evaluate the association between an early age of onset of OC symptoms in OCD children and adolescents and the morbid risks of OCD and tics in their first-degree family members (57). The study investigated 325 first-degree relatives of 106 OCD probands compared with 140 first-degree family members of 44 control probands. The findings of this study were consistent with earlier reports indicating that the familial aggregation of OCD is largely concentrated among families with early-onset OCD probands, with the highest morbid risks reported thus far. The ratio of the rates of OCD in case and control relatives (estimated λ) was 25.2. Other interesting findings were the significantly higher rates of TS and chronic tics among case relatives and the fact that a diagnosis of

TABLE 3-3. *Molecular findings associated to the tic-related obsessive-compulsive disorder phenotype*

Study	Methodology	Sample size	Gene polymorphism
Cruz et al. (66)	Association study	49 OCD-tics and 12 OCD + tics	DRD4 (7 repeat variant) more frequent in OCD plus tics
Nicolini et al. (65)	Allelic Association study	54 OCD without tics, 12 OCD with tics, 54 controls	TaqIA2 allele of the DRD2 and excess of homozygosity for A2A2 in OCD + tics; allele 7 of DRD4 higher in OCD + tics; haplotype A2R7 higher in OCD + tics
Nicolini et al. (64)	Association study	67 OCD 54 controls	DRD2 (A2A2 genotype) more frequent in OCD + tics
Cavallini et al. (29)	Candidate gene study A principal component analysis was performed and derived 13 factors.	180 OCD, 21 with tics; 112 controls	Long/long haplotype of the functional polymorphism in the promoter region of the serotonin transporter locus at 17q11 had a significant association with factor 5 (including counting and repeating rituals) in patients with tics
Millet et al. (63)	TDT and Association study	49 OCD (17 with tics) versus 63 controls	DRD4 (allele 2 variant): inverse association only with OCD without tics;
Urraca et al. (67)	TDT	51 trios with OCD (with and without tics)	Tendency for higher frequency of micro opioid receptor gene in OCD + tics

OCD, obsessive-compulsive disorder; TDT, transmission disequilibrium test

tics in the relatives was the best predictor for this relative to have OCD (57). Table 3-2 shows the risks for OCD, tics, or TS among the first-degree relatives in some of the most recent family studies using adult probands. In conclusion, genetic epidemiologic studies suggest that some forms of OCD are genetically transmitted. Among those, the tic-related OCD is associated with an earlier age of onset of OC symptoms and higher genetic loading.

Molecular Genetic Studies

Molecular genetic studies in OCD have been largely based on a candidate gene approach, in which the frequencies of variants (polymorphisms) of candidate genes are genotyped in a population of OCD probands and compared to the frequencies of the same polymorphisms in subjects recruited from either the general population or family-based controls (58,59). Most studies conducted to date have included candidate genes related to the serotoninergic and dopaminergic systems, based on the fact that

serotonin reuptake inhibitors and dopamine antagonists are effective in the treatment of OCD patients (60–67).

Table 3-3 displays several molecular studies that emphasize the association between OCD and tics. Unfortunately, these results initially raised great enthusiasm, but most of them have not been replicated in subsequent studies.

ENVIRONMENTAL FACTORS

Interestingly, although the morbid risks in the relatives of OCD patients are usually increased, the diagnoses of tics and OCD are concentrated in approximately 50% of families of adult OCD probands (49) and in 57% of the families of children and adolescents with OCD (68). These findings reinforce the ideas that some forms of OCD are familial whereas others are not and that environmental factors play an important role in the final expression of some of the OCD phenotypes.

Epigenetic Risk and Protective Factors

A variety of risk factors including prenatal and perinatal adverse events, gender-specific hormonal factors, pregnancy and birth, psycho-social stressors, and post-infectious immune-based factors have been associated with the expression of OCD (69,70). For example, peri-natal difficulties might predispose to an earlier onset of OCD in males (71), as well as being associated with chronic tic disorders (72). In one study of individuals with TS, delivery complications (especially forceps deliveries) and fetal exposure to high levels of coffee, cigarettes, or alcohol also predicted OCD in the same TS probands (72). This same study found that females with TS experience the onset of complex tics more often than males with TS. Additionally, the fact that males are more frequently affected with early onset OCD than females has raised the hypothesis that androgenic steroids during critical periods in fetal development could play a role in the later development of tic-related OCD (73). Finally, stressful life events or potentially triggering events may also represent additional factors modulating the expression of OCD (74–79). Frequently reported triggers include a recent move, sexual or marital problems, and the illness or death of a near relative (74–78).

Role of Streptococcal Infection and Rheumatic Fever

Studies suggest an association between strepto-coccus infection and OCD (80–82). This line of research was developed after the reports of a higher prevalence of OC symptoms in Syden-ham chorea (SC) patients, the neurologic mani-festation of rheumatic fever (RF) (83). Further studies have described a higher prevalence of OCD and/or TS in RF, even without SC, both in active (84,85) and non-active (86) phases. Familial aggregation of OCD/TS has also been described in cases of RF (86a).

Swedo et al. proposed the acronym PANDAS (for the term *Pediatric Autoimmune Neuropsy-chiatric Disorders Associated with Streptococ-cal infection*) to describe prepubertal children in which OCD and/or TS symptoms abruptly begin or exacerbate after a streptococcal infec-tion but who do not develop RF (83). One study compared plasmapheresis with intravenous immunoglobulin and placebo and documented short-term improvement in the active treatment group versus the control group (87). The mech-anism involved in symptom reduction is unclear because plasma exchange removes both anti-bodies and cytokines. As the largest study to date to investigate immunomodulatory treat-ments in OCD and/or TS symptoms, it is signif-icant as well as controversial (88,89).

Familial aggregation of OCD/TS occurs with RF and in PANDAS (90). Relatives of subjects with PANDAS/OCD have the same rate of OCD as relatives of children with OCD, which may suggest that "classic, early onset OCD" shares underlying mechanisms with the OCD triggered by streptococcal infections. In addi-tion, higher rates of RF were also described among parents and grandparents of PANDAS cases compared with controls (83).

The hypothesized mechanism underlying the relationship between streptococcal infection, RF, and the OCD spectrum manifestations is the molecular mimicry between bacteria and host. This assumption has been widely supported by several studies showing higher levels of autoan-tibodies in OCD patients (91). However, there are several unanswered questions about how the infection could be responsible for the neuropsy-chiatric symptoms. Although cross-reactive anti-bodies binding to streptococcal M proteins and to myosin have been identified in the rheumatic heart disease, the same finding has not been demonstrated in SC and/or PANDAS patients. In addition, the presence of T cells at the site of damaged cardiac valve may explain the immune mechanism in rheumatic carditis (92), however, no similar finding has been demonstrated in SC. Even with the suggestion of cross-reactivity found between N-acetyl-glucosamine (a strepto-coccal antigen) and lysoganglioside (a trans-membrane molecule highly frequent in the central nervous system) using SC monoclonal antibodies (93), it is still unclear how antibodies could affect the central nervous system. The selective permeability of the blood brain barrier gives the brain a privileged immunologic status; however, immune-regulatory substances, such as cytokines, or even activated B or T cells, could facilitate antibody access into the brain by disruption of the barrier.

Finally, one recent study (94) found an association between a variant in the myelin oligodendrocyte glycoprotein gene, a component of the myelin sheath, and OCD. The authors suggested that the potentially autoimmune demyelinating role of this molecule, as a target autoantigen, could be a hypothetical inductor of OCD via demyelination in the frontal lobe or other neuroanatomic regions (94). The complexity of this model, in which a true autoimmune mechanism would be causing OCD, as well as the lack of evidence supporting it, warrants more studies to clarify the issue. Nevertheless, the authors of this chapter speculate that PANDAS, classic OCD and TS, and RF share genetic susceptibility or function as risk factors for the other conditions.

NEUROBIOLOGIC SUBSTRATES

The complex interaction of the genetic and environmental factors previously described presumably leads to abnormalities in the structure and functioning of specific brain circuits, providing the neurobiologic substrate for the expression of the tic-related OCD phenotype. Clues to the nature of these neurobiologic mechanisms may be revealed by reviewing previous studies carried out in samples of OCD or TS subjects, using neurochemical, neuroendocrine and neuroanatomic approaches. Due to space constraints, this chapter selectively reviews the studies that have used neuroimaging techniques.

The prevailing neuroanatomic models of OCD propose a critical role for imbalance of cortico-striatal-thalamic circuits in the disorder (95,96). Such models have been supported by functional imaging studies measuring regional cerebral blood flow (rCBF) or glucose metabolism with positron emission tomography (PET) or single photon emission computed tomography. These studies have consistently shown abnormal metabolic activity in the orbitofrontal cortex, anterior cingulate gyrus, caudate nucleus, and thalamus in groups of OCD patients relative to healthy controls (96–99). PET studies of OCD have also shown that both behavior and drug therapies may normalize metabolic activity patterns in the OFC and basal ganglia

(100–102). Similar cortico-striatal-thalamic circuits have been implicated in rCBF PET, and functional magnetic resonance imaging (MRI) studies performed during the provocation of symptoms in OCD subjects exposed to known anxiogenic stimuli (103,104).

Finally, recent functional imaging studies have shown that specific symptom dimensions of OCD may be associated with distinct activity patterns in the cortico-subcortical circuits above. One PET study found increased resting rCBF in the left orbitofrontal cortex and bilateral anterior cingulate gyrus in relation to the severity of washing symptoms in OCD patients, whereas checking and order/symmetry behaviors were correlated with, respectively, increased and decreased rCBF in the striatum (105). In a functional MRI study, the presentation of checking-related pictures to OCD patients was associated with increased activity of the thalamus, putamen/globus pallidus and dorsal cortical regions (106), whereas washing-related pictures led to activation of the left medial frontal gyrus, right anterior cingulate gyrus and bilateral orbitofrontal cortex (106). Lastly, a PET study of resting glucose metabolism in OCD patients with hoarding symptoms has shown reduced activity in the dorsal anterior cingulate gyrus, as well as in the posterior cingulate gyrus and cuneus in these OCD subjects relative to healthy controls (107).

The results of morphometric studies of adult OCD subjects using MRI have been relatively less consistent, with reports of decreased (108), normal (109) and increased basal ganglia volumes in OCD patients compared to healthy controls (110). A few MRI studies have also reported volumetric abnormalities of the orbitofrontal cortex, anterior cingulate gyrus and temporolimbic structures in OCD patients (111–114). Finally, findings of increased thalamic volumes (115) and amygdala asymmetry have been described in children with OCD (116), reversible after paroxetine treatment.

Neuroimaging studies of subjects with TS have been less numerous, and several of these studies have devoted particular attention to the investigation of the basal ganglia. morphometric studies using MRI have shown abnormal volumes and asymmetry in the caudate nucleus, putamen, and globus pallidus in samples of TS patients compared with healthy volunteers (117–119), although negative findings have also been reported (120). Morphometric MRI studies of TS patients have also found anatomical changes in the corpus callosum, and in frontal, parietal, and occipital cortices (121–123), suggesting that the pathophysiology of TS may also involve structural abnormalities of distributed brain systems. In PET studies investigating glucose metabolism at rest, a pattern of increased motor cortical activity and decreased activity in basal ganglia, thalamic and hippocampal regions has been described in TS patients in comparison to healthy controls (124). Further evidence for the involvement of the basal ganglia in TS is given by neurochemical, PET, and single photon emission computed tomography studies, which have found increased density of presynaptic dopamine transporters and postsynaptic dopamine D2 receptors in the striatum in TS patients relative to controls (125,126), as well as greater dopamine release in the putamen (127). These data are consistent with the efficacy of dopamine antagonists for the treatment of TS. Finally, PET and functional MRI studies have helped to delineate the brain functional systems directly engaged during the emergence of tics in TS. The occurrence of tics has been found to correlate directly with functional activity in a distributed set of brain regions, including the primary motor and medial premotor cortices, supplementary motor area, anterior cingulate gyrus, dorsolateral-rostral prefrontal cortex, inferior parietal cortex, caudate-putamen, Broca's area, superior temporal gyrus, insula, and claustrum (128). Separate investigations of different forms of tics have shown that vocal tics predominantly activate prerolandic and postrolandic language regions, as well as the insula, caudate, thalamus and cerebellum; motor tics, on the other hand, are associated with increased activity predominantly in the sensorimotor cortex (128). It has also been shown that voluntary tic suppression is associated with deactivation of the putamen and globus pallidus, coupled to activation of the prefrontal cortex and caudate nucleus (129).

In conclusion, the data just reviewed indicate that the pathophysiology of both OCD and TS involve abnormalities in cortico-striatum-thalamic-cortical neuronal loops. Despite similarities in the involvement of the basal ganglia in both disorders, differences in the cortico-striatal projections are implicated in each condition. Whereas ventral frontal regions, including the orbitofrontal cortex, are more consistently involved in OCD, the functional circuitry of TS appear to encompass other cortical regions, including motor and sensorial cortical areas and their projections to dorsolateral striatal regions.

In future neuroimaging studies, it will be important to verify whether specific portions of the cortico-striatal-thalamic circuits described previously are particularly affected in those subjects who present with both OCD symptoms and tics. These studies should help to delineate more specifically the neurobiological substrate for the tic-related OCD phenotype.

TREATMENT IMPLICATIONS

This chapter has presented different lines of investigation supporting the existence of a separate tic-related OCD phenotype. It is expected that such refinements in the assessments of different OC phenotypes might lead to greater clarity concerning treatment strategies for individual subjects. Therefore, one may ask the following questions: 1) Does the presence of tics or TS influence the severity of OCD? 2) Is the tic-related OCD associated with worse OCD treatment response? 3) To what extent does the tic-related OCD have a distinctive pattern of response to various psychopharmacological agents? 4) Do environmental factors such as streptococcal infection, associated with the expression of OCD and TS, imply in different approaches to OCD treatment? and 5) Does the presence of tics or TS influence the severity of OCD?

According to a recent study by the authors of this chapter (22a), OCD patients with chronic tics or TS do not differ from OCD patients without tics in terms of severity of OC symptoms. However, the opposite seems to be true: the presence of OCD is associated with worse tic severity in TS patients (15).

Is Tic-Related OCD Associated with Worse Treatment Response?

Approximately 30% to 40% of OCD patients do not show significant improvement after adequate trials with first-line treatments (130,131). Some authors have suggested that the presence of tics may predict a worse response to selective serotonin reuptake inhibitor (SSRI) monotherapy (132,133). Nevertheless, results from a systematic, blind study developed by the authors of this chapter with 41 OCD patients treated for 14 weeks with clomipramine did not confirm the presence of tics and/or TS as predictors of poor treatment response, i.e., patients with and without tics responded equally (134). One possible explanation for the greater improvement in this subgroup of OCD patients with tics could be the additional noradrenergic properties of clomipramine (previous studies used SSRIs), which could have had a positive effect on tics and/or worsened OC symptoms (135). However, in another study of our group, in refractory and respondent OCD cases, tics were equally described in both groups (135a).

To What Extent Does the Tic-Related OCD Phenotype Show a Distinctive Response Pattern to Psychopharmacologic Agents?

Current general guidelines for the treatment of OCD consider cognitive-behavioral therapy (136) and SSRIs as the first-line treatments for OCD (137). As mentioned previously, approximately one third of patients do not respond to SSRI monotherapy, and require augmentation strategies. In the available literature, few treatment studies include patients with OCD and co-morbid TS; the presence of TS is, in fact, often an exclusion criterion in OCD clinical trials. Consequently, the question of the extent to which TS related OCD has a different pattern of response to psychopharmacologic agents remains unanswered. Basically, treatment of OCD in TS should start with the first-line therapies for OCD, plus a first-line treatment for tics or TS when necessary.

Addition of conventional antipsychotics to SSRIs may improve OC symptoms in unresponsive OCD plus tics patients. McDougle (138), in an open study with pimozide added to fluvoxamine in 17 patients with OCD plus tics or schizotypal personality, found that 53% responded to the combination treatment. McDougle et al. (133), in a controlled trial with haloperidol, found that its addition to fluvoxamine was especially effective for OCD patients with co-morbid tic disorders.

Atypical antipsychotics with mixed effects on dopamine and serotonin have also been tested in treatment-resistant OCD without tics. Risperidone has been reported to reduce OCD symptoms when used to augment SSRIs in two open studies (107,139) and one double-blind, placebo-controlled study (140). Similar findings were found with open (141,142) and controlled double-blind studies (143,144) using olanzapine as an augmenter. Shapira et al. (145) reported the only controlled study that found negative results with olanzapine in association with an SSRI in OCD resistant cases. The addition of quetiapine, another atypical antipsychotic, to ongoing SSRI therapy has also been found to be effective in patients with refractory OCD (146), but not in low doses (147). An open trial with amisulpride (148) also suggests that it may be useful when combined with an SSRI.

Interestingly, however, all the atypical antipsychotics mentioned previously were helpful for the treatment-resistant OCD patients regardless of the presence of tics. Therefore, for OCD patients with tics or TS resistant to conventional treatment, the best available evidence suggests augmentation with typical antipsychotics, although this finding needs further replication.

Do Environmental Factors such as Streptococcal Infection Associated with OCD and TS Expression Imply Different Approaches to Treatment?

The hypothesis of the existence of a subgroup of OCD and/or TS with an abrupt onset and symptom exacerbation associated with streptococcal infections, and with the presence of RF with or without SC, has encouraged the conduct of trials using therapies directed against a presumed postinfectious autoimmune process.

These trials have included reports of improvement of OC symptoms and tics with plasma exchange and intravenous immunoglobulins (87). Such findings will need, however, further replication before such strategies can be recommended in clinical settings. One double-blind, crossover study with oral penicillin has also been conducted in 37 PANDAS children (149). The authors postulated that, as in RF prophylaxis, penicillin would be effective in preventing streptococcal-triggered OCD symptoms and tics in children with PANDAS (149). This study, however, found no change in OCD or tic symptom severity during the active (penicillin V) and the placebo phase.

CONCLUSIONS AND FUTURE DIRECTIONS

In this chapter, different approaches used to better describe the tic-related OCD phenotype were presented, including categorical and dimensional approaches, in addition to others suggesting the broadening of the OCD diagnostic boundaries.

A dimensional conceptualization may be the most efficacious in helping to identify the heritable components of OCD. In contrast to the categorical approach, factors or dimensions are not mutually exclusive, so each patient can exhibit one or more symptom dimensions at any one time (150). A limitation for dimensional studies, however, has been the lack of assessment instruments capable of encompassing all the OC symptom dimensions. Thus, instruments capable of assessing some specific phenotypic features of tic-related OCD, such as the presence of sensory phenomena, are also needed for future studies. Meanwhile, two new instruments have been developed recently: the Dimensional Yale-Brown Obsessive-Compulsive Scale (DY-BOCS), for the assessment of OC symptom dimensions, with promising initial psychometric results (151), and the University of São Paulo Sensory Phenomena Scale (USP-SPS), for the assessment of sensory phenomena (available upon request). A validation study of the USP-SPS is currently being conducted.

This chapter also reviewed genetic epidemiology studies that provide compelling evidence to support the relationship between OCD and tic disorders and discussed the role of some common and specific environmental factors, such as streptococcal infection, in the expression of both disorders. These genetic and environmental factors seem to be common to several other OCD spectrum disorders such as BDD, TTM, and "grooming behaviors." This complex gene-environmental interaction presumably plays a crucial role in the formation and/or activity of common structures in cortico-striato-thalamo-cortical circuits, which probably provide the neurobiologic substrate for the expression of the tic-related OCD phenotype. In future studies, it will be also important to understand how different gene effects might result in such a complex pattern of OCD-related phenotypes. OCD segregation analyses (33,50,152,153) have reported divergent results, with some studies suggesting that Mendelian factors alone are not sufficient to fully explain the familial aggregation of OCD, and residual familial effects are necessary to adequately fit the data (50). These segregation analyses in OCD also suggest a quantitative or polygenic transmission model for OCD. In this last form of genetic transmission, the trait is a continuous variable whose value results from the combined effect of many genes. The greater the number of genes, the greater is the value of the quantitative trait. In its purest form, quantitative traits derive from numerous genes each of them of small effect (154). The trait may display a normal distribution around the population mean, which reflects the average number of polygene alleles carried in the population.

The findings of intermediate phenomenologic measures in OCD subjects with chronic tics compared with groups of OCD subjects without tics or OCD plus TS (22a) may be compatible with an additive quantitative genetic model, meaning that the effects of the genes are added to produce a cumulative quantitative effect. From a quantitative point of view, these authors could also speculate that different loadings of susceptibility genes would predispose to the several OCD spectrum disorders. In this model, there would be several thresholds that when reached increase the risk for a specific spectrum disorder. Figure 3-2 is a schematic representation of these ideas.

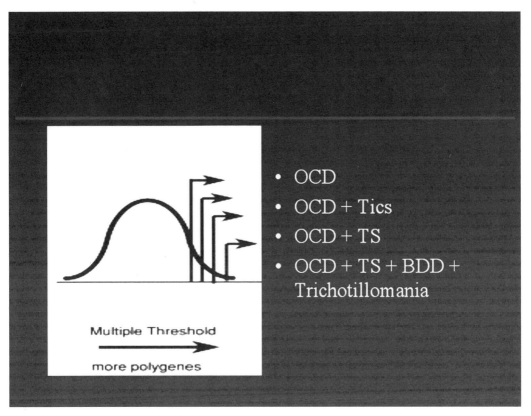

Fig. 3-2. An additive quantitative model for obsessive-compulsive disorder spectrum disorders expression. ADHD, attention deficit hyperactivity disorder; GAD, generalized anxiety disorder; OCD, obsessive-compulsive disorder TS, Tourette syndrome.

This model, however, does not explain the presence of TS, BDD, and TTM alone (i.e., isolated from OCD), suggesting that a more complex model might be involved. Such a model could include a qualitative spectrum of disorders in which different phenotypes would be related to distinct genes, not only different number of genes. Therefore, a mixture of the quantitative (explaining the variation within each group) and qualitative models (explaining the presence of different disorders or subtypes) in interaction with the environment may be a plausible hypothesis to explain the OCD phenotypic variability. Figure 3-1 represents the organization of this idea, suggesting at least two OCD subgroups. One is represented by the tic-related OCD, which would include other OCD spectrum disorders with a common genetic vulnerability that are quantitatively ranked in relationship to each other. The second subgroup, qualitatively different, includes the anxiety-related subgroup. There are possibly several other subgroups, which are not represented in this figure. Therefore, according to this model, different sets of genes predispose to overlapping phenotypes that are in part both quantitative and qualitatively distinct in nature.

Finally, in addition to its importance for genetic studies, it is also hoped that the identification of the core features of the tic-related OCD phenotype will also have clear treatment implications. To date, there is some evidence that the augmentation with typical antipsychotics to ongoing treatment with SSRIs may benefit OCD patients with tics. In the future, the better characterization of the pathophysiologic mechanisms of the tic-related OCD phenotype will contribute more decisively to our ability to find specific pharmacological and environmental based therapies (155).

ACKNOWLEDGMENTS

This work was supported by grants from Fundação de Amparo à Pesquisa do Estado de São Paulo (FAPESP): #99/08560-6 to Drs. Busatto and Miguel, #99/08560-6 to Dr. Mercadante, #98/15013-9 to Dr. Hounie, and #03/07451-6 to Dr. Rosario-Campos, and Mack Pesquisa to Dr. Mercadante. This work was also supported by Conselho Nacional de Desenvolvimento Científico e Tecnológico (CNPQ), Brazil (grant #521369/96-7) to Dr. Miguel.

REFERENCES

1. American Psychiatric Association. *Diagnostic and Statistical Manual of Mental Disorders, 4th ed. (DSM-IV)*. Washington, DC, 1994.
2. Torres AR, Smaira SI. Quadro clínico do transtorno obsessivo-compulsivo. *Rev Bras Psiquiatr*. 2001; 23(suppl. 2):6–9.
3. Miguel EC, Baer L, Coffey BJ, et al. Phenomenological differences appearing with repetitive behaviours in obsessive-compulsive disorder and Gilles de la Tourette's syndrome. *Br J Psychiatry*. 1997;170:140–145.
4. Itard JMD. Memorie sur quelques fonctions involuntaries des appareils de la locomotion de la prehension et de la voix. *Arch Gen Med*. 1825;8:385–407.
5. Kushner HI. A brief history of Tourette syndrome. *Rev Bras Psiquiatria*. 2000;22:76–79.
6. Hounie AG, Petribu K. Sindrome de Tourette—revisão bibliográfica e relato de casos. *Rev Bras Psiquiatria*. 1999;21:50–63.
7. Zohar AH, Pauls DL, Ratzoni G, et al. Obsessive-compulsive disorder with and without tics in an epidemiological sample of adolescents. *Am J Psychiatry*. 1997;154:274–276.
8. Rosario-Campos MC. Peculiaridades do transtorno obsessivo-compulsivo na infância e na adolescência. *Rev Bras Psiquiatria*. 2001;23(suppl. 2):24–26.
9. Gonzalez CH. Aspectos genéticos do transtorno obsessivo-compulsivo. *Rev Bras Psiquiatria*. 2001;23(suppl. 2):38–41.
10. Rasmussen AS, Tsuang MT. Clinical characteristics and family history in DSM-III obsessive compulsive disorder. *Am J Psychiatry*. 1986;143:317–322.
11. Pitman RK. Pierre Janet on obsessive-compulsive disorder (1903). *Arch Gen Psychiatry*. 1987;44:226–232.
12. George MS, Trimble MR, Ring HA, et al. Obsessions in obsessive compulsive disorder with and without Gilles de la Tourette's syndrome. *Am J Psychiatry*. 1993; 150:93–97.
13. Holzer JC, Goodman WK, McDougle CJ, et al. Obsessive-compulsive disorder with and without a chronic tic disorder. A comparison of symptoms in 70 patients. *Br J Psychiatry*. 1994;464:469–473.
14. Petter T, Richter MA, Sandor P. Clinical features distinguishing patients with Tourette's Syndrome and obsessive-compulsive disorder form patients with obsessive-compulsive disorder without tics. *J Clin Psychiatry*. 1998;59:456–459.
15. Swerdlow RN, Zinner S, Farber HR, et al. Symptoms in obsessive-compulsive disorder and tourette syndrome: a spectrum? *CNS Spectrums* 1999;4:21–33.
16. Leckman JF, Goodman WK, North WG, et al. Elevated cerebrospinal fluid levels of oxytocin in obsessive-compulsive disorder: Comparison with Tourette's syndrome and healthy controls. *Arch Gen Psychiatry*. 1994;51(10):782–792.
17. Leckman JF, Goodman WK, Anderson GM, et al. Cerebrospinal fluid biogenic amines in obsessive compulsive disorder, Tourette's syndrome, and healthy controls. *Neuropsychopharmacology* 1995;12:73–86.
18. Swerdlow NR. Obsessive compulsive disorder and tic syndromes. *Med Clin North Am*. 2001;85:735–755.
19. Eapen V, Robertson MM, Alsobrook JP II, et al. Obsessive-compulsive symptoms in Gilles de la Tourette's syndrome and obsessive-compulsive disorder: Differences by diagnosis and family history. *Am J Med Genetics*. 1997;74:432–438.
20. de Groot CM, Bernstein RA. Obsessive characteristics in subjects with Tourette's syndrome are related to symptoms in their parents. *Compr Psychiatry*. 1994; 35:248–251.
21. Miguel EC, Rosário-Campos MC, Prado HS, et al. Sensory phenomena in obsessive-compulsive disorder and Tourette's Disorder. *J Clin Psychiatry*. 2000;61:150–156.
22. Miguel EC, Coffey BJ, Baer L, et al. Phenomenology of intentional repetitive behaviors in obsessive-compulsive disorder and Tourette's syndrome. *J Clin Psychiatry*. 1995;56:246–255.
22a. Diniz JB, Rosario-Campos MC, Hounie AG, et al. Chronic tics and Tourette syndrome in patients with obsessive-compulsive disorder. *J Psychiatr Res*. 2005 (in press).
23. Baer L. Factor analysis of symptom subtypes of obsessive compulsive disorder and their relation to personality and tic disorders. *J Clin Psychiatry*. 1994;55:18–23.
24. Leckman JF, Grice DE, Boardman J, et al. Symptoms of obsessive compulsive disorder. *Am J Psychiatry*. 1997;154:911–917.
25. Hantouche EG, Lancrenon S. Modern typology of symptoms and obsessive-compulsive syndromes: results of a large French study of 615 patients. *Encephale* 1996;22:9–21.
26. Summerfeldt LJ, Richter MA, Anthony MM, et al. Symptom structure in obsessive-compulsive disorder: factor analytic evidence for subgroups. Poster presented at: 150th Annual Meeting of the American Psychiatric Association; 17–21 May 1997; San Diego, CA.
27. Mataix-Cols D, Rauch SL, Manzo PA, et al. Use of factor-analyzed symptom dimensions to predict outcome with serotonin reuptake inhibitors and placebo in the treatment of obsessive-compulsive disorder. *Am J Psychiatry*. 1999;156:1409–1416.
28. Tek C, Ulug B. Religiosity and religious obsessions in obsessive-compulsive disorder. *Psychiatry Res*. 2001; 104:99–108.
29. Cavallini MC, Di Bella D, Siliprandi F, et al. Exploratory factor analysis of obsessive-compulsive patients and association with 5-HTTLPR polymorphism. *Am J Med Genet*. 2002;114:347–353.

30. Foa EB, Huppert JD, Leiberg S, et al. The obsessive-compulsive inventory: development and validation of a short version. *Psychol Assess.* 2002;14:485–496.

31. Mataix-Cols D, Marks IM, Greist JH, et al. Obsessive-compulsive symptom dimensions as predictors of compliance with and response to behavior therapy: results from a controlled trial. *Psychother Psychosom.* 2002;71:255–262.

32. Leckman JF, Pauls DL, Zhang H, et al. Obsessive-compulsive symptom dimensions in affected sibling pairs diagnosed with Gilles de la Tourette syndrome. *Am J Med Genet (Neuropsychiatric Genet).* 2003; 116:60–68.

33. Alsobrook II JP, Leckman JF, Goodman WK, et al. Segregation analysis of obsessive-compulsive disorder using symptom-based factor scores. *Am J Med Genet.* 1999;88:669–675.

34. Zhang H, Leckman JF, Pauls DL, et al. Tourette Syndrome Association International Consortium for Genetics. Genomewide scan of hoarding in sib pairs in which both sibs have Gilles de la Tourette syndrome. *Am J Hum Genet.* 2002;70:896–904.

34a. Paschou P, Feng Y, Pakstis AJ, et al. Indications of linkage and association of Gilles de la Tourette syndrome in two independent family samples: 17q25 is a putative susceptibility region. *Am J Hum Genet.* 2004;75(4):545–560.

35. Bienvenu OJ, Samuels J, Riddle MA, et al. The relationship of obsessive-compulsive disorder to possible spectrum disorders: Results from a family study. *Biol Psychiatry.* 2000;48:287–293.

36. Gonzales CH. In: Familial study in obsessive-compulsive disorder (doctoral thesis). São Paulo, Brazil: Dept. of Psychiatry, Paulista Medical School, Federal University of São Paulo; 2003.

37. Coffey BJ, Miguel EC, Biederman J, et al. Tourette's disorder with and without obsessive-compulsive disorder in adults: are they different? *J Nerv Ment Dis.* 1998;186:201–206.

38. Nestadt G, Addington A, Samuels J, et al. The identification of OCD-related subgroups based on comorbidity. *Biol Psychiatry.* 2003;53:914–920.

39. Chacon P, Rosario-Campos MC, Hounie AG, et al. Comment on "The Identification of OCD-Related Subgroups Based on Comorbidity." *Biol Psychiatry.* 2004;55:960–961.

40. Miguel EC, Leckman JF, Rauch S, et al. The obsessive-compulsive disorder phenotypes: implications for genetic studies. Submitted.

41. Torres AR, Dedomenico AM, Crepaldi AL, et al. Obsessive-compulsive symptoms in patients with panic disorder. *Compr Psychiatry.* 2004;45:219–224.

42. Bellodi L, Cavallini MC, Bertelli S, et al. Morbidity risk for obsessive-compulsive spectrum disorders in first-degree relatives of patients with eating disorders. *Am J Psychiatry.* 2001;158:563–569.

43. Pauls DL, Towbin KE, Leckman JF, et al. Gilles de la Tourette's syndrome and obsessive-compulsive disorder: evidence supporting a genetic relationship. *Arch Gen Psychiatry.* 1986;43:1180–1182.

44. Pauls DL, Raymond CL, Stevenson JM, et al. A family study of Gilles de la Tourette syndrome. *Am J Hum Genet.* 1991;48:154–163.

45. Comings DE, Comings BG. A controlled study of Tourette syndrome. IV. Obsessions, compulsions, and schizoid behaviors. *Am J Hum Genet.* 1987;41:782–803.

46. Eapen V, Pauls DL, Robertson MM. Evidence for autosomal dominant transmission in Tourette's syndrome – United Kingdom cohort study. *Br J Psychiatry.* 1993;162:593–596.

47. Van de Wetering BJ, Heutink P. The genetics of the Gilles de la Tourette syndrome: a review. *J Lab Clin Med.* 1993;121:638–645.

48. Hebebrand J, Klug B, Fimmers R, et al. Rates for tic disorders and obsessive compulsive symptomatology in families of children and adolescents with Gilles de la Tourette syndrome. *J Psychiatr Res.* 1997;31:519–530.

49. Pauls DL, Alsobrook JP, Goodman W, et al. A family study of obsessive-compulsive disorder. *Am J Psychiatry.* 1995;152:76–84.

50. Nestadt G, Samuels J, Riddle M, et al. A family study of obsessive-compulsive disorder. *Arch Gen Psychiatry.* 2000;57:358–363.

51. Grados M, Riddle MA, Samuels JF, et al. The familial phenotype of obsessive-compulsive disorder in relation to tic disorders. *Biol Psychiatry.* 2001;50:559–565.

52. Price RA, Kidd KK, Cohen DJ, et al. A twin study of Tourette syndrome. *Arch Gen Psychiatry.* 1985;42: 815–820.

53. Lenane MC, Swedo SE, Leonard H, et al. Psychiatric disorders in first degree relatives of children and adolescents with obsessive compulsive disorder. *J Am Acad Child Adolesc Psychiatry.* 1990;29:407–412.

54. Riddle M, Hardin M, King R et al. Fluoxetine treatment of children and adolescents with Tourette's and OCD: preliminary clinical experience. *J Am Acad Child Adolesc Psychiatry.* 1990;29:45–49.

55. Leonard HL, Lenane MC, Swedo SE, et al. Tics and Tourette's disorder: a 2- to 7-year follow-up of 54 obsessive-compulsive children. *Am J Psychiatry.* 1992; 149:1244–1251.

56. Reddy PS, Reddy YC, Srinath S, et al. A family study of juvenile obsessive-compulsive disorder. *Can J Psychiatry.* 2001;46:346–351.

57. Rosario-Campos MC, Leckman JF, Curi M, et al. A family study of early-onset obsessive-compulsive disorder. *Am J Med Genet (Neuropsychiatric Genet).* 2005;136(1):92–97.

58. Pato MT, Pato CN, Pauls DL. Recent findings in the genetics of OCD. *J Clin Psychiatry.* 2002;63(suppl. 6): 30–33.

59. Arnold PD, Rosenberg DR, Mundo E, et al. Association of a glutamate (NMDA) subunit receptor gene (GRIN2B) with obsessive-compulsive disorder: a preliminary study. *Psychopharmacology* (Berl). 2004; 174:530–538.

60. Mc Dougle CJ, Goodman WK, Price LH. Dopamine antagonists in tic-related and psychotic spectrum obsessive-compulsive disorder. *J Clin Psychiatry.* 1994; 55(suppl. 3):24–31.

61. Nordstron EJ, Burton FH. A transgenic model of comorbid Tourette's syndrome and obsessive-compulsive disorder circuitry. *Mol Psychiatry.* 2002;7:524, 617–625.

62. Rosenberg DR, Hanna GL. Genetic and imaging strategies in obsessive-compulsive disorder: potential implications for treatment development. *Biol Psychiatry.* 2000;48:1210–1222.

63. Millet B, Chabane N, Delorme R, et al. Association between the dopamine receptor D4 (DRD4) gene and obsessive-compulsive disorder. *Am J Med Genet.* 2003; 116B:55–59.

64. Nicolini H, Cruz C, Camarena B, et al. DRD2, DRD3, and 5HTDA receptor genes polymorphisms in obsessive-compulsive disorder. *Mol Psychiatry*. 1996;1: 461–465.

65. Nicolini H, Cruz C, Páez F, et al. Los genes de los receptores a dopamina D2 y D4 distinguen la presencia clínica de tics en el trastorno obsesivo-compulsivo. *Gac Med Mex*. 1998;8:163–169.

66. Cruz C, Camarena B, King N, et al. Increased prevalence of the seven-repeat variant of the dopamine D4 receptor gene in patients with obsessive-compulsive disorders with tics. *Neurosci Lett*. 1997;231:1–4.

67. Urraca N, Camarena B, Gomez-Caudillo L, et al. Mu opioid receptor gene as a candidate for the study of obsessive compulsive disorder with and without tics. *Am J Med Genet*. 2004;127B:94–96.

68. Rosario-Campos MC, Leckman JF, Curi M, et al. A family study of early-onset obsessive-compulsive disorder. *Am J Med Genet*. In press.

69. Jonnal AH, Gardner CO, Prescott CA, et al. Obsessive and compulsive symptoms in a general population sample of female twins. *Am J Med Genet*. 2000;96: 791–796.

70. Eley TC, Bolton D, O'Connor TG, et al. A twin study of anxiety-related behaviours in pre-school children. *J Child Psychol Psychiatry*. 2003;44:945–960.

71. Lensi P, Cassano GB, Correddu G, et al. Obsessive-compulsive disorder—Familial-developmental history, symptomatology, comorbidity and course with special reference to gender-related differences. *Brit J Psychiat*. 1996;169:101–107.

72. Santangelo SL, Pauls DL, Goldstein J, et al. Tourette's syndrome: what are the influences of gender and comorbid obsessive-compulsive disorder? *J Am Acad Child Adolesc Psychiatry*. 1994;33:795–804.

73. Peterson BS, Leckman JF, Scahill L, et al. Hypothesis: steroid hormones and sexual dimorphisms modulate symptom expression in Tourette's syndrome. *Psychoneuroendocrinol*. 1992;17:553–563.

74. Pollitt J. Natural history of obsessional states. *Brit Med J*. 1957;9:133–140.

75. Ingram IM. Obsessional illness in mental hospital patients. *J Ment Sci*. 1961;107:382–402.

76. Lo WH. A follow-up study of obsessional neurotics in Hong Kong Chinese. *Br J Psychiatry*. 1967;113: 823–832.

77. McKeon J, Roa B, Mann A. Life events and personality traits in obsessive–compulsive neurosis. *Brit J Psychiatry*. 1984;144:185–189.

78. Khanna S, Rajendra PN, Channabasavanna SM. Life events and onset of obsessive–compulsive disorder. *Int J Social Psychiatry*. 1988;34:305–309.

79. Maina G, Albert U, Bogetto F, et al. Recent life events and obsessive-compulsive disorder (OCD): the role of pregnancy/delivery. *Psychiatry Res*. 1999;89:49–58.

80. Swedo SE, Rapapport JL, Cheslow DL. High prevalence of obsessive-compulsive symptoms in patients with Sydenham's Chorea. *Am J Psychiatry*. 1989a; 146:246–249.

81. Swedo SE. Sydehan's Chorea (SC): A model for childhood autoimmune neuropsychiatric disorders. *JAMA* 1994;272:1788–1791.

82. Allen AJ, Leonard HL, Swedo SE. Case study: a new infection-triggered, autoimmune subtype of pediatric OCD and Tourette's syndrome. *J Am Acad Child Adolesc Psychiatry*. 1995;34:307–311.

83. Swedo S. Pediatric autoimmune neuropsychiatric disorders associated with streptococcal infections (PANDAS). *Mol Psychiatry*. 2002;7(suppl. 2):S24–25.

84. Asbahr FR, Negrao AB, Gentil V, et al. Obsessive-compulsive and related symptoms in children and adolescents with rheumatic fever with and without chorea: a prospective 6-month study. *Am J Psychiatry*. 1998;155:1122–1124.

85. Mercadante MT, Busatto G, Prado L, et al. The psychiatric symptoms of rheumatic fever. *Am J Psychiatry*. 2000;157:2036–2038.

86. Hounie AG, Pauls DL, Mercadante MT, et al. Obsessive-compulsive spectrum disorders in rheumatic fever with and without Sydenham's chorea. *J Clin Psychiatry*. 2004;65:994–999.

86a. Hounie AG, Pauls DL, Rosario-Campos MC. Obsessive-compulsive spectrum disorders and rheumatic fever: a family study. *Biol Psychiatry*. 2005. Submitted.

87. Perlmutter S, Leitman S, Garvey M, et al. Therapeutic plasma exchange and intravenous immunoglobulin for obsessive-compulsive disorder and tic disorders in childhood. *Lancet* 1999;354:1153–1158.

88. Kurlan R. Tourette's syndrome and 'PANDAS': will the relation bear out? Pediatric autoimmune neuropsychiatric disorders associated with streptococcal infection. *Neurology* 1998;50:1530–1534.

89. Shulman ST. Pediatric autoimmune neuropsychiatric disorders associated with streptococci (PANDAS). *Pediatr Infect Dis J*. 1999;18:281–282.

90. Lougee L, Perlmutter SJ, Nicolson R, et al. Psychiatric disorders in first-degree relatives of children with pediatric autoimmmune neuropsychiatric disorders associated with streptococcal infections (PANDAS). *J Am Acad Child Adolesc Psychiatry*. 2000; 39:1120–1126.

91. Mercadante MT, Hounie AG, Muniz JB, et al. The basal ganglia and immune-based neuropsychiatric disorders. *Psychiatric Annals* 2001;31:534–540.

92. Guilherme L, Kalil J. Rheumatic fever: The T cell response leading to autoimmune aggression in the heart. *Autoimmun Rev*. 2002;1:261–266.

93. Kirvan CA, Swedo SE, Heuser JS, et al. Mimicry and autoantibody-mediated neuronal cell signaling in Sydenham chorea. *Nat Med*. 2003;9:914–920.

94. Zai G, Bezchlibnyk YB, Richter MA, et al. Myelin oligodendrocyte glycoprotein (MOG) gene is associated with obsessive-compulsive disorder. *Am J Med Genet*. 2004;129B:64–68.

95. Rauch SL, Whalen PJ, Dougherty DD, et al. Neurobiological models of obsessive compulsive disorders. In: Jenike MA, Baer L, Minichiello WE, eds. *Obsessive-Compulsive Disorder: Practical Management*. Boston: Mosby; 1998a;222–253.

96. Saxena S, Brody AL, Schwartz JM, et al. Neuroimaging and frontal-subcortical circuitry in obsessive-compulsive disorder. *Brit J Psychiatry*. 1998;173(suppl.): 35:26–37.

97. Baxter LR Jr, Phelps ME, Mazziotta JC, et al. Local cerebral glucose metabolic rates in obsessive-compulsive disorder. A comparison with rates in unipolar depression and in normal controls. *Arch Gen Psychiatry*. 1987;44:211–218.

98. Swedo SE, Schapiro MB, Grady CL, et al. Cerebral glucose metabolism in childhood-onset obsessive-compulsive disorder. *Arch Gen Psychiatry*. 1989b; 46:518–523.

99. Busatto GF, Buchpiguel CA, Zamignani DR, et al. Regional cerebral blood flow abnormalities in early-onset obsessive-compulsive disorder: an exploratory SPECT study. *J Am Acad Child Adolesc Psychiatry.* 2001;40:347–354.

100. Baxter LR Jr, Schwartz JM, Bergman KS, et al. Caudate glucose metabolic rate changes with both drug and behavior therapy for obsessive-compulsive disorder. *Arch Gen Psychiatry.* 1992;49:681–689.

101. Benkelfat C, Nordahl TE, Semple WE, et al. Local cerebral glucose metabolic rates in obsessive-compulsive disorder. Patients treated with clomipramine. *Arch Gen Psychiatry.* 1990;47:840–848.

102. Schwartz JM, Stoessel PW, Baxter LR Jr, et al. Systematic changes in cerebral glucose metabolic rate after successful behavior modification treatment of obsessive-compulsive disorder. *Arch Gen Psychiatry.* 1996;53:109–113.

103. Rauch SL, Jenike MA, Alpert NM, et al. Regional cerebral blood flow measured during symptom provocation in obsessive-compulsive disorder using oxygen 15-labeled carbon dioxide and positron emission tomography. *Arch Gen Psychiatry.* 1994;51:62–70.

104. Breiter HC, Rauch SL, Kwong KK, et al. Functional magnetic resonance imaging of symptom provocation in obsessive-compulsive disorder. *Arch Gen Psychiatry.* 1996;53:595–606.

105. Rauch SL, Dougherty DD, Shin LM, et al. Neural correlates of factor-analyzed OCD symptom dimensions: a PET study. *CNS Spectr.* 1998b;3:37–43.

106. Mataix-Cols D, Wooderson S, Lawrence N, et al. Distinct neural correlates of washing, checking and hoarding symptom dimensions in obsessive-compulsive disorder. *Arch Gen Psychiatry.* 2004;61:564–576.

107. Saxena S, Brody AL, Maidment KM, et al. Cerebral glucose metabolism in obsessive-compulsive hoarding. *Am J Psychiatry.* 2004;161:1038–1048.

108. Robinson D, Wu H, Munne RA, et al. Reduced caudate nucleus volume in Obsessive-compulsive disorder. *Arch Gen Psychiatry.* 1995;52:393–398.

109. Stein DJ, Coetzer R, Lee M, et al. Magnetic resonance brain imaging in women with obsessive-compulsive disorder and trichotillomania. *Psychiatry Res.* 1997; 74:177–182.

110. Scarone S, Colombo C, Livian S, et al. Increased right caudate nucleus size in obsessive-compulsive disorder: detection with magnetic resonance imaging. *Psychiatry Res.* 1992;45:115–121.

111. Szeszko PR, Robinson D, Alvir JM, et al. Orbital frontal and amygdala volume reductions in obsessive-compulsive disorder. *Arch Gen Psychiatry.* 1999;56:913–919.

112. Rosenberg DR, Keshavan MS. Toward a neurodevelopmental model of obsessive–compulsive disorder. *Biol Psychiatry.* 1998;43:623–640.

113. Szeszko PR, MacMillan S, McMeniman M, et al. Brain structural abnormalities in psychotropic drug-naive pediatric patients with obsessive-compulsive disorder. *Am J Psychiatry.* 2004a;161:1049–1056.

114. Choi JS, Kang DH, Kim JJ, et al. Left anterior subregion of orbitofrontal cortex volume reduction and impaired organizational strategies in obsessive-compulsive disorder. *J Psychiatr Res.* 2004;38:193–199.

115. Gilbert AR, Moore GJ, Keshavan MS, et al. Decrease in thalamic volumes of pediatric patients with obsessive-compulsive disorder who are taking paroxetine. *Arch Gen Psychiatry.* 2000;57:449–456.

116. Szeszko PR, MacMillan S, McMeniman M, et al. Amygdala volume reductions in pediatric patients with obsessive-compulsive disorder treated with paroxetine: preliminary findings. *Neuropsychopharmacology* 2004b;29:826–832.

117. Peterson B, Riddle MA, Cohen DJ, et al. Reduced basal ganglia volumes in Tourette's syndrome using three-dimensional reconstruction techniques from magnetic resonance images. *Neurology* 1993;43:941–949.

118. Peterson BS, Thomas P, Kane MJ, et al. Basal ganglia volumes in patients with Gilles de la Tourette syndrome. *Arch Gen Psychiatry.* 2003;60:415–424.

119. Moriarty J, Varma AR, Stevens J, et al. A volumetric MRI study of Gilles de la Tourette's syndrome. *Neurology* 1997;49:410–415.

120. Singer HS, Reiss AL, Brown JE, et al. Volumetric MRI changes in basal ganglia of children with Tourette's syndrome. *Neurology* 1993;43:950–956.

121. Baumgardner TL, Singer HS, Denckla MB, et al. Corpus callosum morphology in children with Tourette syndrome and attention deficit hyperactivity disorder. *Neurology* 1996;47:477–482.

122. Mostofsky SH, Wendlandt J, Cutting L, et al. Corpus callosum measurements in girls with Tourette syndrome. *Neurology* 1999;53:1345–1347.

123. Peterson BS, Staib L, Scahill L, et al. Regional brain and ventricular volumes in Tourette syndrome. *Arch Gen Psychiatry.* 2001;58:427–440.

124. Eidelberg D, Moeller JR, Antonini A, et al. The metabolic anatomy of Tourette's syndrome. *Neurology* 1997;48:927–934.

125. Wolf SS, Jones DW, Knable MB, et al. Tourette syndrome: prediction of phenotypic variation in monozygotic twins by caudate nucleus D2 receptor binding. *Science* 1996;273:1225–1227.

126. Ernst M, Zametkin AJ, Jons PH, et al. High presynaptic dopaminergic activity in children with Tourette's disorder. *J Am Acad Child Adolesc Psychiatry.* 1999;38:86–94.

127. Singer HS, Szymanski S, Giuliano J, et al. Elevated intrasynaptic dopamine release in Tourette's syndrome measured by PET. *Am J Psychiatry.* 2002;159: 1329–1336.

128. Stern E, Silbersweig DA, Chee KY, et al. A functional neuroanatomy of tics in Tourette syndrome. *Arch Gen Psychiatry* 2000;57:741–748.

129. Peterson BS, Skudlarski P, Anderson AW, et al. A functional magnetic resonance imaging study of tic suppression in Tourette syndrome. *Arch Gen Psychiatry* 1998;55:326–333.

130. Jenike MA, Baer L, Minichiello WE. An overview of obsessive-compulsive disorder. In: Jenike MA, Baer L, Minichiello WE, eds. *Obsessive-Compulsive Disorders—Practical Management.* 3rd ed. St. Louis, MO: Mosby. 1998;3–11.

131. Zohar J, Sasson Y, Amitai K, et al. Pharmacological options for refractory OCD. In: *Proceedings of the 5th International Obsessive-Compulsive Disorder Conference.* Sardinia, Italy: Solvay Pharmaceuticals; 2001: 13–17.

132. McDougle CJ, Goodman WK, Leckman JF, et al. The efficacy of fluvoxamine in obsessive-compulsive disorder: effects of comorbid chronic tic disorder. *J Clin Psychopharmacol.* 1993;13:354–358.

133. McDougle CJ, Goodman WK, Leckman JF, et al. Haloperidol addition in fluvoxamine-refractory

obsessive-compulsive disorder. A double-blind, placebo-controlled study in patients with and without tics. *Arch Gen Psychiatry*. 1994;51:302–308.

134. Shavitt RG, Belotto C, Curi M, et al. Sensory phenomena and treatment response in obsessive-compulsive disorder, submitted.

135. Spencer T, Biederman J, Kerman K, et al. Desipramine treatment of children with attention deficit hyperactivity disorder and tic disorder or Tourette's syndrome. *J Am Acad Child Adolesc Psychiatry*. 1993;32:354–360.

135a. Ferrão YA. In: Clinical characteristics of obsessive compulsive disorder refractory to conventional treatment (doctoral thesis). São Paulo, Brazil: Institute of Psychiatry, Medical School, University of São Paulo, 2004.

136. Van Noppen BL, Steketee G. Individual, group and multifamily cognitive-behavioral treatments. In: Pato MT, Zohar J, eds. *Current Treatments of Obsessive-Compulsive Disorder*. 2nd ed. Washington, DC: American Psychiatric Press. 2001:133–172.

137. Greist JH, Jefferson JW, Kobak KA, et al. Efficacy and tolerability of serotonin transport inhibitors in obsessive-compulsive disorder: a meta-analysis. *Arch Gen Psychiatry*. 1995;52:53–60.

138. McDougle CJ. Update on pharmacologic management of OCD: agents and augmentation. *J Clin Psychiatry*. 1997;58(suppl)12:11–17.

139. Jacobsen FM. Risperidone in the treatment of affective illness and obsessive-compulsive disorder. *J Clin Psychiatry*. 1995;56:423–429.

140. McDougle CJ, Epperson CN, Pelton GH, et al. A double-blind, placebo-controlled study of risperidone addition in serotonin reuptake inhibitor-refractory obsessive-compulsive disorder. *Arch Gen Psychiatry*. 2000;57:794–801.

141. Weiss EL, Potenza MN, McDougle CJ, et al. Olanzapine addition in obsessive-compulsive disorder refractory to selective serotonin reuptake inhibitors: an open-label case series. *J Clin Psychiatry*. 1999;60:524–527.

142. Bogetto F, Bellino S, Vaschetto P, et al. Olanzapine augmentation of fluvoxamine-refractory obsessive-compulsive disorder (OCD): a 12-week open trial. *Psychiatry Res*. 2000;96:91–98.

143. Bystritsky A, Ackerman DL, Rosen RM, et al. Augmentation of SSRI response in refractory OCD using adjunctive olanzapine: a placebo-controlled trial. In: *Proceedings of the 5th International Obsessive Compulsive Disorder Conference*. Sardinia, Italy: Solvay Pharmaceuticals; 2001: 22.

144. Bystritsky A, Ackerman DL, Rosen RM, et al. Augmentation of serotonin reuptake inhibitors in refractory obsessive-compulsive disorder using adjunctive olanzapine: a placebo-controlled trial. *J Clin Psychiatry*. 2004;65:565–568.

145. Shapira NA, Ward HE, Mandoki M, et al. A double-blind, placebo-controlled trial of olanzapine addition in fluoxetine-refractory obsessive-compulsive disorder. *Biol Psychiatry* 2004;55:553–555.

146. Atmaca M, Kuloglu M, Tezcan E, et al. Quetiapine augmentation in patients with treatment resistant obsessive-compulsive disorder: a single-blind, placebo-controlled study. *Int Clin Psychopharmacol*. 2002;17:115–119.

147. Sevincok L, Topuz A. Lack of efficacy of low doses of quetiapine addition in refractory obsessive-compulsive disorder. *J Clin Psychopharmacol*. 2003;23: 448–450.

148. Metin O, Yazici K, Tot S, et al. Amisulpiride augmentation in treatment resistant obsessive-compulsive disorder: an open trial. *Hum Psychopharmacol*. 2003;18: 463–467.

149. Garvey MA, Perlmutter SJ, Allen AJ, et al. A pilot study of penicillin prophylaxis for neuropsychiatric exacerbations triggered by streptococcal infections. *Biol Psychiatry*. 1999;45:1564–1571.

150. Mataix-Cols D, Rosario-Campos MC, Leckman JF. A multidimensional model of obsessive-compulsive disorder. *Am J Psychiatry*. In press.

151. Rosario-Campos MC, Miguel EC, Quatrano S, et al. The Dimensional Yale-Brown Obsessive-Compulsive Scales (D-YBOCS): a new instrument for assessing obsessive compulsive symptom dimensions. Submitted.

152. Nicolini H, Hanna G, Baxter L, et al. Segregation analysis of obsessive-compulsive and associated disorders. Preliminary results. *Ursus Medicus* 1991; 1:25–28.

153. Cavallini MC, Perna G, Caldirola D, et al. A segregation study of panic disorder in families of panic patients responsive to the 35% CO_2 challenge. *Biol Psychiatry*. 1999;46:815–820.

154. Kelsoe JR. Arguments for the genetic basis of the bipolar spectrum. *J Affect Disord*. 2003;73:183–197.

155. Wong ML, Licinio J. From monoamines to genomic targets: a paradigm shift for drug discovery in depression. *Nat Rev Drug Discov*. 2004;3:136–151.

4

Behavioral and Affective Disorders in Tourette Syndrome

Mary M. Robertson[1] and Michael Orth[2]

[1]University College London; St. Georges Hospital Medical School; Department
of Mental Health Sciences, St. Georges Hospital, London, United Kingdom
[2]Department of Neurology, Universitatsklinikum Eppendorf, Hamburg, Germany

This chapter reviews the relevant literature on Tourette syndrome (TS) with respect to behavioral disorders, affective disorders, self-injurious behaviors, and suicide.

BEHAVIORAL DISORDERS IN TOURETTE SYNDROME

For the purpose of this chapter, only oppositional defiant disorder (ODD), conduct disorder (CD) in children, personality disorder (PD) in adults, and non-obscene socially inappropriate behaviors (NOSI) will be examined. Brief mention will be made of "general behavioral problems" and rage attacks.

Conduct Disorder and Oppositional Defiant Disorder Definitions

ODD is characterized by a recurrent pattern of negativistic, defiant, disobedient, and hostile behavior, which persists for at least 6 months. These behaviors include the frequent occurrence of losing temper, arguing with adults, defying or refusing to comply with adult's requests or rules, deliberately annoying people, blaming others for their own mistakes or behaviors, being often touchy, easily annoyed by others, angry, resentful, spiteful, and vindictive; the behavioral disturbance must cause clinical significant impairment in social, academic, or occupational functioning (1).

The essential feature of CD is a repetitive and persistent pattern of overtly aggressive behavior in which the basic rights of others or major-age appropriate societal norms or rules are violated.

There are four main groupings of these behaviors; aggressive conduct that causes or threatens physical harm to persons or animals, conduct which results in property loss or damage, deceitfulness or theft, and finally, serious violations of rules; the behavioral disturbance must cause clinical significant impairment in social, academic or occupational functioning (1).

Oppositional Defiant and Conduct Disorder in Tourette Syndrome: Epidemiologic Studies

In the classic Isle of Wight study in the United Kingdom, reported in the 1970s, Rutter et al. (2) investigated the island's population of 11- and 12-year-old children, including more than 2,000 children. They reported that the presence of tics was significantly associated with disruptive behavior problems. Comings et al. (3) evaluated the frequency of tics and TS in 3,034 children in three schools in greater Los Angeles over a 2-year period. A total of 14 males were diagnosed with TS, but when special educational classes were considered, the prevalence rose to 1/95 for males and 1/759 for females; another two children had probable TS, 10 had possible TS, and 10 had transient tic disorder. These children showed attentional difficulties and obsessive-compulsive behavior (OCB), but also had learning difficulties and/or CD.

In the two-part epidemiologic study of Kadesjo and Gillberg (4), the first part made no mention of either ODD or CD; however, in the second study, of the 58 children who were registered with TS in the catchment area, 21 (36%) were diagnosed with CD (4).

Structured diagnostic interviews were performed on 976 children of ages between 1 and 10 years in the 1975 birth cohort in Upstate New York. Peterson et al. (5) re-assessed 776 subjects as part of a longitudinal study of this cohort 8 years (time two), 10 years (time three) and 15 years (time four) later. Results showed that tics and attention deficit hyperactivity disorder (ADHD) symptoms were associated with OCD after demographic features and co-morbid psychiatric symptoms were controlled. Tics, OCD, and ADHD shared numerous complex associations with demographic and psychopathologic risk factors. Of particular importance in the context of this chapter, tics were significantly associated with conduct problems at baseline and time two supporting the notion that tics in childhood are associated with conduct problems and behavioral abnormalities.

A pilot epidemiological study (6) reported on tics and TS in 166 students ages 13 to 14 years, in one mainstream school in West Essex, United Kingdom. Information was gathered from four sources: parents, teachers, pupils, and the research psychologist. Thirty (18%) pupils were diagnosed as "tic possibles" and five were diagnosed with TS. The tic possibles were rated higher by their teachers on the Strength and Difficulties Questionnaire (P <0.001) than the school children in the same cohort without tics, with the difference being accounted for by ratings of conduct and/or emotional disorder. Of the five youngsters with TS one was also diagnosed with depression. However, this was in addition to four other psychiatric disorders (CD, hyperactivity, substance abuse, and behavioral disorder), indicative of the complexity of the youngster.

Hornsey et al. (7) examined the prevalence of TS in 13 to 14 year-olds in mainstream secondary schools in West Essex using a three-stage ascertainment procedure. First, all 1,012 year nine pupils were screened for tics using validated self-report questionnaires completed by parents, teachers, and pupils. Data were available from at least one informant for 918 (90.7%) subjects. Tics were identified in 189 (18.7%) pupils. Secondly, families were contacted and a semi-structured interview was carried out to determine whether the young person had TS. Finally, to ensure that the diagnosis of TS was correct, all those assessed as having TS were systematically examined by an expert clinician in the field. Seven young people were identified as fulfilling the criteria for TS, giving a minimum prevalence rate of 0.76% and a more realistic rate of 1.85%. Behavioral problems were frequently associated with both the tic and TS group. In particular, with relevance to the chapter, when the total population ($N = 918$) was compared with the tic possible group ($N = 42$), Hornsey et al. reported that significantly more tic possibles (26%) than the total population (11%) had been referred to child mental health clinics ($P = 0.001$). On the Strength and Difficulties Questionnaire (8,9), significantly more tic possibles (28%) than the total population (12%) had probable CD ($P = 0.001$) and probable mental disorder ($P = <0.001$), (tic possible, 37%: whole population, 17%).

Kurlan et al. (10) undertook a community-based epidemiologic study to investigate the behavioral spectrum of tic disorders, using direct interviews by a trained neuropsychological technician, to determine the prevalence of tic disorders and any co-morbid psychopathology in a group of youngsters age 9 to 17 years. Standardized schedules and rating scales were employed. In addition, parents and teachers completed the Child Behavior Checklist (CBCL). Of the 1,596 children who were interviewed, 339 were identified as having tic disorders and 72 were diagnosed with TS. Children with tics, compared with children without tics, were younger, more likely to be male, and have special educational placement. There was substantial agreement (81%) between the parent and the technician for the presence of tics. Significantly more children with tics had various psychopathologies including ODD (17.4%). Moreover, subjects with more severe tics had an increased frequency of scoring in the pathologic range on the CBCL subtests of somatic complaints, aggressive behavior, and externalizing symptoms. Children with tics scored higher on the CBCL total score (537.0 ± 59.8 versus 522.4 ± 50.3: $P = 0.01$). Subjects with TS ($N = 72$) had an increased frequency of several psychopathologies on the CBCL, including delinquent problems, aggressive behavior, externalizing symptoms, and ODD. The authors acknowledged that they had a low response rate (11%)

of selected subjects who agreed to participate and thus their selected sample may not have been random.

After an initial pilot study including 232 children, Lanzi et al. (11) undertook a definitive epidemiologic study. The study population comprised 2,347 primary school children age 5 to 12 years, from Pavia (total population 80,073) in Northern Italy. Specially trained teachers observed the children, and videotapes were also employed. A total of 68 children (56 boys age 6 to 11 years) were identified with tic disorders. A total of 16 of 2,347 (0.68%) had TS. Of importance is that a significant correlation was found between the presence of tic disorders and impaired school performance (Mantel-Haenszel chi square for trend 41.8: *P* <0.00001).

In contrast to the eight investigations just reviewed, which did find behavioral difficulties with TS or tic subjects in community and epidemiologic studies, only three studies (12–14) to the best of the knowledge of the authors reported that persons with tics in the community did not have an increase in behavioral problems.

Studies of Members of Tourette Syndrome Associations and/or Postal Surveys

Stefl (15), in a mailed questionnaire survey to all known affiliates of the TS Association in Ohio, reported that many individuals had "behavior problems." Approximately 53% had received some form of counselling for these problems. Neither counselling nor medication helped the problems. Champion et al. (16) examined the responses to a postal questionnaire survey by 210 patients with TS about their tics and the possible disruption they caused the individuals. More than 40% of respondents reported

problems in dating and difficulties in making and keeping friends.

Tourette Syndrome Specialist Clinic Studies

Comings and Comings (17) undertook an early controlled study in which 246 patients with TS, were compared with 17 patients with ADHD, 15 patients with ADD plus TS, and 47 random control patients; the results suggested that ODD and CD were more common in TS subjects than in control individuals. Coffey and Park (18) investigated 100 youngsters with TS in a specialist center. Lifetime prevalence for associated diagnoses included ODD (52%) and CD (16%). Coffey et al. (19) studied 156 consecutively referred youths with TS (age 5 to 20 years) at a specialist center. All subjects were assessed by clinical interview by a child and adolescent psychiatrist using standardized schedules including the Schedule for Affective Disorders and Schizophrenia for School-Age Children-Epidemiologic version. Nineteen (12%) of the cohort required psychiatric hospitalization (Table 4-1). Results showed that significantly more TS individuals with CD required hospitalization (*P* = 0.04).

Freeman et al. (20) investigated 3,500 TS individuals in 22 countries, and reported that 15% had co-morbid ODD/CD, although 37% of patients had a history of anger control problems and 26% currently had these problems. Twenty percent had social skills problems and 6% had sexually inappropriate behaviors. Mahone et al. (21) used the Behavior Rating Inventory of Executive Function to examine 21 patients with only TS, 18 with only ADHD, 17 with TS plus ADHD, and 20 controls for measures of psychoeducational competence, performance, and measures of executive function. The TS plus ADHD and ADHD groups were rated as more

TABLE 4-1. *Hospitalization significantly associated with conduct disorder*

Diagnosis	Patients not hospitalized, *N* (%)	Hospitalized patients, *N* (%)	*P* values
Conduct disorder	18 (13.3)	6 (31.6)	0.04
Oppositional defiant disorder	77 (57)	13 (72.2)	n.s.
Total	95	19	

n.s., nonsignificant
Adapted from Coffey BJ, Biederman J, Geller DA, et al. Distinguishing illness severity from tic severity in children and adolescents with Tourette's disorder. *J Am Acad Child Adolesc Psychiatry*. 2000;39:556–561.

impaired (P <0.0001) than the other two groups on the five primary indices.

In a study investigating the psychological morbidity and caregiver burden in parents of children with TS, comparing them with parents of children with asthma, Cooper et al. (22) reported that 76.9% of the parents of children with TS compared with 34.6% of parents of children with asthma achieved "caseness" on the General Health Questionnaire, which was significant: forward logistic regression indicated that the child diagnosis (TS/asthma) was the only factor that significantly predicted caseness (OR 6.3 [95% CI 1.9–21.3]). In addition, the mothers of children with TS demonstrated significantly greater caregiver burden in all areas except financial burden (i.e., in the domains of relationships, activities, and well-being). Relationship, well-being, and total scores were positively correlated with General Health Questionnaire caseness. Fathers of children with TS also demonstrated significantly greater relationship, well-being, and total burden. In addition to TS, the children also had ADHD (73%), OCB (54%), ODD (58%), and CD (15%). When the parents of the children with TS ($N = 22$) and asthma ($N = 15$) were asked which aspects of the child's illness most affected their lives, only a subgroup of each category answered. Nevertheless, the most common theme in the 22 parents of children with TS was behavioral problems ($N = 8$). In contrast, behavioral problems were only reported by 1 child with asthma who also had co-morbid ADHD.

Channon et al. (23) undertook a study primarily investigating executive function, memory, and learning in patients with TS. The groups studied were TS only ($N = 14$), TS plus ADHD ($N = 9$) and TS plus OCD ($N = 6$) and controls ($N = 21$), using a variety of measures including the parent form of the CBCL. Results showed that the TS plus ADHD group scored significantly higher than the control group ($P = 0.0001$) and the TS alone group ($P = 0.004$); the TS plus OCD group scored significantly higher than the control group ($P = 0.041$). These results are in accord with those reported by Carter et al. who found behavioral problems more commonly in children with TS plus ADHD

whereas TS only children were similar to unaffected controls (24).

Recently, Sukhodolsky et al. (25) examined the association of disruptive behaviors in 207 children between the ages of 7 and 18 years (mean, 11 years) with social, adaptive, and family functioning in TS with and without ADHD. Probands had either TS alone ($N = 42$), TS plus ADHD ($N = 52$), or ADHD alone ($N = 52$), or were controls ($N = 61$); groups were age, gender, and race matched. The intelligence of the groups was not significantly different. Measure included parents' and teachers' ratings as well as the Vineland Adaptive Behavior Scales, CBCL, Family Environment Scale, Conners Teaching Rating Scale, Schedule for Tourette and Other Behavioral Syndromes, Schedule for Affective Disorders and Schizophrenia for School-Aged-Children—Present and Lifetime Version, Yale Global Tic Severity Scale, and the Children's Yale-Brown Obsessive Compulsive Scale. After ratings, two clinicians independently assigned diagnoses. The results showed that the children with TS only did not differ from unaffected controls on any ratings of behavior or conduct problems. In contrast, on the indices of disruptive behavior the children with TS plus ADHD were rated significantly above unaffected controls and similar to children with ADHD only. Specifically, in the TS-only group six had ODD and none had CD, whereas in the TS plus ADHD group 17 had ODD and two had CD; in the ADHD group 16 had ODD and two had CD. In the children with TS, of 22 correlations, only two were significant without controlling for the probability of type one error. The CBCL Aggressive Behavior Scale was positively related to Yale Global Tic Severity Scale phonic tic severity, and the Conners Teaching Rating Scale was also positively related to the Yale Global Tic Severity Scale total tic severity.

It does seem, in conclusion, that in most studies in which the disorders are being specifically looked for and diagnostic criteria used, a substantial number of individuals with tics and TS, both in clinics and in the community, have been demonstrated to have behavior problems, and often warranting a diagnosis of ODD or CD. The presence of ODD and CD may account for at least some of the morbidity associated with TS. The lack of behavioral impairment in some studies of children with "pure" TS and similarities in impairment between children with TS plus ADHD and ADHD alone suggest that the frequent presence of ADHD in TS may account for the increase in behavioral morbidity (23,25). Clearly, more research in the area is needed comparing "TS-only" individuals and comparing them with TS plus ADHD, TS plus OCD, ADHD, and healthy controls because the presence of ODD and CD in youngsters with TS has management and prognostic implications.

Definition of Personality Disorder

PD is an enduring pattern of inner experience and behavior that deviates markedly from the expectations of the individual's culture. This pattern is manifested in two (or more) of the following areas: a) cognition (i.e., the ways of perceiving and interpreting self, other people, and events), b) affectively (i.e., the range, intensity, lability, and appropriateness of emotional response, and c) interpersonal functioning. Moreover, the enduring pattern is inflexible and pervasive across a broad range of personal and social situations (1).

Studies of Personality Disorder in Tourette Syndrome

To the best of the knowledge of the authors of this chapter, there have been only two documentations of PD in TS patients. The first study to report PDs in TS populations, examined 36 patients with TS (26). No standardized interviews were utilized, but the authors were experienced psychiatrists who were also familiar with TS. Of the 36 TS patients, 27 were diagnosed as having a PD (two hysterical, three inadequate, four schizoid, six passive-aggressive, one obsessive-compulsive, and 11 other). The only study of PD using standardized interviews and measures, was that of Robertson et al. (27) who examined 39 adult TS patients of moderate severity with 34 age- and sex-matched controls (79% male). The TS patients and controls were examined using the Structured Clinical Interview for DSM-III-R Personality Disorders II, to

systematically determine axis II PD. All subjects also completed a self-rated scale for PD. Results showed that, using this structured interview, 25/39 (64%) of TS patients had one or more DSM-III-R PDs, compared with only 2/34 (6%) of control subjects which was highly statistically significant (chi 2 = 22.7; P <0.0001). The TS subjects were also more likely to have an increasing number of PDs (chi 2 = 23.8; P = 0.0006). The types of PDs included borderline (N = 11), depressive, obsessive-compulsive, paranoid, passive-aggressive (N = 9 PD in each group), avoidant (N = 8), antisocial, narcissistic (N = 4 each group) hysterical, schizoid (N = 3 each group), and schizotypal or self-defeating (N = 2 each group).

Thus in conclusion, it appears that in TS clinics TS patients may exhibit a variety of PDs. The cause of this increase in PD in TS clinic patients may well be the result of the long-term outcome of childhood ADHD, referral bias, or because of other childhood psychopathology (as discussed later in text). Thus, it does appear that at least some clinic TS populations have PDs, which has both treatment and prognosis implications (27).

Non-Obscene Socially Inappropriate Behaviors and Other Behavior Problems in Tourette Syndrome

Kurlan et al. (28) surveyed 87 adolescent (older than age 13 years) or adult patients with TS from clinics at Rochester, New York and the National Hospital for Neurology and Neurosurgery (London) regarding the presence, characteristics, and functional impact of NOSI behaviors, using a standardized self-report questionnaire. The mean age of the patients was 28 years (SD = 14; range, 14 to 82 years). Reported behaviors included insulting others (22%), other NOSI comments (5%), and NOSI actions (14%). More often individuals described having an urge to carry out these behaviors (30%, 26%, and 22%, respectively), which they attempted to suppress. The contents of insults included aspersions on weight (30%), intelligence (30%), general appearance (27%), breath or body odor (23%), parts of the anatomy (21%), race/ethnic background (20%), and height (13%).

NOSI was usually directed at a family member or a familiar person, at home or in a familiar setting. The uttering of insults resulted in social difficulties: verbal arguments (30%), school problems (21%), fistfights (13%), job problems (9%), removal from a public place (8%), and legal trouble or arrest (5%). NOSI was closely associated with ADHD and of importance within the context of this chapter, CD (P <0.005). It was suggested that NOSI may represent part of a more general dysfunction of impulse control in patients with TS.

Channon et al. (23) examined real-life-type problem solving in 21 patients with "pure" TS, chosen specifically without any other co-morbid diagnosis such as depression, ADHD, OCD, learning disability or any other illness or injury which might have affected brain function. They were compared with 21 healthy controls that were examined and found not to be significantly different in age, years of education, or National Adult Reading Test (NART) intelligence quotient. The subjects were examined on a Predicaments Task, which consists of sixteen brief scenarios involving everyday awkward situations, with the subjects being videotaped. All responses for the study were rated by a rater blinded to the identity and group membership of the participants and a second rater who was not blinded. The two raters agreed for 90.2% of ratings. All differences were resolved by reference to an additional blind rater. Results showed that the TS subjects were found to perform below the matched control group on the problem-solving task, both in generating a range of potential problem solutions and they also performed more poorly on aspects of executive function. In particular the TS group rated the main character in situations and themselves to be significantly more awkward than did the control group (F = 5.14, df = 1.39, P = 0.029). Thus, it does seem that subjects with TS have a variety of NOSI behaviors, and that they also deem themselves to be more awkward in social settings than their healthy counterparts.

Rage Attacks

Relatively recently, explosive outbursts (also referred to as *rage attacks* or *anger attacks*) have been described in a substantial proportion (possibly as high as one third) of patients with TS (19,29–31). These explosive outbursts are of unknown etiology, sudden onset, and have no clear predisposing/precipitating immediate factors. If there are such factors, the attacks are out of proportion to them. Often the child with these attacks is apologetic and remorseful afterwards. In recent studies, these attacks in people with TS have been demonstrated to be associated with ADHD, OCD, and increased family expressed emotion (30,31). In a study of 105 children with TS age 7 to 17 years, the rage attacks were highly and specifically associated with, in particular, ODD, and it has been suggested that this episodic rage may be associated with disturbed serotonergic function (32).

The Impact of Childhood Psychopathology on Adolescent and Adult Functioning and Psychopathology

In children and adolescents with TS there is a high incidence of co-morbid psychopathology including ADHD, CD/ODD, or a combination of these disorders. Childhood behavior may be an important determinant for the individual's development and eventually for their lives as adults. Robins (33) was one of the first to suggest that adult antisocial behavior requires childhood antisocial behavior, that a variety of antisocial behaviors in childhood is a better predictor of adult antisocial behavior than is any particular behavior, and that adult antisocial behavior is better predicted by childhood behavior than by family background or social class. Zoccolillo et al. (34) investigated the effect of childhood CD on adult social functioning. Results showed that most subjects with CD had pervasive (but not necessarily severe) social difficulties compared with peers without CD. Of the 35 males with CD in childhood, 40% were rated as having an antisocial PD as an adult, compared with only 4% of those without CD. Similarly, for females, of the 26 with childhood CD 35% showed adult antisocial PD, compared with none in those children without childhood CD. Babinski et al. (35) showed that childhood conduct problems as well as hyperactivity-impulsivity independently, jointly predict a greater likelihood of having an arrest record for males but not females. Stevenson and Goodman (36) reported that children as young as age 3 years, with high activity level, management difficulties, and temper tantrums, had significantly prominent adult conviction and criminality on follow-up many years later as adults in the criminal records office. Finally, Fombonne et al. (37,38) reported that children who had early CD resulted in higher rates of adult drug misuse and dependence, alcoholism, suicidal behaviors, adult PDs, criminal offenses and more pervasive social dysfunction in adulthood.

These studies may have important implications for patients with TS; it is conceivable that the co-morbidities predict some of the adult psychopathologies and maladaptive social functioning (e.g., PD), rather than the TS *per se* (25). It remains to be investigated in longitudinal studies if early recognition and treatment of co-morbidity, for example, of ADHD can improve the long-term outcome of patients with TS.

AFFECTIVE DISORDERS

Depression and Depressive Symptomatology

In the DSM-IV-TR (1), a major depressive episode or major depressive disorder (MDD) is when five or more symptoms have been present during the same 2-week period and represent a change from previous functioning. At least one of the symptoms is either depressed mood or loss of interest or pleasure. The other symptoms can include: depressed mood, markedly diminished interest or pleasure in all or almost all activities, significant weight loss or weight gain not attributable to diet, insomnia or hypersomnia nearly every day, psychomotor agitation or retardation, fatigue or loss of energy every day, feelings of worthlessness or excessive or inappropriate guilt, diminished ability to think or concentrate or indecisiveness, recurrent thoughts of death, recurrent suicidal ideation or a suicide attempt or plan. The symptoms must cause distress or impairment and are not accounted for by substance abuse or bereavement (1).

Depression is common, with a lifetime risk of 7.5% to 10%, with rates even higher in women. It is also common in children, with prevalence estimates varying between 1.8% and 8.9%. It may be a mild disorder, or severe, where the lifetime suicide risk is about 15%. It is important to understand that depression is a spectrum disorder, with a variety of types of depression being described (39,40). Winokur (41) suggests that MDD is not a disease but a syndrome, which is clinically homogeneous, but etiologically heterogeneous.

The etiology of depression is often multifactorial, with a wide variety of contributory factors including genetic predisposition, psychosocial variables including serious adverse or negative life events, adverse childhood circumstances (e.g., parental loss, stress or abuse in childhood) and adverse current social circumstances (39,40). Although MDD, depressive illness, and depressive symptomatology have been frequently investigated in TS, the relationship between the two disorders remains somewhat unclear. In the opinion of the authors, the importance of depression in TS individuals has not been sufficiently highlighted, even though it has important treatment, and probably prognostic, implications.

Uncontrolled Studies in Clinic Populations

Following the first description of depression in TS patients by Shapiro et al. in 1973 (42), two further cases with TS and depression were reported in the 1970s (43,44). There have been several uncontrolled studies (45–51), which have reported depressive symptomatology or MDD in their TS cohorts (Table 4-2).

In summary, in approximately 4,930 documented patients with TS, mood disturbances have been reported from 13% to as high as 76%. The main diagnosis was that of a major depressive illness.

Coffey et al. (19) studied 156 consecutively referred youths with TS (age 5 to 20 years) at a specialist center. All subjects were assessed by clinical interview by a child and adolescent psychiatrist using standardized schedules including the Schedule for Affective Disorders

TABLE 4-2. *Uncontrolled studies showing depressive symptomatology or major depressive disorder in patients with Tourette syndrome*

Author	Year	Patients, N	Symptomatology or illness
Stefl (15)	1984	>400	Mood swings (30%)
Ferrari et al. (45)	1984	10	Depression common in parents
Erenberg et al. (46)	1987	99	Mood swings (52%)
Robertson et al. (47)	1988	90	Major depressive disorder (17%)
Wand et al. (48)	1993	446	Mood swings (27%)
Chee and Sachdev (49)	1994	50	Depression (18%)
Rosenberg et al. (50)	1995	200	30%
Coffey and Park (18)	1997	100	Mood (76%) Major depressive disorder (64%) Dysthymia (2%)
Freeman et al. (20)	2000	3,500	Depressed (20%)
Teive et al. (51)	2001	44	Depressed (20%)

TABLE 4-3. *Hospitalized versus non-hospitalized patients with mood disorders and Tourette syndrome*

Diagnosis	Non-hospitalized patients, N (%)	Hospitalized patients, N (%)	P value
Major depressive disorder	59 (43.4)	17 (89.5)	0.001
Bipolar affective disorder	13 (9.6)	11 (57.9)	0.001
Dysthymia	10 (7.4)	0	n.s.
Any mood disorder	68 (50)	18 (94.7)	0.001

n.s., nonsignificant
Adapted from Coffey BJ, Biederman J, Geller DA, et al. Distinguishing illness severity from tic severity in children and adolescents with Tourette's disorder. *J Am Acad Child Adolesc Psychiatry.* 2000;39:556–561.

and Schizophrenia for School-Age Children-Epidemiologic version. Nineteen (12%) of the cohort required psychiatric hospitalization. Significant univariate predictors of hospitalization included MDD. While tic severity was marginally significant as a predictor of psychiatric hospitalization ($P < 0.05$), major depression ($P < 0.016$) was a robust predictor of psychiatric hospitalization, even after statistical adjustment for co-linearity and correction for all other variables assessed. Table 4-3 indicates the figures for the hospitalized versus non-hospitalized patients.

Controlled Studies in Clinic Populations

Several controlled investigations have also found TS individuals to be more depressed than control subjects. Thus, Grossman et al. (52) examined 29 patients with TS and compared them with 29 controls matched for age and gender, using the Minnesota Multiphasic Personality Inventory. Univariate and multivariate analyses indicated that the subjects with TS scored higher on five scales including Depression. Comings and Comings (53) undertook a controlled study in which they examined 246 TS patients, 17 patients with ADHD, 15 with TS plus ADHD, and 47 controls, using the National Institutes of Mental Health Diagnostic Interview Schedule questions for a life history of MDD and a modified Beck Depression Inventory (BDI). Among the controls, only 2.1% had depression scores greater than nine and none had depression scores greater than 10. In contrast, among the TS patients, 22.9% had a score greater than nine, and the scores went up as high as 18 (the maximum score), which was significant ($P < 0.0005$). There were no differences in the frequency of depression in the patients with or without ADHD. There was a good correlation between the depression and the BDI score ($r = 0.63$). There was minimal correlation between the number of tics (i.e., a measure of severity) and either the depression score (r = 0.63) or the BDI score (r = 0.193). Comings and Comings (53) suggested that depressive symptoms were an integral part of TS, rather than being secondary to motor or vocal tics.

Pitman et al. (54) examined 16 patients with TS, 16 with OCD, and 16 controls. They employed the Yale Schedule, which includes the Diagnostic Interview Schedule. Nineteen patients were depressed; seven of the TS patients, 11 with OCD, and only one control. When the TS group was compared with controls (i.e., seven versus one), it reached significance (*P* <0.05); when the OCD group was compared with controls (i.e., 11 versus one), it was also significant (*P* <0.001).

Studies Employing Genetic, Neuroimaging, and Laboratory Techniques

Pauls et al. (55) interviewed 338 biological first-degree relatives of 85 TS probands, 92 biological first-degree relatives of 27 unaffected control probands, and 21 non-biological first-degree relatives of 6 adopted TS probands. The relatives of the unaffected probands and adopted TS probands served as a control sample of the whole data set. The authors examined rates of MDD, which were significantly higher for TS probands than controls. MDD was also significantly increased among relatives of TS probands. When this association was examined further, however, the rates of MDD in relatives of TS plus MDD probands was higher than control subjects, but the rates of MDD in relatives of TS-MDD probands was no higher than controls (55). This finding is compatible with MDD being genetic in its own right, but not with the suggestion that TS and MDD are genetically related. Braun et al. (56) analyzed F-18 fluorodeoxyglucose positron emission tomography scans, which were carried out in 18 medication-free TS patients. Several psychobehavioral features, including depression, were associated with significant increases in metabolic activity in the orbitofrontal cortices. Similar increases, although less robust, were observed in the putamen.

Chappell et al. (57) measured cerebrospinal fluid corticotrophin-releasing factor in medication-free TS patients (*N* = 21), OCD (*N* = 20), and healthy controls (*N* = 29). TS patients had significantly higher levels of cerebrospinal fluid corticotrophin-releasing factor than both other groups. In the context of this review, group differences in cerebrospinal fluid corticotrophin-releasing factor were unrelated to a variety of factors including depression and anxiety.

Diler et al. (58) undertook a [99m]technetiumECD single photon emission computed tomography brain imaging study in 38 children with TS (age 7 to 14 years) and compared them with a control group of 18 control children (age 9 to 14 years) to assess the patterns of regional cerebral perfusion. The Children's Depression Inventory was employed to assess any affective disorder. Although no depressed patients were included in the study, the depression scores were negatively correlated with all regional cerebral perfusion values, especially in the temporal areas.

Controlled Studies Reporting Depression in Younger Tourette Syndrome Patients

Spencer et al. (59) examined 32 TS children, 39 with chronic tics and 38 well control children, who were matched for age and gender. Results showed that nine (29%) of TS subjects, and 13 (33%) of tic children had severe major depression, which was significantly greater than the one (3%) in a well child (chi 2 = 12.4; *P* = 0.002); there were no significant differences found with regards to dysthymia.

Wodrich et al. (60) reported that 33 TS children who were referred to a specialist service for emotional and behavior problems were assessed by the Personality Inventory for Children, which the parents had completed. The TS children were compared with 66 control subjects from the same practice. The ages of the groups of youngsters were not significantly different. Depression, anxiety, and "peculiar behavior" were particularly frequent in children with TS. Depression occurred most frequently (73%), compared with 38% in the control group. The mean depression score was 74.9 (SD = 17.7). The authors concluded that "depression, anxiety, tension and excessive worry" might be characteristic of individuals with TS in comparison with control children of the same specialist service. A possible limitation of this study is that it relied on parents completing a questionnaire about their children; the children did not personally complete the questionnaire.

Carter et al. (24) examined 16 children with TS only, 33 children with TS plus ADHD, and 23 children who had no psychiatric diagnoses, who served as the control group. All children completed the Kovacs Child Depression Inventory. Mean CDI scores for the groups were as follows: TS plus ADHD (10.97), TS alone (8.19), and controls (4.43); the TS children scored significantly higher than the control children.

Findley et al. (61) developed the Yale Children's Global Stress Index. During the investigation, they used several standardized rating scales, including the Children's Depression Rating Scale (Revised). The study groups consisted of TS/OCD patients ($N = 33$) and unaffected controls ($N = 25$). The TS/OCD patients had significantly higher depression ratings than controls. Thus the depression score for 33 TS/OCD subjects was 26.9 (SD = 7.6), compared to a depression score of 18.2 (SD = 1.7) for the controls ($P <0.0001$).

The study by Sukhodolsky et al. (25) included 42 children with TS only, 52 with TS plus ADHD, 52 with ADHD only, and 61 controls. In the TS only group, six had depression compared with 10 in the TS plus ADHD group, and 15 in the ADHD group; this finding was statistically significant (Table 4-4).

Community-Based Studies in Young Tourette Syndrome Patients

In the longitudinal epidemiologic study referred to earlier, Peterson et al. (5) reassessed a cohort of children in the community with tics, and at time three (10 years after first assessment which took place between the ages of 1 and 10 years); depression was significantly associated with the presence of tics.

Kurlan et al. (10), as described earlier, undertook a large prevalence investigation and interviewed 1,596 children between the ages of 9 and 17 years in Rochester, New York, and Monroe County, New York. To assess associated psychobehavioral disorders the researcher administered a structured psychiatric interview to each subject and his or her parent independently using the Diagnostic Interview Schedule for Children, which yielded DSM-IV psychiatric diagnoses. The parents also completed the CBCL, and teachers completed the teacher version of the CBCL. The authors acknowledged that the low response rate (11%) may have resulted in a non-random sample; however, children with tics (using the Diagnostic Interview Schedule for Children) had a significantly higher frequency of ten psychiatric diagnoses, including major depression. The diagnoses clustered among four categories, including one of mood disorders. Among children with tics psychopathology was common ranging from 8.9% to 38.4%; mood disorders were less common (1.2% to 9.7%).

TABLE 4-4. *Controlled studies in which Tourette syndrome patients were more depressed than controls or depression variables were correlated with laboratory findings*

Patient age group	Study	Year	Patients with TS or OCD, N
Adult	Grossman et al. (52)	1986	TS, 29
	Comings and Comings (53)	1987	TS, 246
	Pitman et al. (54)	1987	TS, 16
	Pauls et al. (55)	1994	TS, 85
	Braun et al. (56)	1995	TS, 18
	Chappell et al. (57)	1996	TS, 21
Children	Spencer et al. (59)	1995	TS, 32
	Wodrich et al. (60)	1997	TS, 33
	Carter et al. (24)	2000	TS, 16
	Diler et al. (58)	2002	TS, 38
	Findley et al. (61)	2003	TS/OCD, 33
	Sukhodolsky et al. (25)	2003	TS only, 42

OCD, obsessive compulsive disorder; TS, Tourette syndrome.

Thus in both community studies, individuals with TS were rated as having more depression.

The National Hospital/University College London Collaborative Studies

There have been, to date, 12 published studies from The National Hospital for Neurology and Neurosurgery, Queen Square in London, University College London, and collaborators, which have either specifically examined depressive symptomatology and depressive illness in people with TS, or included depression measures as one part of a study. The authors' group has investigated adult and young TS subjects, both in descriptive clinical, controlled, and community settings. The TS subjects were all assessed using the National Hospital Interview Schedule (62), or earlier versions of the instrument. All TS subjects fulfilled the appropriate DSM and World Health Organization criteria, and depression was assessed using a variety of standardized self-report scales. In some studies the presence of MDD and its correlates was also examined, using International Classification of Diseases (ICD) (World Health Organization diagnostic schemes).

Specialist Tourette Syndrome Clinic Studies

The first study (47) investigated 90 consecutively referred TS clinic patients; of these the 54 adult TS patients were investigated employing standardized psychiatric rating scales including the BDI, and the depression subscales of the Mood Adjective Checklist (MACL) and the Crown Crisp Experiential Index (CCEI) (formerly known as the Middlesex Hospital Questionnaire). On all three measures the TS patients' scores were substantially higher than normative data. BDI and Crown Crisp Experiential Index depression subscales were significantly higher in females, older patients, and those exhibiting echophenomena. People with coprolalia had higher scores on the Crown Crisp Experiential Index depression subscale, whereas the MACL depression scores did not relate to any demographic or TS variable. Depression was not related to medication; using the MACL (the only scale employed to differentiate between

depression and fatigue), patients currently taking medication scored higher on the MACL fatigue subscale, but not on the MACL depression subscale. All 90 patients (adult and children) had full mental state examinations undertaken and 15/90 (17%) were judged clinically to have depressive symptoms severe enough to constitute a depressive illness (ICD diagnosis, World Health Organization). Of importance is that 43/90 probands (48%) had a positive family history of psychiatric illness, of which the most common disorder was depression (the family history was by history, and, not direct examination, and therefore likely to be an underestimate).

In the first controlled study, Channon et al. (63) primarily studied attentional deficits and neuropsychological functioning in 19 TS patients (mean age, 32.4 years; range, 18 to 65) and a mean full scale intelligence quotient of 107.42. They were examined using the Wechsler Adult Intelligence Scale-Revised, the Paced Auditory Serial Addition Test (PASAT) test and a variety of psychiatric rating scales including the self-report BDI. The mean BDI scores for the TS subjects were 10.74 (SD 10.01), whereas the mean for the matched healthy control group was 3.15 (SD = 4.17), which was significantly different (t = 3.02; df = 37, P <0.01). Of interest is that the performance on various neuropsychological tests including the letter cancellation and trail-making tests did not correlate with depressed mood.

In the second controlled study, Robertson et al. (64) investigated 22 TS adult patients (age between 18 and 65 years), and compared them with 19 patients with MDD, and 21 controls, using the BDI. The mean BDI score for controls was 2.71, for TS patients was 12.09, and for MDD patients was 25.32. Analysis of variance showed a significant difference in BDI scores between the three groups. Post-hoc t-tests showed that both the TS and depressed patients scored significantly higher than the controls; the depressed subjects also scored significantly higher than the TS subjects.

In the third controlled study (27) 39 consecutive TS clinic patients comparing them with 34 control subjects (matched for age and gender) using the BDI, as part of the larger investigation into PDs in TS, already discussed. The mean score of the Yale Global Tic Severity Scale in TS subjects was 26.2 (range, 11 to 55), indicative of moderate severity. The mean BDI score for the TS cases was 12.3, while that of the control subjects was 0.7 (t = 6.6; P <0.001; 95% CI, 8.1–15.1), indicating that TS subjects were significantly more depressed.

The fourth controlled study was undertaken by Robertson et al. (65) who studied 57 young people with TS aged 15 years or younger and compared them with a control group of 75 school pupils in mainstream education, who served as age and gender matched controls. All subjects completed standardized rating scales including the Birleson Depression Self-Rating Scale for children. The mean age of the TS group was 11.3 years (SD 2.4) and the mean age of the control group was 10.7 years; there was no significant difference between the two groups. The mean age at onset was 6 years and the mean age at diagnosis was 10 years. The mean Birleson Depression Self-Rating Scale score for the 57 TS group was 8.2 (range, 0 to 19; 95% CI 7.0 to 9.4) and that of the controls was 5.8 (range, 0 to 14; 95% CI 5.2 to 6.4). This was significantly different (T = 3.79; P <0.001).

The fifth controlled study (66) compared data on 87 consecutive TS referrals to the National Hospital for Neurology and Neurosurgery and the Queen Elizabeth Psychiatric Hospital (Birmingham) with 52 healthy controls using the BDI. The TS subjects' mean score on the BDI was 11.5 (SD = 8.0) while the controls' mean score was 4.6 (SD = 3.4), which was significant (T = 4.96, P <0.0001).

Thus, in five separate controlled studies of adult and young people with TS, including 224 TS patients, the TS patients had significantly higher BDI and Birleson Depression Self-Rating Scale scores than the controls.

In an investigation primarily into quality of life in clinic patients with TS (67), depression scores on the BDI significantly influenced the quality-of-life domains. Nineteen patients (21%) had high scores on the BDI (>19) indicating the presence of depression. Patients with depression had significantly lower scores on all subscales of the 36 item Short Form Health Survey except for physical functioning, indicating

worse quality of life, in comparison with patients without depression. Patients with depression had significantly higher TS severity scores on the Yale Global Tic Severity Scale than patients without depression (P = 0.01).

Eapen et al. (68) reported on a further cohort of 91 consecutive adult clinic TS subjects at the National Hospital for Neurology and Neurosurgery, using the BDI, the MACL, and the Crown Crisp Experiential Index. Of the cohort, 58 (63%) were males. The mean age was 29 years (range, 16 to 68; SD = 12.5). The mean age at onset of TS was 7.3 years, and the mean age at diagnosis was 20.8 years (range, 2 to 18; SD = 3.7). The mean number of years from onset to diagnosis was 13.4 (SD = 12.5). Forty-five (49.5%) had a family history of psychiatric disorder, including the following: depression (N = 24), manic depressive disorder (N = 6) and suicidal behavior (N = 6). The mean score on the BDI was 11.1 (range, 0 to 43; SD = 10.4); on the BDI 45.2% were judged to have a depressed score (N >10). The mean score on the MACL depression scale was (4.6 [SD = 5.6]) and the mean score on the Crown Crisp Experiential Index (CCEI) depression scale was 5.8 (SD = 4.0). On clinical mental state examination by trained psychiatrists, 11 (12.1%) had MDD (ICD diagnosis, World Health Organization). Logistic regression analysis was performed in order to examine the independent effects of various psychopathology ratings scores on ADHD, OCB, self-injurious behavior, aggression, and coprophenomena. When all the variables were included in the model and not controlling for the effects of other variables, there was no significant correlation between ADHD and the depression (BDI and MACL) scores. OCB was significantly correlated with depression scores (BDI and CCEI). Aggression was found to correlate with the depression scores (BDI and MACL). Similar analysis for coprophenomena found a significant correlation with the CCEI depression score. SIB was found to correlate with depression scores (BDI and CCEI). Principal component factor analysis using varimax rotation was performed on psychopathology scores derived from the various rating scales employed. This analysis yielded two components, which accounted for 72% of the variance. The first component was interpreted as the "obsessionality component" and the second the "anxiety/ depression component"; this deserves further exploration.

Community-Based Studies

Few studies have examined TS cases from community for depression or psychopathology. In the first community study of the investigators, a cohort of mild TS cases (relatives of a TS proband in a family study), the authors examined a multiply affected British pedigree spanning six generations and consisting of 122 members (69). The authors personally interviewed 85 individuals and obtained information on 25 via family members. Fifty individuals were diagnosed as "cases"; 48 were mild, one was moderate (proband), and one was severe (with a previous diagnosis of schizophrenia). The adults completed the CCEI, and the scores of the TS cases on the depression subscale were no different from the scores of family members who were non-TS cases.

The second was the pilot epidemiologic study already mentioned (6) which reported on tics and TS in 166 students age 13 to 14 years, in one mainstream school in West Essex, United Kingdom. Information was gathered from four sources: parents, teachers, pupils and the research psychologist. Thirty (18%) pupils were diagnosed as "tic possibles" and five were diagnosed as having TS. Using the Depression Self-Rating Scale, depression (with a score of >12) was diagnosed in 50 (34%) of the total population and in seven (29%) of the tic possibles; this difference was not significant. Of the five children with TS, one was diagnosed as having depression. However, this finding was in addition to four other psychiatric disorders (CD, hyperactivity, substance abuse, and behavioral disorder), indicative of the complexity of the case.

The third study was the already mentioned definitive investigation of the prevalence of TS in 918/1012 (90.7%) 13 to 14 year-olds in mainstream secondary schools in West Essex (7). In comparing the tic possible and TS groups with the total population for behavioral problem and depression symptoms, the tic positives ($N = 42$) and TS group ($N = 7$) had more behavioral problems, however the tic possible group ($N = 42$) had Birleson Depression Self-Rating Scale scores similar to the whole group and the TS groups (9.3 [SD = 3.45] versus 9.4 [SD = 4.8] versus 9, respectively) (7). Therefore, children with tics have more difficulties than their peers, but this study did not include depressive symptomatology.

In summary, in all three community studies, individuals with tics or TS did not have increased depression scores compared with subjects without TS. All the TS cases in the community studies were mildly affected and mostly unknown to the clinical services. Thus, tics and TS do not appear to invariably carry a risk for depression, rather the increased risk for depression seen in clinic samples may be the result of referral bias and attributable to the severity of TS, co-morbid psychopathology such as OCD, or other unknown factors.

ETIOLOGY OF DEPRESSION IN TOURETTE SYNDROME

There is now good evidence from controlled and uncontrolled studies to support the view that MDD, depressive illness, and depressive symptomatology are common in TS patients. Depression in TS is highly likely to be multifactorial in origin, as is the depression in non-TS populations [e.g. (41,70,71)].

What exactly are the factors contributing to the depression seen in patients with TS? TS can be a very distressing condition, particularly if tics are moderate to severe. This depression in TS could therefore be explained, at least in part, by the fact that people with TS have a chronic, socially disabling and stigmatizing disease. Another reason, which might play a part in the etiology of depression in clinic TS patients is that, in TS, co-morbidity with OCD is high (as discussed elsewhere in this book). The most common complication of OCD, ranging from 13%–75%, is depression (72). In the Pisa-San Diego collaborative study, MDD was the most common co-morbid disorder in OCD patients, occurring in 38% of subjects (73).

The depression in clinic TS patients may also be due to the side effects of both typical and atypical neuroleptic medications. Depression has been reported with, for example, haloperidol (74,75), pimozide (76,77), fluphenazine (78), tiapride (79), sulpiride (80), and risperidone (77,81). Depression has also been reported in patients being treated with other medications such as tetrabenazine (82), the calcium antagonist flunarizine (83); with mecamylamine, both depression (but similar to that found with placebo) and dysphoria were observed (84). As mentioned earlier, Margolese et al. (81) treated 58 patients with TS with risperidone and 17 (29.3%) developed MDD and 13 patients (22.4) became dysphoric while taking risperidone. Nine of the 17 patients who developed MDD had had a previous history of depression prior to taking the risperidone. A positive personal history of MDD was the only factor to significantly ($P <0.001$) predict the development of depression while taking risperidone. Seventy percent of those who developed MDD or dysphoria discontinued taking risperidone as a result of this adverse effect.

It has been clearly demonstrated that children who have been bullied at school may also become depressed (e.g., 85,86); some of the TS children in the clinic have been bullied, teased, and given pejorative nicknames and thus the depression may result from that experience.

The high levels of depression in some of these studies may reflect the fact that patients that attend specialist clinics (including TS patients) often have more than one problem/disorder; this may introduce ascertainment or referral bias. This view would be supported by epidemiologic studies, in which individuals with TS were not rated as having depressed mood when compared with non-TS subjects or controls, and by the study of Sukhodolsky et al. (25) where the "pure" TS subjects (without co-morbidity) were not more depressed than the controls.

Next, ADHD is common in TS (as described elsewhere in this book) and ADHD has been shown to have a high co-morbidity with depression (87,88), and thus many TS patients could be depressed because of the co-morbidity with ADHD. Similarly, OCB is common in TS

(as discussed elsewhere in this book), although there are phenomenologic differences between symptoms in TS and OCD. Depressive symptoms occur in 20% to 30% of patients with OCD (39); the depression therefore could be partly explained by the OCB/OCD co-morbidity. Family members of TS probands may also have a history of depression (e.g., 47,89), although this does not necessarily imply genetic factors.

Finally, it has also been shown that depression is common, with a lifetime prevalence of 7.5% to 10% in adults (90) and 1.8% to 8.9% in children (91); TS may also be more common than was previously recognized [e.g., (4,6, 10,11)]. Thus, the two disorders could co-exist by chance in some instances.

Taken together the literature indicates that depressive symptoms, and even MDD are common in TS. In contrast, there is no evidence to suggest that the reverse was true, i.e., TS is more common in patients with a main diagnosis of MDD (92). The etiology of depression in TS is highly likely multifactorial similar to primary depressive illness and less likely to be caused by a single etiological factor. Further studies may include the assessment of depression in non-clinic TS patients (such as mild relatives of patients in the clinic) as well as studies examining further the precise phenomenology and natural history of depression in the context of TS. Similar to OCB/OCD, the phenomenology of depressive symptoms may differ between TS and those in MDD. In depressed TS patients, this may help address factors of particular relevance to the etiology of their depression and thus improve its recognition but also treatment and outcome.

Bipolar Affective Disorder

The bipolar affective disorders (BADs) are characterized by recurrent episodes of altered mood and activity, involving upswings as well as downswings. Recent classification systems (DSM-IV-TR and ICD) have therefore had to define both individual episodes and pattern of recurrence. Individual episodes include MDD, manic episode, hypomanic (less severe) episode, and mixed episode, in which features of mania and major depression alternate rapidly (39).

There are two types of bipolar disorder included in DSM-IV-TR (1), bipolar I and bipolar II. Bipolar I disorder is characterized by a single manic episode and no past MDD episodes. Bipolar II disorder is diagnosed if there are recurrent MDD episodes with hypomanic episodes. A manic episode is defined as a distinct period of abnormally and persistently elevated, expansive, or irritable mood, lasting for 1 week (or any duration if hospitalization is necessary). Symptoms include inflated self-esteem or grandiosity, decreased need for sleep, more talkative than usual, distractibility, increased goal-directed activity, psychomotor agitation, and excessive involvement in pleasurable activities that have a high potential for painful consequences (1).

The lifetime prevalence of BAD is about 1%, with females being more commonly affected. Peak age at onset is in the early 20s. Several studies have shown higher prevalence rates in higher social classes, probably reflecting differences in access to diagnosis and treatment. There is clear evidence of a strong familial component; neuroendocrine abnormalities with monoamine excess have been described. Some studies suggest that manic illness may be precipitated by severe stress, and there may be a puerperal trigger factor (39).

Several studies have suggested a relationship between TS and BAD. Thus, Comings and Comings (53) reported in the controlled study mentioned above that none of the controls had a mania score greater than or equal to four, compared with 19.1% of the TS patients (P <0.0005).

The North Dakota group has been particularly prolific in their documentations of the co-occurrence of TS and BAD. Thus, Burd and Kerbeshian (93) documented the case of a TS patient who also had BAD, in whom the frequency and intensity of motor and vocal tics were correlated positively with the presence of manic symptoms, and inversely with depressive symptoms. They then reported three boys younger than age 14 years who had both TS and BAD, who early in life had also had ADHD

(94) and five cases of TS and Down syndrome, one of whom also had BAD (95). Kerbashian and Burd (96) also documented four patients who had TS, BAD, and autistic disorder, having surveyed 200 TS patients' charts. They suggested that the occurrence of the four patients with TS plus BAD plus autistic disorder in a population of 638,800 (1990 census in North Dakota) co-occurred at greater than chance. Had the occurrence been by chance, the total population would have to have been 15 billion. The group described five patients with a peek-a-boo fragile site at 16q22-23 and a variety of diagnoses (97). Three of the five had TS and two had BAD.

In addition to these case reports, Kerbeshian et al. (98) studied 205 TS patients in the North Dakota TS Surveillance Project and 15 (7%) had co-morbid BAD. The estimated risk of developing BAD in individuals with TS was more than four times higher than that expected by chance, but failed to reach statistical significance; males with TS were at a greater risk for BAD than females.

Spencer et al. (59), in the study mentioned earlier, found BAD to occur in 4 (13%) of 32 TS children and 11 (28%) of 39 tic children, compared with only one (3%) healthy child; this finding was statistically significant (chi 2 = 10.0, P = 0.006).

Berthier et al. (99) examined 30 adult TS patients with co-morbid TS and BAD, who were selected from a consecutive series of 90 TS patients. They thus reported that BAD occurred in a third of TS patients; the full spectrum of BAD was found, including bipolar I disorder, bipolar II disorder, schizoaffective bipolar disorder, and cyclothymic disorder. BAD mainly occurred in TS patients with mild tics and was associated with a wide variety of other psychopathologies (99). In this context, Comings and Comings (53) had already proposed that a gene leading to the expression of TS may additionally represent a locus for BAD.

Horrigan and Barnholl (100) presented five cases treated with guanfacine (0.5 mg/day) who developed states similar to hypomania or mania. Four of the cases (one female and three males) had TS, ADHD, and other disorders. The fifth patient was a male with ADHD and various other developmental disorders. Taking careful histories revealed that all of the youngsters with TS had clear risk factors (clinical and/or familial) for BAD, such as cyclothymia, cyclical mood disorder, MDD, bipolar II disorder, dysthymic disorder, intermittent explosive disorder, and alcohol abuse. The non-TS individual was adopted and thus there was no reliable family history.

In the study mentioned earlier, Coffey et al. (19) studied 156 youths with TS at a specialist center, subjects being assessed by standardized schedules. Nineteen (12%) of the cohort required psychiatric hospitalization. Significant univariate predictors of hospitalization included bipolar disorder. Bipolar disorder (P <0.001) was a robust predictor of psychiatric hospitalization, even after statistical adjustment for colinearity and correction for all other variables assessed.

Shytle et al. (101) documented two patients with TS who also had BAD. They treated the patients with mecamylamine (2.5 to 7.5 mg daily). The first patient was a 35-year-old woman who had severe TS, OCB, anxiety, and premenstrual syndrome; in this patient mecylamine helped in mood stabilization. The second patient was a 16-year-old boy who had TS, ADHD, and academic difficulties; manic symptoms were noticed after stopping the mecylamine. Restarting the mecylamine improved his symptoms.

In conclusion, the literature suggests that BAD may well be overrepresented in TS individuals. How TS and BAD relate to each other etiologically remains unclear. It appears that both share a number of neurophysiologic features, including abnormalities in noradrenergic, dopaminergic, and serotonergic neurotransmission (98).

Secondly, treatment with various agents has precipitated BAD/mania in vulnerable individuals, and this factor may well contribute to the apparent association of TS and BAD. Thus, treatment with stimulants (which are frequently used in the treatment of ADHD even in the context of TS), independent of ADHD, has also been documented to produce BAD (102). Jonkers and de Haan (103) reported the case of a 42-year-old woman diagnosed 10 years previously with BAD whose symptoms had never required hospitalization and who had never had prominent anxiety. Because of difficulties

including a prolonged depression, she was treated with a variety of agents. Finally, olanzapine was started at 5 mg/day and during week five of treatment, she developed panic-anxiety and severe obsessive-compulsive symptoms. Olanzapine was discontinued, and lithium was introduced as well as alprazolam and behavior therapy. The obsessive-compulsive symptoms reduced and she enjoyed full remission in 3 months. In the OCD literature, the development of mania or hypomania has been well documented in response to treatment with selective serotonin reuptake inhibitors or tricyclic antidepressants (72).

Third, it is also suggested by the present authors that the role of the co-morbidity encountered in TS patients, may be very important with regards to the association between TS and BAD. In this context, ADHD (as discussed elsewhere in this book) is common in people with TS and has been shown to be associated with BAD (87, 104–107). Hazell et al. (108), in contrast, compared males with ADHD plus mania when they were 9 to 13 years old ($N = 25$); although ADHD had been associated with mania in children, their results cast doubt on juvenile mania leading to adult BAD. Nevertheless it does appear that ADHD and BAD are associated in many individuals and cohorts. In addition, OCD is common in TS (72,109,110), and CD as described earlier in this chapter, have also been reported in association with BAD (111–114).

Fourth, psychosocial factors, such as stressful life events and social rhythm disruption, may also be important in the episodes of both depression and mania (115). In summary and conclusion, it seems that TS and BAD may be related in some individuals. However, study numbers are relatively small and thus more investigations are required. It is, however, unclear at the present time why there may well be BAD overrepresented in patients with TS, and more research is needed.

Suicide in Patients with Tourette Syndrome

Suicide may be defined as intentional self-inflicted death; deliberate self-harm represents intentionally self-inflicted self-harm without a fatal outcome. There are approximately 1/10,000 suicides per year or 1% of all deaths are from suicide per year. Sociologic and biochemical factors are thought to be relevant in the context of suicide, which is often associated with psychiatric disorders such as MDD, schizophrenia, alcoholism, substance abuse, PD, or a family history of suicide (39). Given the evidence that MDD and depressive symptomatology are so common in people with TS it is surprising that there are only a few reports of suicide in people with TS.

One of us reported two individuals with TS who committed suicide (116). The first patient was a 33-year-old man with TS who was treated with sulpiride and became depressed. There was no family history of depressive spectrum disorders. After becoming depressed, he took an overdose and cut his wrists. He was treated, improved, and 1 month later committed suicide. The second patient was a 19-year-old woman from the Netherlands who found her TS symptoms unbearable. She necessitated many hospital admissions. Her parents also found her TS symptoms unbearable and even discussed the option of suicide with her. She committed suicide at the age of 27 years. The senior author (MMR) has also had other patients who completed suicide (Robertson, unpublished data 2005). The only other documentation of completed suicide was that of Margolese et al. (81) in a patient treated with risperidone, although few details were given. Hence, two of the three documented suicides seem to have been precipitated by medication. Other studies described patients committing deliberate self-harm (117, 118), and, in some instances, these behaviors can be dangerous (attempted hanging twice) (119). Some of these behaviors may border on self-injurious behaviors, in which death is not wished and the patients report that they just "have to" hurt themselves. Self-injurious behaviors can be very dangerous but are usually distinct from suicidal ideation and suicide attempts.

Self-Injurious Behaviors in Tourette Syndrome

The self-injurious behaviors encountered in people with TS are on the whole not associated with a desire to die, rather merely to inflict injury,

TABLE 4-5. *Summary of studies reporting self-injurious behaviors in Tourette syndrome patients**

Author	Patients with Tourette syndrome, N	Patients with self-injurious behaviors, %
Moldofsky et al., 1974 (121)	15	53
Van Woert et al., 1977 (122)	111	43
Nee et al., 1980 (123)	50	48
Caine et al., 1988 (12)	41	17
Stefl, 1984 (15)	555	34
Robertson et al., 1989 (124)	90	30
Total	862	225

*Although not entirely comparable (e.g., Stefl undertook a questionnaire study, Caine et al. was an epidemiologic investigation, and Robertson et al. conducted the study in a tertiary clinic), the table does indicate that a substantial percentage of patients with Tourette syndrome in a variety of settings exhibit self-injurious behaviors. Collated from Robertson MM. Self-injurious behavior and Tourette syndrome. *Adv Neurol.* 1992;58:105–114.

and they often have an obsessional quality to them. In his original paper in 1885, Georges Gilles de la Tourette described two patients who had self-injurious behaviors; one bit his tongue and the other bit his lower lip (120). Self-injurious behaviors in TS include picking at sores and scabs, punching the abdomen, hitting self, biting (lips, teeth, tongues), filing of teeth, head banging, tongue or cheek biting, pummelling of the body, eye injuries, tooth extraction, touching of hot surfaces, sticking pins under skin or violent head shaking (120–123) (Table 4-5).

These self-injurious behaviors often seem to respond to an internal urge and may be aimed to relieve an inner tension similar to the sensations that precede complex tics or compulsive behaviors. It is thus not surprising that a relationship of self-injurious behavior with OCD has been reported (124,125). However, when self-injurious behaviors were differentiated according to their severity (e.g., scratching, picking at scabs, or hitting versus cutting or eye poking), less severe behaviors correlated with obsessions and compulsions whereas the more severe behaviors were associated more with impaired impulse control (125). However, in TS, self-injurious behaviors may also occur in the context of an underlying mood disorder, in particular depression; in addition, self-injurious behaviors may follow in the wake of substance abuse and ADHD or PDs. Hence, in a given patient, the relationship of self-injurious behavior to other psychiatric disorders needs to be clearly established because this relationship may have implications for management. Self-injurious behaviors can cause severe distress to patients, may entail the danger of incurring lasting physical injuries, and can be difficult to treat.

CONCLUSIONS

In conclusion, the incidence of behavioral disorders and depression seems to be higher in TS patients compared with controls. The strongest evidence for this assumption stems from studies assessing patients seen in specialist centers. However, as indicated by several epidemiologic studies in the community, children with TS are burdened by more behavioral problems than non-affected youngsters. It is worth noting that some studies clearly demonstrate that co-morbid disorders, in particular CD/ODD, OCD, and ADHD, contribute to the behavioral difficulties to a greater extent than TS itself. It is therefore important to specifically assess individuals with TS regarding associated conditions. This may have important treatment implications, such as for depression, even though the incidence of suicide may be lower in depressed TS patients than in other patients with depression. Whether this indicates that the depression in TS patients may be less dangerous or that suicide in TS may be under recognized is not clear and merits further research.

It is also not clear what the common co-occurrence of various behavioral disorders with TS indicates about the underlying etiology of either of these disorders. The complexity of TS and its associated conditions and psychopathologies [for review see Robertson (126)] clearly complicates research addressing these issues (Fig. 4-1). A better description and differentiation of endophenotypes may further understanding in this respect. A better description of

1. Multifactorial—depression

2. Adult psychopathology as a result of the childhood comorbid psychopathology (ADHD, ODD, CD) rather than the TS per se
   — Personality disorder

3. As a result of Referral Bias
   — Conduct disorder
   — Oppositional defiant disorder
   — Personality disorder

4. Due to comorbidity with ADHD
   — Oppositional defiant disorder
   — Conduct disorder

5. Impulsivity + rage—but not fulfilling criteria for ADHD
   — More research needed

6. Secondary to medication
   — Dysphoria
   — Depression

7. Due to comorbidity (ADHD, OCD, CD)
   — Bipolar affective disorder (BAD)

FIG. 4-1. Suggested relationships between psychopathology and tourette syndrome.

endophenotypes could also help design treatment trials examining drugs directed at particular subsets of symptoms more specifically.

Suggestions for Future Research

There is no doubt that more controlled studies are required in the areas of both behavioral disorders and affective disorders in TS. It is imperative that more controlled studies are employed with both diagnoses being made by an expert using a structured reliable and valid interview (e.g., to diagnose DSM MDD) and self-rating scales used as well (e.g., BDI) so that the results can be compared with the literature to date. This author also suggests that, with regard to depressive disorders, scales such as the Newcastle and Levine Pilowsky Scales are used so that the phenomenology of the depression can be accurately assessed. In addition, it is important that the "pure" TS clinic individuals be compared with TS plus ADHD and TS plus OCD, patients with MDD and healthy controls, so that it can be determined what precisely is caused by TS and what can be accounted for by the co-morbid disorders. In addition family histories must be obtained in a standardized way (e.g., depression, BAD, alcoholism) to enable the family history to be assessed alongside the phenomenology of the affective disorders.

ACKNOWLEDGMENTS

The author would like to thank both the UK and USA Tourette Syndrome Associations for their ongoing support.

REFERENCES

1. American Psychiatric Association. *Diagnostic and Statistical Manual of Mental Disorders. DSM-IV.* Washington, DC: American Psychiatric Association, 1994.

2. Rutter M, Tizard J, Yule W, et al. Research report: Isle of Wight Studies, 1964–1974. *Psychol Med.* 1976; 6:313–332.

3. Comings DE, Himes JA, Comings BG. An epidemiologic study of Tourette's syndrome in a single school district. *J Clin Psychiatry.* 1990;51:463–469.

4. Kadesjo B, Gillberg C. Tourette's disorder: epidemiology and comorbidity in primary school children. *J Am Acad Child Adolesc Psychiatry.* 2000;39:548–555.

5. Peterson BS, Pine DS, Cohen P, et al. Prospective, longitudinal study of tic, obsessive-compulsive, and attention-deficit/hyperactivity disorders in an epidemiological sample. *J Am Acad Child Adolesc Psychiatry.* 2001;40:685–695.

6. Mason A, Banerjee S, Eapen V, et al. The prevalence of Tourette syndrome in a mainstream school population. *Dev Med Child Neurol.* 1998;40:292–296.

7. Hornsey H, Banerjee S, Zeitlin H, et al. The prevalence of Tourette syndrome in 13-14-year-olds in mainstream schools. *J Child Psychol Psychiatry.* 2001;42:1035–1039.

8. Goodman R. The Strengths and Difficulties Questionnaire: a research note. *J Child Psychol Psychiatry.* 1997;38:581–586.

9. Goodman R. The extended version of the Strengths and Difficulties Questionnaire as a guide to child psychiatric caseness and consequent burden. *J Child Psychol Psychiatry.* 1999;40:791–799.

10. Kurlan R, McDermott MP, Deeley C, et al. Prevalence of tics in schoolchildren and association with placement in special education. *Neurology* 2001;57:1383–1388.

11. Lanzi G, Zambrino CA, Termine C, et al. Prevalence of tic disorders among primary school students in the city of Pavia, Italy. *Arch Dis Child.* 2004;89:45–47.

12. Caine ED, McBride MC, Chiverton P, et al. Tourette's syndrome in Monroe County school children. *Neurology* 1988;38:472–475.

13. Zohar AH. The epidemiology of obsessive-compulsive disorder in children and adolescents. *Child Adolesc Psychiatr Clin N Am.* 1999;8:445–460.

14. Costello EJ, Angold A, Burns BJ, et al. The Great Smoky Mountains Study of Youth. Goals, design, methods, and the prevalence of DSM-III-R disorders. *Arch Gen Psychiatry.* 1996;53:1129–1136.

15. Stefl ME. Mental health needs associated with Tourette syndrome. *Am J Public Health.* 1984;74:1310–1313.

16. Champion LM, Fulton WA, Shady GA. Tourette syndrome and social functioning in a Canadian population. *Neurosci Biobehav Rev.* 1988;12:255–257.

17. Comings DE, Comings BG. A controlled study of Tourette syndrome. II. Conduct. *Am J Hum Genet.* 1987;41:742–760.

18. Coffey BJ, Park KS. Behavioral and emotional aspects of Tourette syndrome. *Neurol Clin.* 1997;15:277–289.

19. Coffey BJ, Biederman J, Geller DA, et al. Distinguishing illness severity from tic severity in children and adolescents with Tourette's disorder. *J Am Acad Child Adolesc Psychiatry.* 2000;39:556–561.

20. Freeman RD, Fast DK, Burd L, et al. An international perspective on Tourette syndrome: selected findings from 3,500 individuals in 22 countries. *Dev Med Child Neurol.* 2000;42:436–447.

21. Mahone EM, Koth CW, Cutting L, et al. Executive function in fluency and recall measures among children with Tourette syndrome or ADHD. *J Int Neuropsychol Soc.* 2001;7:102–111.

22. Cooper C, Robertson MM, Livingston G. Psychological morbidity and caregiver burden in parents of children with Tourette's disorder and psychiatric comorbidity. *J Am Acad Child Adolesc Psychiatry.* 2003;42: 1370–1375.

23. Channon S, Pratt P, Robertson MM. Executive function, memory, and learning in Tourette's syndrome. *Neuropsychology* 2003;17:247–254.

24. Carter AS, O'Donnell DA, Schultz RT, et al. Social and emotional adjustment in children affected with Gilles de la Tourette's syndrome: associations with ADHD and family functioning. Attention Deficit Hyperactivity Disorder. *J Child Psychol Psychiatry.* 2000;41:215–223.

25. Sukhodolsky DG, Scahill L, Zhang H, et al. Disruptive behavior in children with Tourette's syndrome: association with ADHD comorbidity, tic severity, and functional impairment. *J Am Acad Child Adolesc Psychiatry.* 2003;42:98–105.

26. Shapiro AK, Shapiro ES, Bruun RD, et al. *Gilles de la Tourette syndrome.* New York: Raven Press, 1978.

27. Robertson MM, Banerjee S, Hiley PJ, et al. Personality disorder and psychopathology in Tourette's syndrome: a controlled study. *Br J Psychiatry.* 1997;171:283–286.

28. Kurlan R, Daragjati C, Como PG, et al. Non-obscene complex socially inappropriate behavior in Tourette's syndrome. *J Neuropsychiatry Clin Neurosci.* 1996; 8:311–317.

29. Bruun RD, Budman CL. Paroxetine treatment of episodic rages associated with Tourette's disorder. *J Clin Psychiatry.* 1998;59:581–584.

30. Budman CL, Bruun RD, Park KS, et al. Rage attacks in children and adolescents with Tourette's disorder: a pilot study. *J Clin Psychiatry*. 1998;59:576–580.

31. Budman CL, Bruun RD, Park KS, et al. Explosive outbursts in children with Tourette's disorder. *J Am Acad Child Adolesc Psychiatry*. 2000;39:1270–1276.

32. Budman CL, Rockmore L, Stokes J, et al. Clinical phenomenology of episodic rage in children with Tourette syndrome. *J Psychosom Res*. 2003;55:59–565.

33. Robins LN. Sturdy childhood predictors of adult antisocial behavior: replications from longitudinal studies. *Psychol Med*. 1978;8:611–622.

34. Zoccolillo M, Pickles A, Quinton D, et al. The outcome of childhood conduct disorder: implications for defining adult personality disorder and conduct disorder. *Psychol Med*. 1992;22:971–986.

35. Babinski LM, Hartsough CS, Lambert NM. Childhood conduct problems, hyperactivity-impulsivity, and inattention as predictors of adult criminal activity. *J Child Psychol Psychiatry*. 1999;40:347–355.

36. Stevenson J, Goodman R. Association between behavior at age 3 years and adult criminality. *Br J Psychiatry*. 2001;179:197–202.

37. Fombonne E, Wostear G, Cooper V, et al. The Maudsley long-term follow-up of child and adolescent depression. 1. Psychiatric outcomes in adulthood. *Br J Psychiatry*. 2001;179:210–217.

38. Fombonne E, Wostear G, Cooper V, et al. The Maudsley long-term follow-up of child and adolescent depression. 2. Suicidality, criminality and social dysfunction in adulthood. *Br J Psychiatry*. 2001;179:218–223.

39. Katona C, Robertson MM. *Psychiatry at a Glance*. London: Blackwell Science, 2000.

40. Robertson MM. Diagnosing Tourette syndrome: is it a common disorder? *J Psychosom Res*. 2003;55:3–6.

41. Winokur G. All roads lead to depression: clinically homogeneous, etiologically heterogeneous. *J Affect Disord*. 1997;45:97–108.

42. Shapiro AK, Shapiro E, Wayne HL, et al. Tourette's syndrome: summary of data on 34 patients. *Psychosom Med*. 1973;35:419–435.

43. Goforth EG. A single case study. Gilles de la Tourette's syndrome. *J Nerv Ment Dis*. 1974;158:306–309.

44. Penna MW, Lion JR. Gilles de la Tourette's syndrome and depression: a case report. *Dis Nerv Syst*. 1975; 36:41–43.

45. Ferrari M, Matthews WS, Barabas G. Children with Tourette syndrome: results of psychological tests given prior to drug treatment. *J Dev Behav Pediatr*. 1984; 5:116–119.

46. Erenberg G, Cruse RP, Rothner AD. The natural history of Tourette syndrome: a follow-up study. *Ann Neurol*. 1987;22:383–385.

47. Robertson MM, Trimble MR, Lees AJ. The psychopathology of the Gilles de la Tourette syndrome. A phenomenological analysis. *Br J Psychiatry*. 1988;152:383–390.

48. Wand RR, Matazow GS, Shady GA, et al. Tourette syndrome: associated symptoms and most disabling features. *Neurosci Biobehav Rev*. 1993;17:271–275.

49. Chee KY, Sachdev P. The clinical features of Tourette's disorder: an Australian study using a structured interview schedule. *Aust N Z J Psychiatry*. 1994;28:313–318.

50. Rosenberg LA, Brown J, Singer HS. Behavioral problems and severity of tics. *J Clin Psychol*. 1995; 51:760–7.

51. Teive HA, Germiniani FM, Della Coletta MV, et al. Tics and Tourette syndrome: clinical evaluation of 44 cases. *Arq Neuropsiquiatr*. 2001;59:725–728.

52. Grossman HY, Mostofsky DI, Harrison RH. Psychological aspects of Gilles de la Tourette syndrome. *J Clin Psychol*. 1986;42:228–235.

53. Comings BG, Comings DE. A controlled study of Tourette syndrome. V. Depression and mania. *Am J Hum Genet*. 1987;41:804–821.

54. Pitman RK, Green RC, Jenike MA, et al. Clinical comparison of Tourette's disorder and obsessive-compulsive disorder. *Am J Psychiatry*. 1987;144:1166–1171.

55. Pauls DL, Leckman JF, Cohen DJ. Evidence against a genetic relationship between Tourette's syndrome and anxiety, depression, panic and phobic disorders. *Br J Psychiatry*. 1994;164:215–221.

56. Braun AR, Randolph C, Stoetter B, et al. The functional neuroanatomy of Tourette's syndrome: an FDG-PET Study. II: Relationships between regional cerebral metabolism and associated behavioral and cognitive features of the illness. *Neuropsychopharmacology* 1995; 13:151–168.

57. Chappell P, Leckman J, Goodman W, et al. Elevated cerebrospinal fluid corticotropin-releasing factor in Tourette's syndrome: comparison to obsessive compulsive disorder and normal controls. *Biol Psychiatry*. 1996;39:776–783.

58. Diler RS, Reyhanli M, Toros F, et al. Tc-99m-ECD SPECT brain imaging in children with Tourette's syndrome. *Yonsei Med J*. 2002;43:403–410.

59. Spencer T, Biederman J, Harding M, et al. The relationship between tic disorders and Tourette's syndrome revisited. *J Am Acad Child Adolesc Psychiatry*. 1995; 34:1133–1139.

60. Wodrich DL, Benjamin E, Lachar D. Tourette's syndrome and psychopathology in a child psychiatry setting. *J Am Acad Child Adolesc Psychiatry*. 1997; 36:1618–1624.

61. Findley DB, Leckman JF, Katsovich L, et al. Development of the Yale Children's Global Stress Index (YCGSI) and its application in children and adolescents with Tourette's syndrome and obsessive-compulsive disorder. *J Am Acad Child Adolesc Psychiatry*. 2003;42:450–457.

62. Robertson MM, Eapen V. The National Hospital Interview Schedule for the assessment of Gilles de la Tourette syndrome. *International Journal of Methods in Psychiatric Research* 1996;6:203–226.

63. Channon S, Flynn D, Robertson MM. Attentional deficits in the Gilles de la Tourette syndrome. *Neuropsychiatry Neuropsychol Behav Neurol*. 1992;5: 170–177.

64. Robertson MM, Channon S, Baker J, et al. The psychopathology of Gilles de la Tourette's syndrome. A controlled study. *Br J Psychiatry*. 1993;162:114–117.

65. Robertson MM, Banerjee S, Eapen V, et al. Obsessive compulsive behavior and depressive symptoms in young people with Tourette syndrome. A controlled study. *Eur Child Adolesc Psychiatry*. 2002;11:261–265.

66. Rickards H, Robertson M. A controlled study of psychopathology and associated symptoms in Tourette syndrome. *World J Biol Psychiatry*. 2003;4:64–68.

67. Elstner K, Selai CE, Trimble MR, et al. Quality of Life (QOL) of patients with Gilles de la Tourette's syndrome. *Acta Psychiatr Scand*. 2001;103:52–59.

68. Eapen V, Fox-Hiley P, Banerjee S, et al. Clinical features and associated psychopathology in a Tourette syndrome cohort. *Acta Neurol Scand.* 2004;109: 255–260.

69. Robertson MM, Gourdie A. Familial Tourette's syndrome in a large British pedigree. Associated psychopathology, severity, and potential for linkage analysis. *Br J Psychiatry.* 1990;156:515–521.

70. Zimmerman M, Coryell W, Pfohl B, et al. The validity of four definitions of endogenous depression. II. Clinical, demographic, familial, and psychosocial correlates. *Arch Gen Psychiatry.* 1986;43:234–244.

71. Strober M, Schmidt-Lackner S, Freeman R, et al. Recovery and relapse in adolescents with bipolar affective illness: a five-year naturalistic, prospective follow-up. *J Am Acad Child Adolesc Psychiatry.* 1995; 34:724–731.

72. Perugi G, Toni C, Frare F, et al. Obsessive-compulsive-bipolar comorbidity: a systematic exploration of clinical features and treatment outcome. *J Clin Psychiatry.* 2002;63:1129–1134.

73. Perugi G, Akiskal HS, Ramacciotti S, et al. Depressive comorbidity of panic, social phobic, and obsessive–compulsive disorders re-examined: is there a bipolar II connection? *J Psychiatr Res.* 1999;33:53–61.

74. Caine ED, Polinsky RJ. Haloperidol-induced dysphoria in patients with Tourette syndrome. *Am J Psychiatry.* 1979;136:1216–1217.

75. Bruun RD. Dysphoric phenomena associated with haloperidol treatment of Tourette syndrome. *Adv Neurol.* 1982;35:433–436.

76. Regeur L, Pakkenberg B, Fog R, et al. Clinical features and long-term treatment with pimozide in 65 patients with Gilles de la Tourette's syndrome. *J Neurol Neurosurg Psychiatry.* 1986;49:791–795.

77. Bruggeman R, van der Linden C, Buitelaar JK, et al. Risperidone versus pimozide in Tourette's disorder: a comparative double-blind parallel-group study. *J Clin Psychiatry.* 2001;62:50–56.

78. Bruun RD. Subtle and underrecognized side effects of neuroleptic treatment in children with Tourette's disorder. *Am J Psychiatry.* 1988;145:621–624.

79. Chouza C, Romero S, Lorenzo J, et al. [Clinical trial of tiapride in patients with dyskinesia (author's transl)]. *Sem Hop.* 1982;58:725–733.

80. Robertson MM, Schnieden V, Lees AJ. Management of Gilles de la Tourette syndrome using sulpiride. *Clin Neuropharmacol.* 1990;13:229–235.

81. Margolese HC, Annable L, Dion Y. Depression and dysphoria in adult and adolescent patients with Tourette's disorder treated with risperidone. *J Clin Psychiatry.* 2002;63:1040–1044.

82. Jankovic J, Glaze DG, Frost JD, Jr. Effect of tetrabenazine on tics and sleep of Gilles de la Tourette's syndrome. *Neurology* 1984;34:688–692.

83. Micheli F, Gatto M, Lekhuniec E, et al. Treatment of Tourette's syndrome with calcium antagonists. *Clin Neuropharmacol.* 1990;13:77–83.

84. Silver AA, Shytle RD, Sheehan KH, et al. Multicenter, double-blind, placebo-controlled study of mecamylamine monotherapy for Tourette's disorder. *J Am Acad Child Adolesc Psychiatry.* 2001;40:1103–1110.

85. Salmon G, James A, Smith DM. Bullying in schools: self reported anxiety, depression, and self esteem in secondary school children. *BMJ.* 1998;317:924–925.

86. Bond L, Carlin JB, Thomas L, et al. Does bullying cause emotional problems? A prospective study of young teenagers. *BMJ.* 2001;323:480–484.

87. Biederman J, Newcorn J, Sprich S. Comorbidity of attention deficit hyperactivity disorder with conduct, depressive, anxiety, and other disorders. *Am J Psychiatry.* 1991;148:564–577.

88. Milberger S, Biederman J, Faraone SV, et al. Attention deficit hyperactivity disorder and comorbid disorders: issues of overlapping symptoms. *Am J Psychiatry.* 1995;152:1793–1799.

89. Montgomery MA, Clayton PJ, Friedhoff AJ. Psychiatric illness in Tourette syndrome patients and first-degree relatives. *Adv Neurol.* 1982;35:335–339.

90. Kessler RC, Zhao S, Blazer DG, et al. Prevalence, correlates, and course of minor depression and major depression in the National Comorbidity Survey. *J Affect Disord.* 1997;45:19–30.

91. Angold A, Costello EJ. Developmental epidemiology. *Epidemiol Rev.* 1995;17:74–82.

92. Eapen V, Laker M, Anfield A, et al. Prevalence of tics and Tourette syndrome in an inpatient adult psychiatry setting. *J Psychiatry Neurosci.* 2001;26:417–420.

93. Burd L, Kerbeshian J. Gilles de la Tourette's syndrome and bipolar disorder. *Arch Neurol.* 1984; 41:1236.

94. Kerbeshian J, Burd L. Tourette disorder and bipolar symptomatology in childhood and adolescence. *Can J Psychiatry.* 1989;34:230–233.

95. Kerbeshian J, Burd L. Comorbid Down's syndrome, Tourette syndrome and intellectual disability: registry prevalence and developmental course. *J Intellect Disabil Res.* 2000;44:60–67.

96. Kerbeshian J, Burd L. Case study: comorbidity among Tourette's syndrome, autistic disorder, and bipolar disorder. *J Am Acad Child Adolesc Psychiatry.* 1996; 35:681–685.

97. Kerbeshian J, Severud R, Burd L, et al. Peek-a-boo fragile site at 16d associated with Tourette syndrome, bipolar disorder, autistic disorder, and mental retardation. *Am J Med Genet.* 2000;96:69–73.

98. Kerbeshian J, Burd L, Klug MG. Comorbid Tourette's disorder and bipolar disorder: an etiologic perspective. *Am J Psychiatry.* 1995;152:1646–1651.

99. Berthier ML, Kulisevsky J, Campos VM. Bipolar disorder in adult patients with Tourette's syndrome: a clinical study. *Biol Psychiatry.* 1998;43:364–370.

100. Horrigan JP, Barnhill LJ. Guanfacine and secondary mania in children. *J Affect Disord.* 1999;54:309–314.

101. Shytle RD, Silver AA, Sanberg PR. Comorbid bipolar disorder in Tourette's syndrome responds to the nicotinic receptor antagonist mecamylamine (Inversine). *Biol Psychiatry.* 2000;48:1028–1031.

102. DelBello MP, Soutullo CA, Hendricks W, et al. Prior stimulant treatment in adolescents with bipolar disorder: association with age at onset. *Bipolar Disord.* 2001;3:53–57.

103. Jonkers F, De Haan L. Olanzapine-induced obsessive-compulsive symptoms in a patient with bipolar II disorder. *Psychopharmacology* (Berl) 2002;162:87–88. Epub 2002 Apr 4.

104. Hazell PL, Lewin TJ, Carr VJ. Confirmation that Child Behavior Checklist clinical scales discriminate juvenile mania from attention deficit hyperactivity disorder. *J Paediatr Child Health.* 1999;35:199–203.

105. Faraone SV, Glatt SJ, Tsuang MT. The genetics of pediatric-onset bipolar disorder. *Biol Psychiatry.* 2003;53:970–977.

106. Tramontina S, Schmitz M, Polanczyk G, et al. Juvenile bipolar disorder in Brazil: clinical and treatment findings. *Bicl Psychiatry.* 2003;53:1043–1049.

107. Wilens TE, Biederman J, Wozniak J, et al. Can adults with attention-deficit/hyperactivity disorder be distinguished from those with comorbid bipolar disorder? Findings from a sample of clinically referred adults. *Biol Psychiatry.* 2003;54:1–8.

108. Hazell PL, Carr V, Lewin TJ, et al. Manic symptoms in young males with ADHD predict functioning but not diagnosis after 6 years. *J Am Acad Child Adolesc Psychiatry.* 2003;42:552–560.

109. Chen YW, Dilsaver SC. Comorbidity for obsessive-compulsive disorder in bipolar and unipolar disorders. *Psychiatry Res.* 1995;59:57–64.

110. Freeman MP, Freeman SA, McElroy SL. The comorbidity of bipolar and anxiety disorders: prevalence, psychobiology, and treatment issues. *J Affect Disord.* 2002;68:1–23.

111. Kutcher SP, Marton P, Korenblum M. Relationship between psychiatric illness and conduct disorder in adolescents. *Can J Psychiatry.* 1989;34:526–529.

112. Kovacs M, Pollock M. Bipolar disorder and comorbid conduct disorder in childhood and adolescence. *J Am Acad Child Adolesc Psychiatry.* 1995;34:715–723.

113. Lewinsohn PM, Klein DN, Seeley JR. Bipolar disorders in a community sample of older adolescents: prevalence, phenomenology, comorbidity, and course. *J Am Acad Child Adolesc Psychiatry.* 1995;34:454–463.

114. Biederman J, Mick E, Wozniak J, et al. Can a subtype of conduct disorder linked to bipolar disorder be identified? Integration of findings from the Massachusetts General Hospital Pediatric Psychopharmacology Research Program. *Biol Psychiatry.* 2003;53:952–960.

115. Malkoff-Schwartz S, Frank E, Anderson B, et al. Stressful life events and social rhythm disruption in the onset of manic and depressive bipolar episodes: a preliminary investigation. *Arch Gen Psychiatry.* 1998;55:702–707.

116. Robertson MM, Eapen V, van de Wetering BJ. Suicide in Gilles de la Tourette's syndrome: report of two cases. *J Clin Psychiatry.* 1995;56:378.

117. Dillon JE. Self-injurious behavior associated with clonidine withdrawal in a child with Tourette's disorder. *J Child Neurol.* 1990;5:308–310.

118. Whelan R, Dearlove OR. Management of clonidine overdose in a child with Tourette syndrome. *Dev Med Child Neurol.* 1995;37:469.

119. Cruz R. Clomipramine side effects. *J Am Acad Child Adolesc Psychiatry.* 1992;31:1168–1169.

120. Robertson MM. Self-injurious behavior and Tourette syndrome. *Adv Neurol.* 1992;58:105–114.

121. Moldofsky H, Tullis C, Lamon R. Multiple tic syndrome (Giles de la Tourette's syndrome). *J Nerv Ment Dis.* 1974;159:282–292.

122. Van Woert MH, Yip LC, Balis ME. Purine phosphoribosyltransferase in Gilles de la Tourette syndrome. *N Engl J Med.* 1977;296:210–212.

123. Nee LE, Caine ED, Polinsky RJ, et al. Gilles de la Tourette syndrome: clinical and family study of 50 cases. *Ann Neurol.* 1980;7:41–49.

124. Robertson MM, Trimble MR, Lees AJ. Self-injurious behavior and the Gilles de la Tourette syndrome: a clinical study and review of the literature. *Psychol Med.* 1989;19:611–625.

125. Mathews CA, Waller J, Glidden D, et al. Self injurious behavior in Tourette syndrome: correlates with impulsivity and impulse control. *J Neurol Neurosurg Psychiatry.* 2004;75:1149–1155.

126. Robertson MM. Heterogeneous psychopathology of Tourette syndrome. In: Bedard M-A, Agid Y, Chouinard S, et al., eds. *Mental and behavioral dysfunction in movement disorders.* Totowa, NJ: Humana Press, 2003.

5

Tics Associated with Other Disorders

Joseph Jankovic and Nicte I. Mejia

Parkinson's Disease Center and Movement Disorders Clinic, Department of Neurology, Baylor College of Medicine, Houston, Texas

Tics are abrupt, repetitive movements (motor tics) or sounds (phonic tics), commonly preceded by a premonitory sensation of an urge, tension, discomfort, or other sensory phenomena (1,2). Tourette syndrome (TS), amply reviewed in this volume, is the most frequent cause of tics. However, it is important to recognize that tic-like phenomena may be observed in a variety of other conditions (3) including sporadic, genetic, and neurodegenerative disorders, or may be caused by other etiologies such as drugs, infection, stroke, and head trauma (4,5) (Table 5-1).

This review is organized according to tic mimickers (phenomenology) and tics secondary to other causes (etiology), sometimes referred to as *tourettism* (Table 5-2). These authors have undertaken this task in a belief that a study of tics secondary to other causes may not only help differentiate TS from tourettism, but also provide insights into the pathogenesis of primary tics and TS.

TIC MIMICKERS

Dystonia

Dystonia is a neurologic syndrome characterized by involuntary, sustained, patterned, and often repetitive muscle contractions of opposing muscles, causing twisting movements, abnormal postures, or both (6). Both dystonia and tics may share clinical phenomenology in that both may be rapid, patterned, and repetitive. The term *dystonic tic* has been used to characterize tics that are transiently sustained, such as oculogyric tics, blepharospasm, and rotatory movements of the scapula; indeed, dystonic movements of the scapula are nearly always due to tics (7). Dystonic movements as a manifestation of dystonia may not be easily differentiated from dystonic tics in patients with TS, but the latter are typically preceded by premonitory sensations (8). The differentiation between dystonia and tics is further complicated by the occasional coexistence of both in the same individual. These authors initially reported nine patients in whom motor tics preceded the onset of their primary dystonia (9). In a recent review of 155 patients with tics and other associated diagnoses, 31 (20.0%) patients had dystonia as the associated disorder. Of these patients, 24 (15.4%) initially met diagnostic criteria for TS and were later found to develop dystonia; three (1.9%) patients were first diagnosed with primary dystonia and later developed tics; three (1.9%) had co-existent tics and dystonia without a clear understanding of which occurred first; and one (0.6%) had onset of tics and dystonia at the same time (Fig. 5-1) (5).

Families affected with TS and dystonia have been described; Nemeth et al. reported a three-generation family in which five patients presented with dystonia and three also had TS, manifested chiefly by facial tics (10). In addition to primary dystonia, tics may be associated with a variety of secondary dystonias. For example, three members of a large Danish family with dopa-responsive dystonia and the X251R mutation in the *GCH1* gene were also affected with TS (11).

Botulinum toxin (BTX) is a safe and effective treatment option for patients with TS and associated dystonia. Of the 107 patients with TS and

TABLE 5-1. *Tic mimickers*

- Dystonia: sustained, patterned
- Chorea: continuous, random
- Myoclonus: brief unsuppressible movements
- Hyperexplexia: excessive startle
- Akathisia: inner feeling of restlessness
- Rituals: repetitive actions in obsessive compulsive disorder
- Restless leg syndrome: subjective crawling sensation, leg movement more than arm movement
- Stereotypies: repetitive, coordinated movements (autism)

dystonia in the database of the authors of this chapter, 17 were diagnosed with oromandibular dystonia, bruxism, or both; in 10 patients the focal dystonia was severe enough to interfere with swallowing, chewing, or speech, requiring BTX injections. Over a period of 3.0 ± 1.9 years (range, 0.3 to 9.7) BTX was administered in a total of 71 injection visits to the 10 patient's masseter, submentalis, and lateral pterygoid muscles for jaw-closing dystonia, jaw-opening dystonia, and jaw-deviation dystonia. The latency to onset of benefit was 4.6 days (range, 1 to 21) and the mean total duration of response to BTX was 14.4 ± 12.0 weeks (range, 12 to 50). The mean peak effect on a scale of 0 to 4 (total abolishment of dystonia) was 3.15 ± 0.9. Of these 10 patients, five encountered notable premonitory sensory symptoms and four derived significant relief of these symptoms from BTX injections. Complications such as

dysphagia and dysarthria were reported in five of all treatment visits (16.1 %) (12).

Myoclonus

Myoclonus is a lightning-like movement produced by a sudden and brief contraction (positive myoclonus) or a muscle inhibition (negative myoclonus). Similar to a tic, myoclonus is a jerk-like movement; however, in contrast to a tic, myoclonus is usually not suppressible and is not preceded by premonitory sensations. Because of the phenomenologic overlap, myoclonus is frequently misdiagnosed as a tic and vice versa. In a review of 155 patients with tics and associated disorders, two (1.2%) patients meeting criteria for TS developed myoclonus later in life; one (0.6%) developed myoclonus and the other (0.6%) developed segmental myoclonus and dystonia. One other (0.6%) patient had onset of myoclonus, tics, and essential tremor at the same time, without a clear etiologic relationship between the diagnoses (Fig. 5-1) (5).

Myoclonus may be caused by a variety of genetic and secondary causes. Progressive myoclonus epilepsy of Unverricht-Lundborg type (EPM1), one of the major types of progressive myoclonus epilepsy, is an autosomal recessive disorder with onset between age 6 to 15 years, characterized by stimulus-sensitive

TABLE 5-2. *Other causes of tics*

Dystonia	Primary and secondary dystonia
Heredodegenerations	Huntington disease
	Neuroacanthocytosis
	Neurodegeneration with brain iron accumulation, pantothenate kinase associated neurodegeneration)
	Wilson disease
Infectious	Encephalitis (measles, herpes virus), mycoplasma pneumoniae
Post-Infectious	Sydenham chorea, Pediatric Autoimmune Neuropsychiatric Disorders Associated with Streptococcal infection)?
Drugs	Amphetamines, methylphenidate and other central nervous system stimulants (cocaine), carbamazepine, phenytoin, phenobarbital, lamotrigine, levodopa
	Dopamine receptor-blocking drugs (tardive tourettism)
Toxins	Carbon monoxide, wasp venom, mercury
Developmental	Static encephalopathy, mental retardation syndromes, autistic disorders (Asperger syndrome, Rett syndrome), fetal alcohol syndrome
Metabolic	Lesch-Nyhan syndrome, phenylketonuria, citrullinemia
Other Genetic or Chromosomal Disorders	Down syndrome, Klinefelter's syndrome, XYY, Fragile X, Triple X and 9p mosaicism, partial trisomy 16, 9p monosomy, Beckwith-Wiedemann syndrome, Duchenne muscular dystrophy, Ehler-Danlos syndrome, congenital adrenal hyperplasia
Other	Head trauma, peripheral trauma, stroke, malignancies, neurocutaneous syndromes, schizophrenia, psychogenic

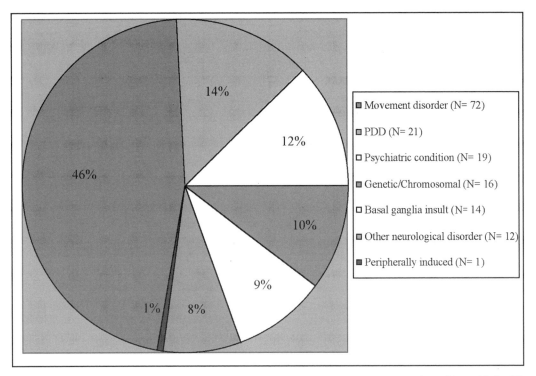

14%

12%

46%

10%

9%

1% 8%

- Movement disorder (N= 72)
- PDD (N= 21)
- Psychiatric condition (N= 19)
- Genetic/Chromosomal (N= 16)
- Basal ganglia insult (N= 14)
- Other neurological disorder (N= 12)
- Peripherally induced (N= 1)

FIG. 5-1. Associated diagnoses in 155 patients with tics and coexistent disorders. (From Mejia NI, Jankovic J. Secondary tics and tourettism. *Rev Bras Psiquiatr.* 2005. In press. With permisison.)

myoclonus and tonic-clonic seizures (13). One (0.6%) of the patients in the recent series of 155 patients with tics and associated disorders (5), diagnosed with EPM1, was initially misdiagnosed as TS because her upper facial myoclonus was wrongly attributed to blinking tics. Similar to juvenile myoclonic epilepsy, EPM1 is also frequently exacerbated by phenytoin. The gene responsible for EPM1 is localized to 21q22.3, and encodes cystatin B, a cysteine protease inhibitor (14). Interestingly, cystatin B mutations are now known to account for both Mediterranean myoclonus and for "Baltic" myoclonus, which were previously thought to represent separate entities. Myoclonus is also exhibited in Lafora disease, an autosomal recessive form of progressive myoclonus epilepsy caused by several different mutations in the EPM2A gene, which codes for laforin (a protein with unknown function, but similar to a family of enzymes known as phosphatases). This disorder is characterized clinically by the onset of myoclonic and photoconvulsive seizures in late childhood and early teens, progressively intractable seizures,

dementia, and death within 10 years after onset; microscopically, Lafora bodies (polyglucosan inclusions) may be found in brain tissue, staining strongly with periodic acid-Schiff (15). Generalized and multifocal myoclonus may also be seen in patients with anoxic brain insult, Alzheimer disease, and Creutzfeldt-Jakob disease. Also, myoclonus may be a postinfectious disorder, as part of the opsoclonus-myoclonus syndrome (16).

Chorea

Chorea, defined as involuntary, abrupt, irregular, continuous, dance-like movements that randomly migrate from one body part to the other, presents in Huntington disease (HD), Sydenham chorea, and other disorders, and is another hyperkinetic movement disorder that may mimic tics. Furthermore, some patients with HD and Sydenham chorea exhibit both phonic and motor tics.

CAUSES OF TICS

Although TS is the most common cause of tics, there are many other etiologies of tics and

TS-like features (tourettism). To better understand the spectrum of causes of tourettism, the authors of this chapter evaluated 1,452 patients with tics seen at Baylor College of Medicine since 1981, 1,138 (78.3%) of whom met the diagnostic criteria for TS without having a coexistent disorder other than the commonly associated attention deficit hyperactivity disorder, obsessive-compulsive disorder, or other behavioral co-morbidities well established to be associated with TS. Information was reviewed for 155 patients (101 male patients = [65.1%]), mean age 40.5 ± 20.2 years, who presented with tics but did not meet diagnostic criteria for TS or had TS-like features with coexistent neurologic disorders. Tics were associated with insults to the basal ganglia ($N = 14$; 9.0%), pervasive developmental disorders ($N = 21$; 13.5%), genetic and chromosomal disorders ($N = 16$; 10.3%), other movement disorders ($N = 72$; 46.4%), psychogenicity ($N = 19$; 12.2%), peripheral trauma ($N = 1$; 0.6%), and other non-movement related neurologic disorders ($N = 12$; 7.7%). These groups of patients will be discussed later in the respective sections (Fig. 5-1) (5).

Huntington Disease

HD is an autosomal dominant neurodegenerative disorder, caused by expanded CAG repeats in the *huntigtin* gene on chromosome 4. It is characterized by chorea, cognitive decline, and behavioral changes. The diagnosis of tics in HD patients may be difficult because of overlapping phenomenology of tics and chorea (both are abrupt, brief, jerk-like and multifocal movements) and because TS and HD, particularly in early stages, share common features such as involuntary vocalizations, disinhibited and impulsive behaviors, affective disorders, poor attention, obsessive-compulsive features, and family history (4). Several cases of adult-onset tics have been reported to be the presenting or coexisting features of HD. Kerbeshian et al. reported a 40-year-old man with childhood-onset TS who eventually evolved into HD (17). The authors of this chapter also reported a 40-year-old man who, except for depression, was well until he presented with tics including facial grimacing, head jerking, sniffing, and coughing (18). Besides a family history of a neurodegenerative disorder, the diagnosis of HD was supported by magnetic resonance imaging evidence of caudate and cortical atrophy and confirmed by DNA analysis.

Neuroacanthocytosis

This autosomal recessive disorder has been linked to chromosome 9q21 and homozygous mutations in the *CHAC* (chorea-acanthocytosis) gene (19). It is a relatively uncommon movement disorder, typically manifested by chorea, stereotypy, parkinsonism, and self-mutilatory behaviors such as lip and tongue biting. The authors of this chapter first drew attention to the occurrence of both motor and phonic tics, including coprolalia and, because of a variety of other neurologic features, proposed changing the term for this disorder from *choreo-acanthocytosis* to *neuroacanthocytosis* (20). Besides movement disorders, patients with neuroacanthocytosis often exhibit personality, psychiatric, and cognitive changes, seizures, dysarthria, dysphagia, areflexia, and amyotrophy associated with evidence of axonal neuropathy, elevated serum creatine kinase, and more than 3% acanthocytes on peripheral blood smear. Tics are present in more than 40% of patients; other movement disorders associated with neuroacanthocytosis include chorea (58%), dystonia (47%), orofacial dyskinesia (53%), parkinsonism (34%), and involuntary vocalizations (47%) (4,21). In the series of 155 patients with tics and associated disorders, two (1.2%) had neuroacanthocytosis (Fig. 5-1) (5).

Neurodegeneration with Brain Iron Accumulation

Neurodegeneration with brain iron accumulation (NBIA) (previously termed *Hallervorden-Spatz disease*) is a severely incapacitating neurodegenerative disorder that presents usually in the second or third decade of life with progressive dementia, dystonia, rigidity, and spasticity. Some patients also exhibit simple and complex tics, stereotypies, self-mutilatory behavior, and obsessive-compulsive disorder (22). The NBIA gene was originally linked to 20p12.3-p13 (23) and later a 7-bp deletion and various missense mutations were identified in *PANK-2* gene, which codes for pantothenate kinase (essential for the regulation of coenzyme A biosynthesis) (24). The disorder with the clinical phenotype of NBIA associated with mutations in the *PANK-2* gene is now referred to as *pantothenate kinase associated neurodegeneration* (PKAN) (25). The diagnosis of NBIA is aided with magnetic resonance imaging, which may show marked hypointensity (deposition of iron) surrounded by an area of hyperintensity (gliosis and axonal spheroids) in the globus pallidus internal segment ("eye-of-the-tiger" sign) and hypointensity of substantia nigra reticulata on transverse relaxation time-weighted images (26). Case studies have found tics to be a rare presenting symptom of NBIA, but a 20-year-old man with NBIA who initially developed generalized seizures, anxiety, cognitive impairment, and memory impairment was reported to also have multiple complex motor tics (such as leg crossing) and vocal tics (27).

Pervasive Developmental Disorders

Pervasive developmental disorders (PDD) such as infantile autism, Asperger syndrome, Rett syndrome, and mental retardation, may have a variety of features typically associated with TS, including attention deficit hyperactivity disorder, disinhibition, poor impulse control, and obsessive-compulsive features (4). In one series of patients with PDD, 16 of 41 (39.0%) patients later developed TS symptoms (28). Asperger syndrome, an autistic disorder with impairment in reciprocal social interaction, circumscribed interest in one topic, verbal and nonverbal communication problems, motor clumsiness, and repetitive behavior and rigid thinking, is observed to coexist with stereotypies (29). Twenty-one (13.5%) of the 155 patients with tics and associated disorders in a recent review were diagnosed with pervasive developmental disorders (Fig. 5-1) (5), including Asperger syndrome (N = 13 [8.3%]), mental retardation (N = 4 [2.5%]), autism (N = 3 [1.9%]), and Savant syndrome (autism in which extraordinary skills, such as musical or mathematical, exist; N = 1 [0.6%]) (30). The authors of this chapter have previously

described tics and other TS features in seven Asperger syndrome patients (31). Rett syndrome, associated in more than 80% of cases with mutations in the X-linked gene encoding methyl-CpG binding protein 2, may also exhibit features of TS. Occurring almost exclusively in girls, this autistic disorder is characterized by gradual social withdrawal, psychomotor regression, loss of acquired communication skills, and hand clumsiness that is gradually replaced by stereotypical hand movements (32). In a study of 32 Rett girls, the authors of this chapter suggested that the occurrence of the stereotypies, dystonia, and tics in this condition were age-related (33).

Other Genetic and Chromosomal Disorders

Multiple other genetic and chromosomal disorders have been reported to manifest with tics. Among these are X-linked mental retardation, Albright hereditary osteodystrophy, Duchenne muscular dystrophy, factor VIII hemophilia, fragile X syndrome, Lesch-Nyhan syndrome, triple X and 9P mosaicism, 47 XXY karyotype, Down syndrome, Klinefelter syndrome, partial trisomy 16, 9p monosomy, Beckwith-Wiedemann syndrome, tuberous sclerosis, congenital adrenal hyperplasia secondary to 21-hydroxylase deficiency, neurofibromatosis, and phenylketonuria (Table 5-2) (4). In a series by the authors of this chapter, some of the genetic and chromosomal disorders observed to coexist with tics included Down syndrome (N = 5, 3.2%), corpus callosum dysgenesis (N = 1 [0.6%]), mental retardation due to craniosynostosis (N = 1 [0.6%]), Arnold-Chiari malformation (N = 1 [0.6%]), Klinefelter disease (N = 1 [0.6%]), neurofibromatosis (N = 1 [0.6%]), congenital heart disease (N = 1 [0.6%]), progressive myoclonus EPM1 (an autosomal recessive type of progressive epilepsy; N = 1 [0.6%]), and Sandifer syndrome (flexion movement involving chiefly the neck and trunk, associated with either esophageal reflux or hiatal hernia; N = 1 [0.6%]) (Fig. 5-1) (5).

Stroke and Other Brain Lesions

Tourettism has been well documented with lesions of the basal ganglia. A 43-year-old man developed tics including tongue clicking and protrusion, eye closure, sniffing, and frowning, as well as palilalia after a four-artery angiography, which presumably caused a stroke involving the basal ganglia (34). A 66-year-old man with post-anoxic hemiballism and coprolalia, but without motor or phonic tics, was also described (35). A 62-year-old woman presented with an acute onset of dysphasia and a suppressible "urge" to shake her right arm after developing lacunar infarcts in the right superior cerebellar peduncle and left basal ganglia, has also been reported (36). The authors of this chapter reported two boys who presented with hemidystonia, cranial-cervical tics, attention deficit hyperactivity disorder, and obsessive compulsive disorder, 2 weeks after suffering right hemispheric basal ganglia strokes at age 8 years (5,37). The temporal relationship between the stroke and TS-like symptoms, as well as the absence of phonic tics and family history of TS symptoms in these patients argued strongly in favor of a cause and effect relationship, and against a simple coincidental occurrence of a stroke and idiopathic TS.

Trauma

Only a few reports of patients who developed tics after closed head injuries have been documented in the literature. A 27-year-old man without family history of tics developed multiple motor tics following closed head trauma with loss of consciousness (38). Majumdar et al. (39) reported a 7-year-old girl who developed motor and phonic tics 15 months after being struck by a car and sustaining a severe head injury. Magnetic resonance imaging later showed encephalomalacia in the left putamen, globus pallidus, head of the caudate, and the internal capsule. Head trauma coexisted in four (2.5%) of the 155 patients with tics and associated diagnoses that these authors recently reported (Fig. 5-1) (5). Two patients with pre-existing tics, referred to the Baylor College of Medicine Movement Disorders Clinic, had well documented marked exacerbation of their motor tics after the head trauma (40). In addition to head trauma, the authors of this chapter have studied patients with peripheral trauma resulting

in focal, often dystonic, tics that superficially resemble segmental myoclonus (5,41).

Infections

The encephalitic lethargica pandemic that occurred in Europe between 1916 and 1927 is one of the first reported infectious events to be associated with tics such as complex vocalizations of blocking, compulsive shouting (klazomania), echolalia, palilalia, and oculogyric crises; autopsy data revealed neurofibrillary tangles and neuronal loss in the globus pallidus, hypothalamus, midbrain tegmentum, periaqueductal gray matter, striatum, and the substantia nigra (42,43). Dale et al. (44) reported a 4-year-old patient who developed motor tics, palilalia, and attention deficit hyperactivity disorder shortly after developing acute varicella zoster striatal encephalitis. Herpes simplex and HIV encephalitis, mycoplasma pneumoniae, and Lyme infections have also been reported to be associated with motor and phonic tics (4). In the review of 155 patients with tics and associated diagnoses, three (1.9%) patients presented tics after an infectious process (Fig. 5-1), including a rubella virus infection ($N = 1$ [0.6%]), an unspecified viral infection ($N = 1$ [0.6%]), and a *Mycoplasma pneumoniae* infection ($N = 1$ [0.6%]) (5). Besides specific brain infections, postinfectious disorders can be associated with a variety of movement disorders, including tics. Group A beta-hemolytic streptococcus infections and complications such as Sydenham chorea (45,46) and Pediatric Autoimmune Neuropsychiatric Disorders Associated with Streptococcal infection (PANDAS) has also been reported to coexist with TS and obsessive compulsive disorder (47). Even though the lack of disease-specific anti-neuronal antibodies in patients with PANDAS and TS, as well as other inconsistencies, have cast doubt on the association of PANDAS and TS (48), the series of 155 patients with tics and associated disorders included one (0.6%) patient with PANDAS who developed tics (Fig. 5-1) (5).

Drugs and Toxins

Amphetamines, cocaine, heroin, methylphenidate, pemoline, levodopa, antidepressants, carbamazepine, phenytoin, phenobarbitol, lamotrigine, dextroamphetamine, and other dopamine blocking agents (dopamine receptor-blocking drugs, neuroleptics) have been reported to induce or exacerbate tics (4). The authors of this chapter reported a 22-year-old patient with TS who had been in remission until age 20 years and then had recurrence of tics due to cocaine (49). Tardive tourettism due to exposure to dopamine receptor-blocking drugs or neuroleptics also has been reported. Three (1.9%) patients in the series of 155 patients with tics and associated disorders were diagnosed with tardive tourettism (Fig. 5-1) (5). Bharucha and Sethi (50) described a 45-year-old schizophrenic man who developed tics after a 10-year treatment with dopamine receptor-blocking drugs (fluphenazine, perphenazine, thiothixene). Finally, tics have been reported as a result of exposure to certain toxins such as carbon monoxide, wasp venom, and mercury (4); one (0.6%) of the 155 patients in the review of tics and associated disorders presented with tics after exposure to toluene, xylene, and carbon monoxide (5).

Psychogenic Tics

Although once considered to be of psychological origin, the perception about the cause of TS began to change when, in the 1960s, neuroleptics were found to be effective in suppressing tics. Indeed, psychogenic causes, previously also categorized as conversion, somatization, or hysteria, are very rarely thought to play a role in the etiology of tics, even in patients seen in specialized, tertiary referral clinics. Out of 14,568 patients in the movement disorders clinic of these authors between 1990 and 2003, only 23 (0.16%) fulfilled the diagnostic criteria for psychogenic tics (51). The diagnosis of psychogenic tics depends not only on exclusion of organic causes, but also on the presence of characteristic clinical features. Psychogenic tics are typically incongruent with the typical presentation of classical tics, inconsistency over time, additional atypical signs, multiple somatizations, obvious psychiatric disturbance, disappearance with distraction, absence of premonitory sensations, deliberate slowing, and complete resolution with suggestion, physiotherapy, or placebo. Sixteen of the 155 (10.3%) patients in the series

of secondary tics presented with psychogenic tics and one (0.6%) had a combination of psychogenic tics and dystonia (5). Conversely, in two cases TS preceded the onset of psychogenic dystonia ($N = 1$ [0.6]) and psychogenic tremor ($N = 1$ [0.6%]) (Fig. 5-1) (5). Management of patients with psychogenic movement disorders is challenging and beyond the scope of this review, however if management is individualized and targeted to not only the motor symptoms, but also to the underlying psychopathology, and conducted by a skilled clinician, can markedly improve the long-term prognosis (52).

CONCLUSION

This chapter has reviewed cases and reports of well-documented tics and other features of TS in association of a variety of causes and disorders. Although an association between these disorders and tics does not necessarily define a cause-and-effect relationship, these reports may provide clues to the pathogenic mechanisms underlying idiopathic tic disorders and TS.

REFERENCES

1. Jankovic J. Tourette's syndrome. *N Engl J Med.* 2001; 345:1184–1192.
2. Leckman J, Peterson B, King R, et al. Phenomenology of tics and natural history of tic disorders. In: Cohen DJ, Jankovic J, Goetz CG, ed. *Tourette Syndrome, Advances in Neurology*, vol. 85. Lippincott Williams & Wilkins: Philadelphia; 2001:1–14.
3. The Tourette Syndrome Classification Study Group. Definitions and classification of tic disorders. *Arch Neurol.* 1993;50:1013–1016.
4. Jankovic J, Kwak C. Tics in other neurological disorders. In: Kurlan R. *Handbook of Tourette's Syndrome and Related Tic and Behavioral Disorders.* Marcel Dekker: New York, NY; 2004.
5. Mejia NI, Jankovic J. Secondary tics and tourettism. *Rev Bras Psiquiatr.* 2005. In press.
6. Jankovic J, Fahn S. Dystonic disorders. In: Jankovic J, Tolosa E, eds. *Parkinson's Disease and Movement Disorders, 4th edition.* Lippincott Williams & Wilkins: Philadelphia; 2002:331–357.
7. Jankovic J, Stone L. Dystonic tics in patients with Tourette's syndrome. *Mov Disord.* 1991;6:248–252.
8. Kwak C, Dat Vuong K, Jankovic J. Premonitory sensory phenomenon in Tourette's syndrome. *Mov Disord.* 2003;18:1530–1533.
9. Stone L, Jankovic J. The coexistence of tics and dystonia. *Arch Neurol.* 1991;48:862–865.
10. Nemeth A, Mills K, Elston J, et al. Do the same genes predispose to Gilles de la Tourette syndrome and dystonia? Report of a new family and review of the literature. *Mov Disord.* 1999;14:826–831.

11. Romstad A, Dupont E, Krag-Olsen B, et al. Dopa-responsive dystonia and Tourette syndrome in a large Danish family. *Arch Neurol.* 2003;60:618–622.

12. Silay Y, Jankovic J. Botulinum toxin treatment for oromandibular dystonia and bruxism in patients with Tourette syndrome. *Neurology.* 2005 (suppl 1): A76. Presented at the 57th Annual Meeting of the AAN, Miami, FL, April 2005.

13. Lehesjoki AE, Koskiniemi M. Progressive myoclonus epilepsy of Unverricht-Lundborg type. *Epilepsia* 1999; 40(suppl 3):23–28.

14. Di Giaimo R, Riccio M, Santi S, et al. New insights into the molecular basis of progressive myoclonus epilepsy: a multiprotein complex with cystatin B. *Hum Mol Genet.* 2002;11:2941–2950.

15. Ianzano L, Young EJ, Zhao XC, et al. Loss of function of the cytoplasmic isoform of the protein laforin (EPM2A) causes Lafora progressive myoclonus epilepsy. *Hum Mutat.* 2004;23:170–176.

16. Pranzatelli MR, Travelstead AL, Tate ED, et al. B- and T-cell markers in opsoclonus-myoclonus syndrome: immunophenotyping of CSF lymphocytes. *Neurology* 2004;62:1526–1532.

17. Kerbeshian J, Burd L, Leech C, et al. Huntington's disease and childhood onset Tourette syndrome. *Am J Med Genet.* 1991;39:1–3.

18. Jankovic J, Ashizawa T. Tourettism associated with Huntington's disease. *Mov Disord.* 1995;10:103–105.

19. Rampoldi L, Danek A, et al. Clinical features and molecular basis of neuroacanthocytosis. *J Mol Med.* 2002; 80:475–491.

20. Spitz M, Jankovic J, Killian J. Familial tic disorder, parkinsonism, motor neuron disease, and acanthocytosis: a new syndrome. *Neurology* 1985;35:366–377.

21. Saiki S, Hirose G, Sakai K, et al. Chorea-acanthocytosis associated with tourettism. *Mov Disord.* 2004;19:833–836.

22. Nardocci N, Rumi V, Combi M, et al. Complex tics, stereotypies, and compulsive behavior as clinical presentation of juvenile progressive dystonia suggestive of Hallervorden-Spatz disease. *Mov Disord.* 1994;9:369–371.

23. Taylor T, Litt M, Kramer P, et al. Homozygosity mapping of Hallervorden-Sptz syndrome 20p12.3-p13. *Nat Genet.* 1996;14:479–481.

24. Zhou B, Westaway S, Levinson B, et al. A novel pantothenate kinase gene (PANK2) is defective in Hallervorden-Spatz syndrome. *Nat Genet.* 2001;28:345–349.

25. Thomas M, Hayflick SJ, Jankovic J. Clinical heterogeneity of neurodegeneration with iron accumulation-1 (Hallervorden-Spatz Syndrome) and Pantothenate Kinase Associated Neurodegeneration (PKAN). *Mov Disord.* 2004;19:36–42.

26. Hayflick S, Westaway S, Levinson B, et al. Genetic, clinical, and radiographic delineation of Hallervorden-Spatz syndrome. *N Engl J Med.* 2003;348:33–40.

27. Carod-Artal FJ, Vargas AP, Marinho PB, et al. Tourettism, hemiballism and juvenile parkinsonism: expanding the clinical spectrum of the neurodegeneration associated to pantothenate kinase deficiency (Hallervorden-Spatz syndrome). *Rev Neurol.* 2004;38:327–331.

28. Comings D, Comings B. Clinical and genetic relationships between autism, pervasive developmental disorder and Tourette syndrome: a study of 19 cases. *Am J Med Genet.* 1991;39:180–191.

29. Vokmar F, Klin A, Pauls D. Nosological and genetic aspects of Asperger syndrome. *J Autism Dev Disord.* 1998;28:457–463.

30. Heaton P, Wallace GL. Annotation: the savant syndrome. *J Child Psychol Psychiatry.* 2004;45:899–911.

31. Ringman J, Jankovic J. The occurrence of tics in Asperger syndrome and autistic disorder. *J Child Neurol.* 2000;15:394–400.

32. Jankovic J. In: Fernandez-Alvarez E, Arzimanoglou A, Tolosa E, eds. *Paediatric Movement Disorders.* John Libbey Eurotex Limited; Montrouge, France: 2005: 247–260.

33. Fitzgerald P, Jankovic J, Glaze D, et al. Extrapyramidal involvement in Rett's syndrome. *Neurology* 1990;40: 293–295.

34. Bleeker H. Gilles de la Tourette's syndrome with direct evidence of organicity. *Psychiatr Clin.* 1978;11: 147–154.

35. Masso J, Obeso J. Coprolalia associated with hemiballismus: response to tetrabenazine. *Clin Neuropharmacol.* 1985;8:189–190.

36. Ward C. Transient feelings of compulsion caused by hemispheric lesions: three cases. *J Neurol Neurosurg Psychiatry.* 1988;51:266–268.

37. Kwak C, Jankovic J. Tourettism and hemidystonia secondary to stroke. *Mov Disord.* 2002;17:821–825.

38. Singer C, Sanchez-Ramos J, Weiner W. A case of post-traumatic tic disorder. *Mov Disord.* 1989;4:342–344.

39. Majumdar A, Appleton RE. Delayed and severe but transient Tourette syndrome after head injury. *Pediatr Neurol.* 2002;27:314–317.

40. Krauss JK, Jankovic J. Tics secondary to craniocerebral trauma. *Mov Disord.* 1997;12:776–782.

41. Jankovic J. Can peripheral trauma induce dystonia and other movement disorders? Yes! *Mov Disord.* 2001; 16:7–12.

42. Wolfhart G, Ingvar D, et al. Compulsory shouting (Benedek's "klazomania") associated with oculogyric spasms in chronic epidemic encephalitis. *Acta Psychiatr Scand.* 1961;36:369–377.

43. Howard R, Lees A. Encephalitis lethargica: a report of four recent cases. *Brain* 1987;110:19–33.

44. Dale RC, Church AJ, Isobel H. Striatal encephalitis after varicella zoster infection complicated by tourettism. *Mov Disord.* 2003;18:1554–1556.

45. Cardoso F, Vargas AP, Oliveira LD, et al. Persistent Sydenham's chorea. *Mov Disord.* 1999;14:805–807.

46. Cardoso F. Infectious and transmissible movement disorders. In: Jankovic J, Tolosa E, editors. *Parkinson's disease and movement disorders.* 4th ed. Baltimore: Williams & Wilkins; 2002:930–940.

47. Dale RC, Church AJ, Surtees RA, et al. Encephalitis lethargica syndrome: 20 new cases and evidence of basal ganglia autoimmunity. *Brain* 2004;127:21–33.

48. Singer HS, Loiselle CR, Lee O, et al. Anti-basal ganglia antibodies in PANDAS. *Mov Disord.* 2004;19:406–415.

49. Cardoso F, Jankovic J. Cocaine related movement disorders. *Mov Disord.* 1993;8:175–178.

50. Bharucha KJ, Sethi KD. Tardive tourettism after exposure to neuroleptic therapy. *Mov Disord.* 1995;10:791–793.

51. Thomas M, Jankovic J. Psychogenic movement disorders: diagnosis and management. *CNS Drugs* 2004;18: 437–452.

52. Jankovic J, Cloninger CR, Fahn S, et al. Therapeutic approaches to psychogenic movement disorders. In: Hallett M, Fahn S, Jankovic J, et al., eds. *Psychogenic Movement Disorders: Neurology and Neuropsychiatry.* AAN Enterprises and Lippincott Williams & Wilkins: Philadelphia; 2006:323–328.

6

Preclinical Models Relevant to Tourette Syndrome

Neal R. Swerdlow[1] and Ashley N. Sutherland[2]

[1]Department of Psychiatry, UCSD School of Medicine, La Jolla, California; [2]Department of Psychology,
San Diego State University, San Diego, California

INTRODUCTION: WHAT ROLE MODELS?

Advances in the understanding of Tourette syndrome (TS) are occurring at multiple levels of analysis. Genetic studies have determined that TS is polygenic, and candidate regions of the genome are being targeted for fine mapping. Neuroimaging studies have identified both striatal volumetric and neurochemical abnormalities in TS populations, and efforts are underway to enhance the resolution of these signals, understand their functional implications, and link them to genes. Clinical trials have identified novel pharmacological and behavioral approaches to treating TS. Even neuropathologic studies, hindered by many features of this childhood developmental disorder, are beginning to find cellular pathology that is consistent with regional abnormalities detected via neurochemical imaging. Other areas of TS science, including the putative link between TS and autoimmune processes, remain areas of active investigation.

Progress at each of these levels of analysis would accelerate with the development and implementation of preclinical models of TS. Preclinical models are tools for understanding clinical conditions via experimentation that does not directly involve clinical populations. Three common types of preclinical models involve either healthy human subjects, *infra-human* (animal) subjects, or *in silico* (computer/artificial intelligence) subjects. Of these, animal models are the most widely applied to studying neuropsychiatric disorders, and are the main focus of this chapter.

Preclinical models allow investigators to study the brain and biology at a level that is not accessible in studies of patients. Restrictions in patient studies often reflect ethical concerns. For example, it is not ethical to withhold medications from patients, despite the fact that these medications alter laboratory measures and complicate their interpretation. Obviously, ethical considerations also preclude the use of many invasive experimental procedures in patient populations.

Beyond ethical considerations, another major hurdle in biological studies of TS reflects the fact that TS is relatively rare and more heterogeneous than was once appreciated. TS studies are slowed by difficulties in subject recruitment, and are often "underpowered," with small numbers of subjects, whose similarities in terms of their TS diagnosis are outdistanced by their differences in age, sex, co-morbid diagnoses, medication history, and many other undocumented variables (e.g., history of recurrent streptococcal infections). In contrast, an experimenter can, in a matter of days or weeks, study large numbers of animals that are identical in their genetics, age, sex, home environment, exposure (or lack thereof) to medications or infections. Studies in healthy human subjects can also proceed with a pace and level of subject homogeneity that cannot be achieved in studies with TS subjects.

The utility of animal models in part reflects the fact that humans are more like other animal species than humans may want to admit. Certainly, most genes and brain substrates of relevance to TS are shared among humans, non-human primates, and rodents. Humans share more than 90% of the mouse genome and, whereas, brain structures differ—particularly within later developing cortical regions—much of the basic "wiring diagram" or cortico-striato-pallido-thalamic circuitry is conserved across these species. Therefore, many hypotheses regarding biological mechanisms in TS—from gene to protein to cell to system—can be tested using infrahuman models.

The search for effective treatments for TS is a process that functions semi-independently from efforts to unravel the pathophysiology of this disorder. Most medications for human disorders were developed without a complete understanding of pathogenesis; certainly this is true for TS. One key advantage of preclinical models, particularly those involving rodents, is that they allow novel treatments to be developed rapidly, in a cost-effective "rapid throughput" fashion, and without direct risk to humans. Drug development strategies need not be strictly bound to a comprehensive hypothesis or disease model. Still, as discussed below, these strategies can benefit greatly from advances in the understanding of TS pathophysiology or even from a greater understanding of the normal physiology of systems thought to be involved in the genesis of TS.

Animal Models: Validity

Several schemes are used to assess the validity of animal models. In one common approach, validity is assessed on three levels: face, predictive, and construct.

Face Validity

Face validity is achieved when there is phenomenologic similarity between the model and the clinical condition: the model resembles the condition or specific features of the condition. Shock-induced fighting in rats (a model of aggression), "hallucinatory" behavior in para-chlorophenylalanine-treated cats (a model of hallucinosis), and oral movements in chronic neuroleptic-treated rats (a model of tardive dyskinesia) all bear striking resemblance to human "target" conditions. Inherent in the assessment of face validity, however, is the danger of

anthropomorphism: researchers must be aware that a behavior in one species might reflect species-specific neural, psychological, and social processes that are quite distinct from those underlying the "target" condition in humans. This issue may be most particularly relevant to models for human disorders of higher order cognitive and affective functions, in which true corollaries may not exist within the neural repertoire of a different species. Animal behavior or appearance can also be artificially shaped to resemble human features, via experimental manipulations or constraints. In other words, researchers can create conditions in the laboratory that make a rat's behavior "look like" a human's behavior. This condition sometimes happens inadvertently, based on complex environmental cues. In contrast, animal models may achieve both validity and utility without recreating some of the simpler, observable symptoms of a disorder; for example, it is not likely that researchers will soon provide animal models with face validity for coprolalia.

Most models achieve face validity because a behavior resembles a specific symptom of a disorder. Obviously, symptoms are not disorder-specific. Thus, face valid models do not necessarily address issues that are specifically (or etiologically) related to a single disorder. For example, lack of initiative, interest, or energy characterize both a major depressive episode and the residual phase of a schizophrenia, and thus conditions that impair initiation and goal-directed behaviors in rats model characteristics of both affective and psychotic disorders. In the same way, repetitive, stereotyped movements are characteristic of TS as well as many other conditions. Animal models of stereotyped behaviors might be relevant to some, all, or none of these disorders.

It is clear that there is more to tics than meets the eye (or ear). Motor and phonic events in TS usually follow a sensory or psychic experience—an urge or sense of discomfort. Even the most skilled observers cannot see or hear these premonitory events. As with the more complex psychological experiences associated with a number of different neuropsychiatric disorders, it will likely never be possible for a mouse or rat to tell researchers that they are experiencing a premonitory urge. Thus, while it is possible to create animal models with face validity for motor and phonic tics, there is no way to know (and much reason to doubt) whether these animal behaviors are accompanied by the more complex sensory and psychic antecedents to the tics of TS. It is easy to observe a mouse jerk, jump, or squeak, but much more difficult to ascertain whether an internal experience fueled the event.

It is no surprise then, that it is possible for an animal model to achieve face validity for TS, and yet have no true physiological relevance to the disorder. Examples of such animal models may be the stargazer mouse and the stargazer rat.

The stargazer mutant mouse results from a single recessive gene mutation on chromosome 15. It is characterized by ataxia, repetitive stereotyped head-lifting/neck arching movements ("stargazing"), and lifelong frequent, prolonged seizure activity (1,2). The stargazer rat is an autosomal dominant recessive mutant of the Zucker rat (3). Its phenotype is also characterized by stargazing and head tossing movements, in addition to hyperactivity, deafness, small body size, increased caloric demand, and reduced triglycerides (4). At the level of face validity for TS, both of these animals exhibit repetitive, intense, involuntary head movements that develop early in life, thereby "resembling" common motor tics exhibited by TS patients. However, mechanistic studies attribute the behavioral abnormalities in stargazer mice to cerebellar dysfunction (1,2), and the behavioral abnormalities in stargazer rats to inner ear dysfunction (3). Neither cerebellar dysfunction nor inner ear dysfunction are common problems in TS. Thus, whereas these animal models may ultimately help researchers understand a number of different brain disorders, the most parsimonious view is that they achieve face validity for TS, despite the fact that their underlying brain disturbance has little or no direct physiological connection with this disorder.

Predictive Validity

Predictive validity is achieved if the predictions made by the model can be validated in the clinical condition being modelled. Although they are also used to detect and study conditions or drugs that precipitate or exacerbate a clinical condition, predictive models are most often used to screen drugs for therapeutic potential. The behaviors used in these models often have no resemblance to the human condition. For example, the ability of dopamine antagonists to prevent apomorphine (APO)-induced emesis in dogs (5) predicts the potency of these drugs as antipsychotic and anti-tic agents in humans, despite the fact that canine emesis bears no resemblance to psychosis or tics. Predictive models are assessed by criteria of sensitivity, specificity, relative potency (in the model compared to the clinical setting) and generalizability across different chemical classes (e.g., phenothiazine, butyrophenone, dibenzodiazepine).

Numerous predictive models are used to screen psychopharmacologic agents, including antipsychotics (e.g., conditioned avoidance responding), antidepressants (e.g., Porsolt swim test), and anxiolytics (e.g., Geller-Seifter conflict paradigm). Each model can be evaluated by the above criteria and utilized for its particular strengths. For example, the Geller-Seifter paradigm is not sensitive to the anxiolytic properties of some serotonergic compounds, but predicts quite accurately the anxiolytic properties of benzodiazepines (6). As noted by Willner (7), the validity of any model must be assessed in the context of its utility; it is not necessary for a predictive model to be valid across different chemical classes if that goal is not what the model is being used to accomplish. A corollary to this notion of utility is that predictive validity is only meaningful if the model is relatively free of logistical constraints—temporal, fiscal, or otherwise. In one example of a useful predictive model, several measures of catalepsy in rats and mice accurately predict which putative antipsychotic agents will produce extrapyramidal side effects (EPS) in humans, and by exclusion, identify putative novel antipsychotics that will have minimal extrapyramidal side effects liability (Fig. 6-1) (8). This same model predicts the ability of drugs to suppress motor initiation, a property that is often used (perhaps to the detriment of some patients) to suppress involuntary movements in hyperkinetic disorders, including TS. The ability of nicotine to potentiate the

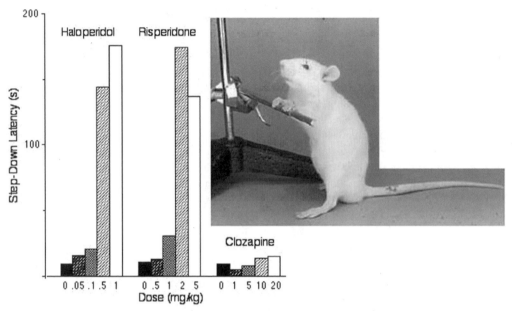

Fig. 6-1. The predictive validity of step-down catalepsy testing in rats (inset) for drugs that suppress motor initiation in humans. Rats are first positioned with their front paws resting on a horizontal bar. Drugs that suppress motor initiation cause a delay in the normal tendency of the rat to step down from the bar. There are many variations in this measure, some of which are automated, and others of which are more suitable for use in mice. [Data replotted from (8).] (From Hoffman DC, Donovan H. Catalepsy as a rodent model for detecting antipsychotic drugs with extrapyramidal side effect liability. *Psychopharmacology* 1995;120:128–133. With permission.)

motor-suppressant effects of haloperidol in this type of catalepsy model has been used by some to predict an augmenting effect of nicotine on the tic-suppressant properties of dopamine antagonists (9–11). This prediction awaits confirmation in controlled clinical trials.

Other predictive animal models for TS assess the ability of drugs to block dopamine agonist-induced repetitive, stereotyped rat behaviors such as rearing, sniffing, and gnawing. As would be expected, dopamine antagonists prevent the expression of amphetamine- or APO-induced stereotyped behaviors (12–14), and the potency of drugs in this model correlate with their affinity for dopamine receptors. This type of "receptor tautology" can limit the utility of an animal model, if the model only identifies drugs with a specific pharmacological profile (based on specific agonist-antagonist relationships). Variants of this predictive model assess the ability of drugs to suppress stereotypy induced by stress (15) or head shakes (in mice) or

shoulder shakes (in rats) stimulated by the 5-hydroxytryptamine type 2A and 2C ($5HT_{2A/2C}$) agonist 1-(2,5-dimethoxy-4-iodophenyl)-2-aminopropane [DOI]) (16,17). A number of drugs are effective in suppressing DOI-induced shakes in rodents via mechanisms that likely do not involve direct 5HT receptor antagonism, including haloperidol, nicotine, mecamylamine, and the reversible anticholinesterase inhibitor, donepezil (16–19). Of these drugs, haloperidol has clear anti-tic properties in humans, nicotine and mecamylamine have been reported to suppress tics in uncontrolled but not controlled studies, and donepezil has not yet been studied for this property (20–24).

Most predictive models focus on acute drug effects. With some notable exceptions, clinical benefit from medications in TS evolves over time. This "disconnect" between the acute effectiveness of drugs in animal models versus need for sustained treatment in the clinical condition characterizes many preclinical models (e.g., the same is true for most models that predict antipsychotic medications [5]). Based on this disconnect, it seems likely that viable TS candidate drugs might be rejected by acute predictive models, that might otherwise be detected using models that employ chronic dosing schedules.

Demonstrating predictive validity in models for TS therapeutics is complicated by the difficulty verifying "true positive" responses in TS clinical trials. Part of this difficulty reflects the normal waxing and waning pattern of TS symptoms (24). Patients typically present for treatment during a period of symptom exacerbation, which—based on a typical sinusoidal pattern of symptoms severity in TS—would naturally be followed by a period of relative remission. As this natural course progresses, symptom reduction is often inappropriately attributed to treatments that were initiated during the exacerbation phase. The process continues, with dose adjustments and, ultimately, medication changes, accompanying successive periods of symptom exacerbation. Although efforts have been made to model the periodicity of tic symptoms *in silico* and *in vivo* (24), the complexity of these models will inevitably present a challenge for rapid through-put drug screening. Clinically, these temporal patterns lead to an abundance of anecdotal reports of positive treatment responses, and to many superstitions—about medications and the physicians who prescribe them—that are based on erroneous causal associations. Perhaps more so than with other common neuropsychiatric disorders, there is an impressive number of idiosyncratic/individualized therapeutic responses and non-responses in TS, making it very difficult to unequivocally reject or endorse the therapeutic potential of any given drug for any given patient, even armed with data from relatively large, controlled clinical trials. Without data supporting efficacy in controlled clinical trials, it is difficult to claim predictive validity based on a drug effect in an animal model.

The example of nicotine is characteristic of the complex interplay of preclinical and clinical information in the development of TS therapeutics. Findings in animal models have long identified interactions of brain nicotinic and dopaminergic systems, suggesting that nicotinic agents might be useful "levers" for modifying dopamine function, and thereby play a therapeutic role in disorders of putative dopaminergic pathology, such as TS. Theories along this line were boosted by case reports, and then case series, suggesting that nicotine gum or transdermal patches could provide long lasting tic suppression in TS patients, or could augment the anti-tic effects of dopamine antagonists (20–23). These uncontrolled clinical reports prompted a number of animal model studies, demonstrating that nicotine could augment the motor-suppressant effects of dopaminergic blockade in rats (10) or block the hyperkinetic effects of serotonergic or other neurochemical manipulations in animal models (discussed previously). With this ping-ponging of clinical-preclinical enthusiasm, patients and families began to ask physicians to prescribe nicotine for TS, and others simply purchased it over-the-counter. This trend led to a number of additional anecdotal reports of positive effects. Indeed, many highly experienced TS clinicians commented on one or more patients who had a remarkable response to nicotine patches. Other studies reported preclinical and anecdotal clinical findings suggesting a potential therapeutic role for the nicotinic antagonist, mecamylamine, in TS (11,25).

Many factors converge to delay the progress of controlled clinical trials in TS, ranging from the difficulties of subject recruitment in pediatric populations, to the relative disinterest of the pharmaceutical industry to support drug development for "rare" disorders. More than 13 years after the initial case report of nicotine effects on tics in TS (21), a placebo-controlled, double-blind study of transdermal nicotine in TS was completed (23). The results were complex. While global clinical benefit was associated with nicotine use, it was difficult to detect significant reductions in tic severity using the "gold standard" Yale Global Tic Severity Scale. Of the 16 different tic measures (four measures taken at four different time points), only three demonstrated statistically significant improvement with nicotine. A subsequent report has also documented some behavioral and neuropsychological benefits of nicotine in a small TS sample (26).

Still, the relatively weak evidence that nicotine leads to statistically significant changes in tic severity in the first large, controlled TS nicotine trial by the same investigative group that had detected and reported positive nicotine effects on tics in several uncontrolled samples, presents a quandary for the field. How are researchers now to interpret the numerous animal model findings with nicotine that were previously viewed as positive predictors or a therapeutic response in TS? Also, because the clinical benefits of nicotine in TS, if any, appear to be most evident in "nonmotor" features of TS, how do researchers interpret models based on nicotine-enhanced motor suppression?

Construct Validity

To demonstrate construct validity, the theoretical rationale behind the model must be consistent with what is known about the "pathophysiologic construct" of the disorder in humans. As with predictive models, those with construct validity need not achieve face validity (or even predictive validity). Unfortunately, there remains substantial ambiguity regarding the psychopathologic constructs of TS, and models with construct validity are limited by the validity of the construct. Nonetheless, as researchers advance to finer levels of resolution in these constructs (e.g., a transition from "basal ganglia disorder" to "ventral striatal hyperdopaminergic disorder" to proteins to genes) models with construct validity must keep pace.

A number of TS animal models may achieve some degree of construct validity. Two examples of constructs used in TS animal models are discussed below. There are many additional reasonable pathophysiological constructs for TS, and these two constructs are neither exclusive of each other, nor are they meant to account for all forms of TS. Nonetheless, for both of these constructs, there are animal models that may achieve construct validity.

Construct One

In some forms, TS may result from immunologically-mediated basal ganglia dysfunction, triggered in vulnerable individuals by one or more pathogens (most often implicated is group A beta-hemolytic streptococcus [GABHS]).

Hallett et al. (27,28) and later Taylor et al. (29) reported evidence that infusion of sera from TS patients into the striatum of rats triggered the expression of repetitive stereotyped movements (e.g., licking, head shaking), and in the case of the Hallett et al. study (27), vocalizations. Hallett et al. (27) also demonstrated that at least some of these behavioral effects could be elicited by intrastriatal infusion of immunoglobulin G isolated from TS sera. There were a number of differences in the methods and results of the Hallett et al. and Taylor et al. studies, but the findings from both of these studies generally suggest that this animal model might be a valid representation of the construct of immune-mediated pathology in TS. Interestingly, a similar conclusion was not reached by a recent study from Loiselle et al. (30). This group performed striatal microinfusions of sera from children with TS (containing elevated levels of antibodies against human putamen), sera from children with Pediatric Autoimmune Neuropsychiatric Disorders Associated with Streptococccus and antibodies to the streptococcal M5 protein. In this "failure to replicate," none of the microinfusions elicited abnormal movements. Obviously, these disparate sets of results must be reconciled before this sera-infusion model can be used to understand mechanisms of, and predict treatments for, TS-related immune-mediated syndromes.

Hoffman et al. (31) took a different approach to modelling immune-mediated pathology in TS and related disorders. In their studies, sera from mice immunized with GABHS was shown to be immunoreactive to cerebellum, globus pallidus, and thalamus. GABHS-immunized mice also exhibited motor hyperactivity that was correlated with brain immunoglobulin G deposits and serum immunoreactivity to GABHS proteins. Ultimately, the authors interpreted their findings to suggest that anti-GABHS antibodies cross-reactive with brain components may play a role in the pathophysiology of TS and related disorders. Compared to the model of Hallett et al. (27) and Taylor et al. (29), this model clearly relates less directly to TS per se (i.e., sera did not originate from TS or Pediatric Autoimmune Neuropsychiatric Disorders Associated with Streptococccus patients), and more directly to mechanisms for GABHS-mediated central nervous system dysfunction.

Construct Two

TS results from cortico-striatal circuit dysfunction caused by genetic and/or epigenetic events in early brain development. While crucial details are lacking, there is at least general agreement that the brain circuitry most likely responsible for tics in TS includes elements of connections between the frontal cortex and basal ganglia, and/or intrinsic basal ganglia circuitry that receives these cortical inputs (32–36). Furthermore, there is reasonable evidence that the processes that trigger these circuit dysfunctions arise early in brain development as the result of genetic and possibly epigenetic events. One attempt to model these general constructs by Campbell, Burton et al. (37–39) has resulted in a "ticcy" transgenic mouse that exhibits amygdala, orbitofrontal, and cortico-striatal glutamate overactivity.

This "D1CT-7" transgenic mouse was developed using a transgene that expresses the intracellular A1 subunit of cholera toxin and causes tonic hyperactivity in two subsets of neurons. One subset are cortical glutamatergic pyramidal neurons containing dopamine receptor subtype-1 (D1) and $5HT_{2A/2C}$ receptors, located in somatosensory insular cortex and piriform cortex, that innervate and excite sensorimotor, orbitofrontal, and deeper-layer corticostriatal neurons. A second subset of hyperactive neurons is amygdala gamma-aminobutyric acid-ergic interneurons that contain D1 receptors, which indirectly trigger amygdala glutamate output. The investigators believe that chronic hyperactivation of these two subsets of neurons trigger juvenile-onset "ticcy" and compulsion-like behavioral abnormalities, including "twitching," "jerking," repetitive climbing, and leaping (37–39), all detected by rating videotaped behavioral samples. The authors describe these behaviors as a model of "co-morbid obsessive compulsive disorder (OCD) plus TS" and evoke convergent support

from findings of stress sensitivity and sexual dimorphism in some aspects of the D1CT-7 phenotype.

As noted previously, construct models are only as valid as their constructs. This model is based on the construct that TS is pathophysiologically linked to tonic hyperactivity within cortical, limbic, and cortico-striatal circuitry. One challenge to the construct validity of this model, therefore, is the fact that most studies of regional brain function in TS report hypoactivity in this circuitry, including reduced glucose uptake in orbitofrontal cortex, caudate, parahippocampus, and midbrain regions (40), as well as reduced blood flow in the caudate nucleus, anterior cingulate cortex, and temporal lobes (41–44). The single greatest consistency across metabolic imaging studies in TS—that of distributed hypometabolism—contrasts sharply with the observed corticostriatal hypermetabolism reported by many groups in patients with OCD (45). The only suggestion of regional activation in TS comes during active tic suppression, which is associated with increased right caudate neuronal activity, as measured by functional magnetic resonance imaging (46); however, tic suppression is also accompanied by bilaterally diminished neuronal activity on functional magnetic resonance imaging measures, evident in the putamen, globus pallidus, and thalamus. The most analogous paradigm in OCD—obsession provocation—is associated with increased metabolic activity at every level of cortico-striato-pallido-thalamic circuitry (47), which in sharp contrast to the pattern observed in TS. Thus, although the basic construct in this model—sustained corticostriatal hyperactivity—may be a valid construct for regional brain dysfunction in OCD, it is harder to argue that it has construct validity for TS.

D1CT-7 mice exhibit a number of other features that are not characteristic of TS patients, including reduced seizure threshold (37). Certain pharmacologic sensitivities of this mouse—including reduced movements with clonidine and dopamine receptor subtype-2 (D2) blockers (38)—appear to be consistent with clinical responsiveness in TS, while their increased sensitivity to n-methyl-D-aspartate (NMDA) antagonists has no known correlate in TS patients. Finally, the authors' prediction from their model that ketanserin should have anti-TS or anti-OCD properties (39) has not been supported by any controlled studies. Thus, the D1CT-7 mouse has some interesting properties that deserve careful study and may reveal a lot about the behavioral and neural circuit response to sustained corticostriatal hyperactivity, but it is premature to say that this model achieves construct validity for TS.

Developing an Animal Model of Tourette Syndrome Based on the Construct of Deficient Sensorimotor Gating

As might be evident from the previous discussion, there are many different routes to the development of an animal model of TS. Most models with face validity arise from the observation that an animal exhibits abnormal movements, followed by a post hoc extrapolation that those movements "resemble" tics. Models with predictive validity arise from the observation that a group of chemicals with anti-tic properties in patients also has a specific, reproducible, and quantifiable impact on a laboratory animal. Models with construct validity arise from efforts to translate across species a biological construct about the pathophysiology of TS. A variant of these approaches to developing TS models has led to one particularly promising set of models for this disorder, based on the conceptual linkage between TS symptoms and deficits in a physiological process called "sensorimotor gating."

As noted previously, the understanding that motor and vocal expression of tics is integrally connected to an internal experience of sensory or psychic information has reshaped the conceptualization of TS. As revealed in the groundbreaking work by Drs. Cohen, Leckman, and others, TS patients report a variety of sensory and mental states associated with their tics (48–54). "Simple" sensory tics are experienced as a recurrent sensation at or near the skin that is typically bothersome or uncomfortable, like an "itch" or a "crawling" feeling. Patients may be unusually aware of, distracted by, and distressed by particular sensory stimuli that most individuals

would not notice, including perceptions of internal (somatic) or external origin. One patient explained, "[Do] you know the scratchy feeling of a tag on your neck when you put on a new shirt? I have tags on every part of every shirt, all the time."

Premonitory urges are more complex phenomena, which may include both sensory and psychic discomfort, that are momentarily relieved by a tic. A variant of these sensory-psychic antecedents to tics may be the discomfort or distress if sensory information is not experienced as "just right," based on complex stimulus properties, including balance and symmetry, texture, or context. The full elaboration of tics, therefore, can involve a sequence of: 1) a sensory event or psychic urge, 2) inner conflict over if and when to yield to the urge, 3) the motor or phonic production, and 4) a transient sensation of relief.

The notion that intrusive sensory and/or psychic information contributes to the genesis of tics in TS converges with a construct applied to a number of neuropsychiatric disorders—that deficient "gating" of sensory, cognitive or motor information is a critical antecedent to the internal experience and external manifestation of symptoms (55). According to this construct, during waking moments, the normal human nervous system receives much more information than it is capable of processing effectively. This information comes from both extrinsic and intrinsic sources—an environment full of complex stimuli, sensations from visceral and somatomotor self-monitoring, and a brain laden with complex thoughts, memories, and feelings. A healthy nervous system employs many mechanisms to suppress, or "gate" irrelevant information in sensory, cognitive, and motor domains, to permit an orderly, hierarchical layering of the most relevant information that forms the contents of consciousness. These automatic ("preconscious") gating mechanisms have been described at levels of analysis that range from psychological/psychoanalytic to cellular/neurobiological (55–57). A breakdown in these gating mechanisms is thought to underlie deficits in cognition, motor function, and affective stability that accompany specific psychiatric disorders. In TS, this breakdown is associated with the perceptual or psychic process experienced as a sensory tic or premonitory urge. Attempts to systematically study deficient gating mechanisms have been extremely productive and have focused heavily on measurements of physiological "surrogates": processes that are assumed to contribute to or correlate with some aspects of sensory, motor, or cognitive gating. One such surrogate gating measure is prepulse inhibition (PPI) of the startle reflex.

The startle reflex is a constellation of responses to sudden, relatively intense stimuli that is classified as a defensive response. In humans, the blink reflex component of startle is measured using electromyography of the orbicularis oculi muscle; in laboratory animals, startle is quantified by assessing the downward force generated by the limbs, reflected from the upward force generated through the contract of the skeletal muscles and shortening of the torso (Fig. 6-2). In PPI, a weak sensory prestimulus inhibits a motor response to a powerful sensory event, a process termed *sensorimotor inhibition* or *sensorimotor gating* (58). PPI occurs when the prepulse and startling stimuli are in the same or different sensory modalities. Virtually all mammals exhibit PPI. It is not a form of conditioning because it occurs on the first exposure to the prepulse and pulse stimuli, and it does not exhibit habituation or extinction over trials.

Although the inhibitory effect of the prepulse on the startle reflex is exerted in the pons, studies have described the limbic cortico-striato-pallido-thalamic circuitry and descending pontine projections that regulate the inhibitory "tone" within the pons, and thus determine the degree to which the prepulse inhibits the subsequent motor response (56). PPI thus appears to reflect the activation of "hard-wired" centrally mediated behavioral inhibitory processes that are regulated by forebrain neural circuitry.

Interest in PPI as a measure of sensorimotor gating was stimulated by observations that disorders with dysfunction in forebrain substrates that regulate PPI (e.g., limbic or frontal cortex, basal ganglia) are characterized by impaired cognitive, sensory, or motor inhibition. PPI is deficient in patients with schizophrenia (59,60),

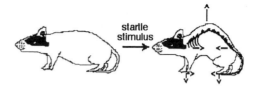

Fig. 6-2. Schematic representation of the postural changes in the whole body startle reflex in rats. Contraction of the skeletal musculature leads to the shortening of the torso, and elevation of the dorsum, and generates an equal-but-opposite force directed through the feet. This downward force is automatically quantified via sensors, with millisecond resolution. In humans, startle is typically quantified via electromyelography, most often of the orbicularis oculi.

Huntington disease (61,62), OCD (63,64), nocturnal enuresis and attention deficit disorder (65), and blepharospasm (66), as well as in patients with TS (67,68). Importantly, converging preclinical and clinical findings make it clear that PPI deficits can reflect disturbances at any one of several levels of cortico-striato-pallido-thalamic circuitry, and are not unique to a single form of psychopathology (56,60). This notion is consistent with models (69) proposing that interacting corticostriatal systems regulate cognitive and behavioral inhibition, and contribute to inhibitory deficits in several different neuropsychiatric disorders.

Sensorimotor inhibition or gating is assessed by a number of paradigms that show strong structural parallels to PPI. In each of these paradigms, including measures of "recovery cycle" (also called *blink excitability* [70]), "paired pulse inhibition" (71), or "intracortical inhibition" (72), the dependent measure is the motor response to a target stimulus ("pulse" or "S2") presented either alone or shortly after the presentation of a lead stimulus ("prepulse" or "S1"). The normal response under specific stimulus conditions is to exhibit a diminished motor response to S2 in the presence of S1, compared with the response to S2 alone. To date, studies utilizing measures of blink excitability, PPI, and intracortical inhibition have all demonstrated inhibitory deficits in TS patients (67,68,70,72) (Fig. 6-3).

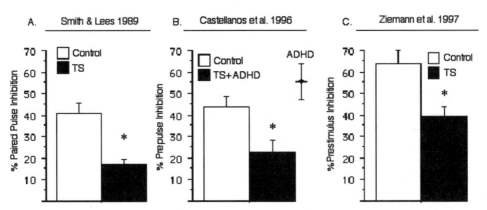

Fig. 6-3. Deficient inhibition in Tourette syndrome patients, as assessed by three different paradigms, including measurements of **A)** blink recovery cycle (70), **B)** prepulse inhibition (67), and **C)** intracortical inhibition (72). Although these paradigms differ in the types of stimuli and the measurement of responses, in each case the response evoked by an intense stimulus is automatically suppressed by a preceding stimulus. In each of these measures, individuals with Tourette syndrome exhibit about half as much inhibition as that exhibited by matched normal comparison subjects. In the cases of recovery cycle and prepulse inhibition, stimuli are electric shocks delivered to the face; in the case of intracortical inhibition, stimuli are transcranial magnetic pulses. Data were replotted for direct comparisons across studies.

Thus, the pathophysiologic construct that TS is a disorder of deficient gating comes directly from clinical observations about premonitory events. The rationale for studying PPI in TS reflects the fact that this measure assesses sensorimotor gating. The finding of impaired PPI in TS patients provides an empiric linkage between the pathophysiologic construct and an experimental measure (Figs. 6-3B and 6-4). Of most direct relevance to the present discussion is the fact that PPI (and to some degree, other related measures) can be studied in laboratory animals, using stimulus parameters and equipment for stimulus delivery and response acquisition that are similar or identical to what is used in humans. In fact, many human startle response characteristics parallel those observed in laboratory animals, including reflex habituation and PPI (*cf.* 73).

As noted previously, animal models must be assessed in terms of their utility—their ability to bypass logistical constraints of human studies and to provide a means to rapidly test mechanistic hypotheses and screen therapeutic compounds. Based on descriptions by Davis (74), measures of startle gating bring several advantages to any animal model (Table 6.1), and thereby enhance its utility.

There are also some disadvantages, or at least special considerations, associated with animal models of startle gating. Indeed, the ease

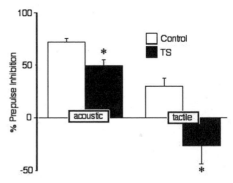

Fig. 6-4. Prepulse inhibition deficits in children with Tourette syndrome (*) versus healthy comparison children in a study (68) extending the findings of Castellanos et al. (67) (Fig. 6-3B). In this study, the preceding stimulus and stimulus were both either acoustic stimuli (*left side of figure*) or tactile air puffs (*right side of figure*). (From Swerdlow NR, Karban B, Ploum Y, et al. Tactile pre-puff inhibition of startle in children with Tourette syndrome: In search of an "fMRI-friendly" startle paradigm. *Biol Psychiatry.* 2001;50:578–585. With permission.)

TABLE 6-1. *Advantages of startle gating models*

1. Fast and efficient: ideal for "rapid throughput" screening
2. Automated, quantifiable, reliable, stable
3. Under tight stimulus control: experimenter can easily "dial-in" desired parameters
4. Controlled by a simple neural circuit
5. Regulated by forebrain circuitry relevant to neuropsychiatric disorders, including Tourette syndrome
6. Neurochemical regulation/pharmacologically predictable
7. Strain and sex differences in gating: accessible to genetic and hormonal manipulations
8. Can be measured across species, from drosophila to human
9. Abnormalities in startle gating in specific neuropsychiatric populations, including Tourette syndrome

of generating large amounts of data with automated measures of PPI make it incumbent on the users of this model to understand the interpretative complexities of this measure because large amounts of misinterpreted data can cause difficulties. The authors of this chapter (75) and others (76) have written about some of the potential pitfalls of interpreting PPI data in humans and laboratory animals. For example, in studies of PPI using acoustic stimuli, the amount of inhibition generated by the weak prepulse is greatly reduced by hearing impairment in either humans (e.g., in pediatric populations at increased risk for recurrent ear infections) or lab animals (e.g., mutant mice with hearing loss). PPI can be calculated in several different ways (e.g., percent scores vs. difference scores, corrected for "no-stimulus" baselines, etc.), some of which, under particular stimulus conditions, can be more or less sensitive to confounding changes in startle magnitude on pulse alone trials. In human studies, there are special considerations that must be given to racial differences in facial musculature (77), sex (78), menstrual phase (79,80), and perhaps even sexual orientation (81); in animal studies, there are strain and substrain differences in PPI and startle reactivity that need to be considered in study design (*cf.* 75). Indeed, the sensitivity of PPI to physiological variables is both part of its strength and part of its weakness as a neurobiological measure.

Prepulse Inhibition Models with Predictive and Construct Validity for Tourette Syndrome

The use of PPI and PPI deficits in models of relevance to TS is categorically different from the use of other behaviors in existing TS models. Most models, even those with construct validity discussed above, utilize one or more dependent measures that are thought to "look like" TS symptoms. In contrast, PPI is used as a dependent measure in TS models because it assesses physiological processes (described collectively as sensorimotor gating) that are empirically known to be deficient in TS patients (67,68), and are also linked conceptually to the internal experience (rather than the observable expression) of the disease. Predictive and construct models using PPI take advantage of the fact that these gating processes, and their impact on PPI, are conserved across species, even if specific symptomatic manifestations of deficient gating are not conserved.

One of the common preclinical uses of PPI has been to identify compounds with antipsychotic potency (73,82, *cf* 83). It has become clear that different applications of this model identify drugs with different clinical properties. For example, dopamine agonists such as APO disrupt PPI in rats, and the ability of drugs to prevent this effect correlates highly with their antipsychotic potency and their D2 affinity (73). Because D2 blockade is one mechanism to suppress tics in TS, this model also predicts the therapeutic potency of dopamine antagonists for TS. Of course, it is not terribly surprising that a model based on a behavior that is stimulated by dopamine agonists would be predictive of antidopaminergic properties. In this manner, the APO-PPI model parallels the APO-emesis model described earlier, an important distinction being that in the PPI model, the behavior induced by the dopamine agonist (reduced PPI) is one that is also exhibited by TS patients. Presumably, compared with the brain mechanisms responsible for canine emesis (e.g., dopamine receptors in the area posterma), those responsible for reduced PPI in this model are linked more closely to the brain mechanisms responsible for reduced PPI in TS.

A variant of this model was recently reported, in which the PPI-disruptive effects of APO were opposed by acute administration of nicotine (84). Several studies have reported effects of nicotine and mecamylamine on PPI in humans and rats that, like many behavioral effects of nicotine, are complex and difficult to reproduce (85–87). As noted above in relation to the effects of nicotine on DOI-induced body shakes, the relevance of detecting activity for nicotine in predictive models for TS is that drugs acting on nicotinic receptors have been reported to provide therapeutic benefit in some TS patients. How this putative clinical utility of nicotine is manifested in TS remains a question of great importance.

An interesting feature of the PPI predictive model is the fact that under some stimulus conditions (low inhibitory drive), low doses of some dopamine agonists can actually enhance PPI. For example, low doses of pergolide, a direct dopamine agonist, significantly increase PPI in rats when either weak prepulses or short prepulse intervals are used (88) (Fig. 6-5). The inhibitory effects of prepulses at short intervals (<60 msec) are thought to be "automatic" or "preattentional" because, unlike longer interval inhibition, PPI with these short prepulse intervals is not enhanced by directed attention (89). Importantly, low doses of pergolide also have therapeutic benefit in TS (90), an effect that would not be predicted by other models predictive of anti-tic properties (e.g., catalepsy testing or active avoidance suppression). Conceivably, the clinical benefit of pergolide in TS may reflect its ability to enhance preattentional inhibitory mechanisms, as suggested by its impact on short interval PPI. Other dopamine agonists, such as levodopa, also have anti-tic efficacy (91), but have not been systematically studied in preclinical PPI models.

The neurochemical regulation of PPI extends beyond dopamine and includes norepinephrine, glutamate, and serotonin, in addition to several neuropeptides (cf. 56,92). PPI in rats is disrupted by cirazoline, an agonist at the alpha-1 norepinephrine receptor (93). Our studies in progress suggest that such effects of cirazoline

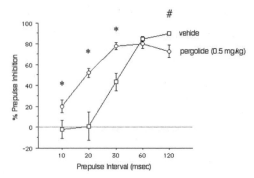

Fig. 6-5. Pergolide, a dopamine agonist with tic-suppressing properties, enhances prepulse inhibition elicited by short prepulse intervals in rats (*). At longer intervals (60 msec) pergolide actually reduces prepulse inhibition (#). (From Swerdlow NR, Platten A, Shoemaker J, et al. Effects of pergolide on sensorimotor gating of the startle reflex in rats. *Psychopharmacology* 2001;158:230–240. With permission.)

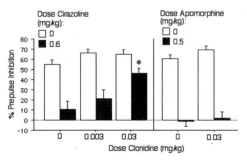

Fig. 6-6. Clonidine, an alpha-2 agonist with tic-suppressing properties, prevents the prepulse inhibition-disruptive effects of the alpha-1 agonist, cerazoline (*) (*left side of figure*). The pharmacologic specificity of this effect is demonstrated by the inability of clonidine to prevent the prepulse inhibition-disruptive effects of the D1/D2 agonist, apomorphine (*right side of figure*). (Data from 94.)

are opposed by the alpha-2 agonist, clonidine, which is an effective anti-tic medication (94) (Fig. 6-6). Thus, it is conceivable that anti-tic properties of noradrenergic agents might be predicted via the ability to reverse the gating-disruptive effects of cirazoline.

Future uses of PPI in predictive models for TS should extend beyond simple pharmacologic challenge studies. For example, immune, neurotoxic, or genetic models for TS (some discussed previously) should be studied using PPI as a dependent measure. If these models result in gating deficits, it might be possible to use PPI in rapid throughput studies to predict interventions that prevent or reverse dysfunction in these models. Future studies may also rely increasingly on different species, with the pharmacology of PPI in mice becoming increasingly sophisticated (and in some ways, distinct from that in rats), while the pharmacology of PPI in higher animals, including infrahuman primates, is yet at earlier stages of exploration. Finally, animal models of PPI might be useful in identifying targets within basal ganglia output circuitry where neurosurgical interventions, such as deep brain stimulation, might be most effective in restoring gating functions.

PPI has also been used in a number of models that have construct validity for TS. As with the predictive models, these construct models were initially developed based on their presumed relevance to schizophrenia. As findings emerge from TS science, however, it is apparent that many of these constructs apply equally well, and in some cases better, to the pathophysiology of TS.

For example, a number of studies have provided evidence for a functional hyperdopaminergic state in TS, and more recent findings have identified increased presynaptic monoaminergic function focused within the ventral striatum (35,95). In rats, infusion of dopamine or dopamine agonists into the ventral striatum disrupt PPI (73,96), and microdialysis studies have demonstrated that the time course and magnitude of reduced PPI after systemic amphetamine administration corresponds tightly to the efflux of dopamine within the ventral striatum (97) (Fig. 6-7). Other studies have demonstrated modest but consistent striatal volume loss in TS (34,98), and in rats, excitotoxic lesions of the striatum—either anteroventral or dorsal posterior regions, and particularly the nucleus accumbens—result in PPI deficits (99–101). Both of these animal models (PPI deficits after intrastriatal drug infusion or lesions) have been used extensively to study cellular and systems-level mechanisms responsible for gating deficits, as well as ways to restore gating after these localized perturbations. Obviously, such studies could have direct relevance to clinical pathology associated with ventral striatal hyperdopaminergia or striatal volume loss.

While surgical and pharmacologic manipulations of the ventral forebrain in rats can mimic neurochemical (increased ventral striatum dopamine), volumetric (reduced striatal volume), and behavioral abnormalities (reduced PPI) seen in TS, construct models must ultimately move researchers past focusing on the nature of the brain insult, to what caused the insult. Constructs for the etiology of TS fall broadly into the same three categories implicated in the etiology of many complex disorders: environment, genes, or both.

The two environmental insults most often implicated in the etiology of TS are early developmental/epigenetic insults and infectious/immune insults. A number of studies have already demonstrated that PPI is sensitive to both of these types of insults. Adult rats demonstrate PPI deficits after *in utero* or early life (e.g., by day seven) exposure to a variety of insults (Table 6-2). Among these are infectious or cytokine-stimulatory agents (102,105–109), suggesting at least generally that immune activation or its consequences on central nervous system function can lead to a disruption in PPI. In at least one model (prenatal exposure to an LPS endotoxin [102]), the impact on PPI exhibits both sensitivity to dopamine blockade and sexual dimorphism, with male rats exhibiting more profound deficits compared to females. Again, these models might provide constructs for a number of different neurodevelopmental disorders, only one of which is TS. To date, neither of the existing "construct" models for TS discussed previously (streptococcal/immune challenge in rats or mice or D1CT-7 transgenic mice) have yet been studied in the PPI paradigm.

As they relate to TS, one weakness in the construct validity of most neurodevelopmental PPI animal models is that the PPI deficits typically emerge only in adulthood. In contrast,

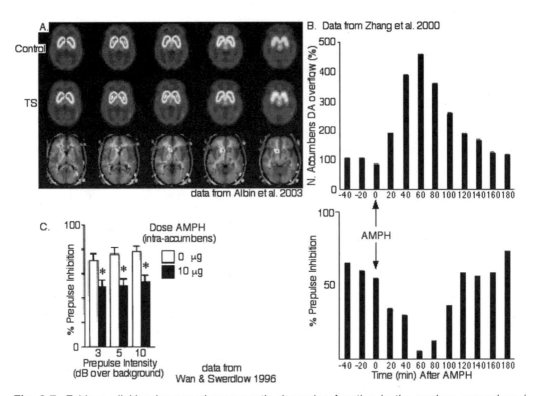

Fig. 6-7. Evidence linking increased presynaptic dopamine function in the nucleus accumbens/ventral striatum with Tourette syndrome (A) and with reduced prepulse inhibition in rats (B,C). (Courtesy of Drs. Kirk Frey and Roger Albin; Data from Albin RL, Koeppe RA, Bohnen NI, et al. Increased ventral striatal monoaminergic innervation in Tourette syndrome. *Neurology* 2003;61:310–315.) **A:** Presynaptic nigrostriatal terminals in Tourette syndrome, depicted by in vivo binding of [11C]dihydrotetrabenzamide (DTBZ) to vesticular monoamine transporter-2 (VMAT2). Top row: Averaged DTBZ binding at 5 levels from dorsal (*left*) to ventral (*right*) striatum in controls. Middle row: DTBZ binding to VMAT2 in TS subjects. Bottom row: Voxel-wise t-statistical map for regions of significantly increased VMAT2 in Tourette syndrome. **B:** Dopamine overflow in the nucleus accumbens measured by microdialysis (*top graph*), and prepulse inhibition (*bottom graph*) in rats after systemic treatment with the dopamine releaser, d-amphetamine. (Data from Zhang J, Forkstam C, Engel JA, et al. Role of dopamine in prepulse inhibition of acoustic startle. *Psychopharmacology* 2000;149:181–188.) Note clear temporal linkage of increasing accumbens dopamine release and decreasing prepulse inhibition. **C:** Reduced prepulse inhibition (*) in rats after direct infusion of d-amphetamine into the accumbens/ventral striatal region. (Data from Wan FJ, Swerdlow NR. Sensorimotor gating in rats is regulated by different dopamine-glutamate interactions in the nucleus accumbens core and shell subregions. *Brain Res.* 1996;722:168–176.)

TS symptoms (and PPI deficits in TS) emerge in childhood. The implications of this difference are not well understood. For example, PPI has a normal maturational course in humans and rats, and PPI levels in rat pups are substantially lower than they are in adult rats. Consequently, the PPI-disruptive effects of early developmental insults might be difficult to detect in pups due to floor effects. This explanation is not fully satisfying because: A) researchers have demonstrated that the PPI-disruptive effects of both APO and phencyclidine can be detected by day 20 in rat pups (well before puberty) (116), and B) the PPI-disruptive effects of some in utero insults (e.g., valproic acid exposure) can be detected in prepubertal rats (109).

One clear construct for the etiology of TS, based on its dense inheritance patterns, is that

TABLE 6-2. *Early developmental insults reported to produce lasting prepulse inhibition deficits in adult rats*

In Utero:
Lipopolysaccharide (LPS) endotoxin (102)
Maternal influenza (105)
Maternal herpes simplex (107)
Leukemia inhibitory factor (108)
Valproic acid (109)
Vitamin D deficiency (110)
Protein deprivation (111)
Cytosine arabinoside (ARA-C) (mitosis inhibitor) (112)

Neonatal:
Lesions of the ventral hippocampus (103,104)
Lesions of the amygdala (103)
Phencyclidine exposure (113)
Maternal deprivation (114)

Post-weaning:
Social isolation rearing (115)

this disorder or a strong vulnerability to manifest it is transmitted via powerful effects of a relatively small number of genes. The hypotheses that deficient sensorimotor gating is a valid explanation for important clinical features of this disorder, and that deficient PPI in rats is a valid construct model for PPI deficits in TS, would be supported by evidence that PPI is heritable, and that this heritability is under powerful control by a small number of genes.

There is relatively little information regarding the heritability of PPI in humans. One study in adult female twins provided evidence that more than 50% of the variance in PPI reflected genetic factors (117), but the use of adult females in this study certainly led to an underestimation of heritability, due to the significant variations in PPI across the menstrual cycle (79,80). In the most extreme case, PPI can be disrupted in humans and rodents by a single gene, and this is the basis for PPI deficits in HD patients (61,62) and in mice transgenic for the HD gene (118). Embryonic transfer studies in mice demonstrate that, unlike other complex behavioral phenotypes, levels of PPI correspond to the genetic strain of the embryo, but not to the strain of the uterine environment or of the rearing mother (119). Thus,

there is reason to believe both that PPI exhibits high heritability and that it can be powerfully controlled by a small number of genes.

Due to the apparently strong genetic control of PPI, it is used as an endophenotype to help identify vulnerability genes in brain disorders (120). The important notion here is that the expression of the clinical phenotype of TS is complex and variable, influenced by a number of non-genetic factors. In contrast, if reduced PPI is a quantitative physiologic trait that is closer to the genes than is the clinical phenotype, it will provide a more powerful signal for identifying TS genes. If this is the case, then it could be of great importance in detecting genes of interest in ongoing TS genetic studies.

The genetic variability of PPI is seen in the range of PPI performance across large numbers of rodent strains (121–123). This variability of a quantitative trait gives investigators a number of useful experimental options. In one example, Amar et al. (124) reported a significant correlation across 10 inbred mouse strains between PPI and frontal cortical activity of glycogen synthase kinase-3 beta, a regulatory enzyme for several levels of intracellular signal transduction pathways. Another way to take advantage of PPI as a quantitative genetic trait is to identify quantitative trait loci that contribute to its regulation. This process has been pursued in both rats (125) and mice (126), with several quantitative trait loci identified. Although more of a "shotgun" approach to linking genes and function, the role of a large number of candidate genes in the regulation of PPI has also been explored using knockout/in and transgenic mice (e.g., 127–129). One promising line of investigation relates to findings of deficient PPI in both human and animal variants of 22q11 deletion syndrome (130). The genetics of PPI will become more relevant to TS if there is concordance between these PPI "genes" and the chromosomal regions of interest identified in ongoing linkage studies with TS sib-pairs and large families (131). As chromosomal "hot spots" are identified and mapped from these ongoing studies, the physiological impact of candidate TS genes on brain function can be studied in genetically engineered rodents, using PPI as a dependent measure.

SUMMARY

Preclinical models, if used appropriately, can greatly accelerate the understanding of neuropsychiatric disorders. A number of animal models have predictive validity for anti-dopaminergic compounds that have traditionally been used to suppress motor and vocal tics in TS. Other models have been proposed that may have construct validity for specific hypotheses of infectious/immune and neural circuit etiologies of TS. A more comprehensive set of models is described, based on the hypothesis that primary symptoms of TS, including sensory tics and premonitory urges, result from dysfunction in brain mechanisms that regulate sensorimotor gating. These models utilize operational measures of central gating mechanisms, including PPI of the startle reflex, to achieve predictive validity across a number of different chemical classes of drugs, and to achieve construct validity across broad domains of neurodevelopmental, immune and genetic etiologies of TS. PPI-based animal models offer a number of strong advantages for predictive and mechanistic studies of TS. Ultimately, the utility of these "deficient gating" models will be judged by their ability to bring us closer to identifying the causes and effective treatments of this disorder.

ACKNOWLEDGMENT

NRS is supported by NIMH Award MH 01436. Much of the material in this review is duplicative of material in other published reviews and data papers (132).

REFERENCES

1. Noebels JL, Qiao X, Bronson RT, et al. Stargazer: a new neurological mutant on chromosome 15 in the mouse with prolonged cortical seizures. *Epilepsy Res.* 1990;7:129–135.
2. Qiao X, Hefti F, Knusel B, et al. Selective failure of brain-derived neurotrophic factor mRNA expression in the cerebellum of stargazer, a mutant mouse with ataxia. *J Neurosci.* 1996;16:640–648.
3. Truett GE, Brock JW, Lidl GM, et al. Stargazer (stg), new deafness mutant in the Zucker rat. *Lab Anim Sci.* 1994;44:595–599.
4. Brock JW, Truett GE, Ross KD, et al. Quantitative analysis of abnormal spontaneous behavior and clinical assessment of the stargazer rat. *Lab Anim Sci.* 1995; 45:276–280.
5. Freedman DX, Giarman NJ. Apomorphine test for tranquilizing drugs: effect of dibenamine. *Science* 1956;124:264–265.
6. File SE. The use of social interaction as a method for detecting anxiolytic activity of chlordiazepoxide-like drugs. *J Neurosci Methods.* 1980;2:219–238.
7. Willner P. Validation criteria for animal models of human mental disorders: learned helplessness as a paradigm case. *Prog Neuropsychopharmacol Biol Psychiatry.* 1986;10:677–690.
8. Hoffman DC, Donovan H. Catalepsy as a rodent model for detecting antipsychotic drugs with extrapyramidal side effect liability. *Psychopharmacology* 1995;120:128–133.
9. Elazar Z, Paz M. Potentiation of haloperidol catalepsy by microinjections of nicotine into the striatum or pons in rats. *Life Sci.* 1999;64:1117–1125.
10. Emerich DF, Zanol MD, Norman AB, et al. Nicotine potentiates haloperidol-induced catalepsy and locomotor hypoactivity. *Pharmacol Biochem Behav.* 1991;38: 875–880.
11. Sanberg PR, Newman MB, Manresa JJ, et al. Mecamylamine effects on haloperidol-induced catalepsy and defecation. *Int J Neurosci.* 2001;109:81–90.
12. Fog R. On stereotypy and catalepsy: studies on the effect of amphetamines and neuroleptics in rats. *Acta Neurol Scand Suppl.* 1972;50:3–66.
13. Randrup A, Munkvad I. Pharmacology and physiology of stereotyped behavior. *J Psychiatr Res.* 1974;11:1–10.
14. Costall B, Naylor RJ. Detection of the neuroleptic properties of clozapine, sulpiride and thioridazine. *Psychopharmacologia* 1975;43:69–74.
15. Knott PJ, Hutson PH. Stress-induced stereotypy in the rat: neuropharmacological similarities to Tourette's syndrome. *Adv Neurol.* 1982;35:233–238.
16. Dursun SM, Handley SL. Similarities in the pharmacology of spontaneous and DOI-induced head-shakes suggest 5HT2A receptors are active under physiological conditions. *Psychopharmacology* (Berlin) 1996;128: 198–205.
17. Tizabi Y, Russell LT, Johnson M, et al. Nicotine attenuates DOI-induced head- twitch response in mice: implications for Tourette's syndrome. *Prog Neuropsychopharmacol Biol Psychiatry.* 2001;25:1445–1457.
18. Hayslett RL, Tizabi Y. Effects of donepezil on DOI-induced head twitch response in mice: implications for Tourette syndrome. *Pharmacol Biochem Behav.* 2003; 76:409–415.
19. Gaynor CM, Handley SL. Effects of nicotine on head-shakes and tryptophan metabolites. *Psychopharmacology* (Berlin) 2001;153:327–333.
20. McConville BJ, Sanberg PR, Fogelson MH, et al. The effects of nicotine plus haloperidol compared to nicotine only and placebo nicotine only in reducing tic severity and frequency in Tourette's disorder. *Biol Psychiatry.* 1992;31:832–840.
21. Sanberg PR, Fogelson HM, Manderscheid PZ, et al. Nicotine gum and haloperidol in Tourette's syndrome. *Lancet* 1988;1:592.
22. Sanberg PR, McConville BJ, Fogelson HM, et al. Nicotine potentiates the effects of haloperidol in animals and

in patients with Tourette's syndrome. *Biomed Pharmacother.* 1989;43:19–23.

23. Silver AA, Shytle RD, Philipp MK, et al. Transdermal nicotine and haloperidol in Tourette's disorder: a double-blind placebo-controlled study. *J Clin Psychiatry.* 2001;62:707–714.

24. Peterson BS, Leckman JF. The temporal dynamics of tics in Gilles de la Tourette syndrome. *Biol Psychiatry.* 1998;44:1337–1348.

25. Silver AA, Shytle RD, Sanberg PR. Mecamylamine in Tourette's syndrome: a two-year retrospective case study. *J Child Adolesc Psychopharmacol.* 2000;10:59–68.

26. Howson AL, Batth S, Ilivitsky V, et al. Clinical and attentional effects of acute nicotine treatment in Tourette's syndrome. *Eur Psychiatry.* 2004;19:102–112.

27. Hallett JJ, Harling-Berg C, Knopf PM, et al. Anti-striatal antibodies in Tourette's syndrome cause neuronal dysfunction. *J Neuroimmunol.* 2000;111:195–202.

28. Hallett J, Kiessling L. Genetics of childhood disorders: XXXV. Autoimmune disorders, part 8: animal models for noninflammatory autoimmune disorders of the brain. *J Am Acad Child Adolesc Psychiatry.* 2002;41:223–225.

29. Taylor JR, Morshed SA, Parveen S, et al. An animal model of Tourette's syndrome. *Am J Psychiatry.* 2002;159:657–660.

30. Loiselle CR, Lee O, Moran TH, et al. Striatal microinfusion of Tourette's syndrome and PANDAS sera: failure to induce behavioral changes. *Mov Disord.* 2004;19:390–396.

31. Hoffman KL, Hornig M, Yaddanapudi K, et al. A murine model for neuropsychiatric disorders associated with group A beta-hemolytic streptococcal infection. *J Neurosci.* 2004;24:1780–1791.

32. Mink JW. Basal ganglia dysfunction in Tourette's syndrome: a new hypothesis. *Pediatr Neurol.* 2001;25:190–198.

33. Swerdlow NR, Young AB. Neuropathology in Tourette syndrome. *CNS Spectr.* 1999;4:65–74.

34. Peterson BS, Thomas P, Kane MJ, et al. Basal ganglia volumes in patients with Gilles de la Tourette syndrome. *Arch Gen Psychiatry.* 2003;60:415–424.

35. Albin RL, Koeppe RA, Bohnen NI, et al. Increased ventral striatal monoaminergic innervation in Tourette syndrome. *Neurology* 2003;61:310–315.

36. Minzer K, Lee O, Hong JJ, et al. Increased prefrontal D2 protein in Tourette syndrome: a postmortem analysis of frontal cortex and striatum. *J Neurol Sci.* 2004;219:55–61.

37. Campbell KM, Veldman MB, McGrath MJ, et al. TS+OCD-like neuropotentiated mice are supersensitive to seizure induction. *Neuroreport* 2000;11:2335–2338.

38. McGrath MJ, Campbell KM, Parks CR, et al. Glutamatergic drugs exacerbate symptomatic behavior in a transgenic model of comorbid Tourette's syndrome and obsessive-compulsive disorder. *Brain Res.* 2000;877:23–30.

39. Nordstrom EJ, Burton FH. A transgenic model of comorbid Tourette's syndrome and obsessive-compulsive disorder circuitry. *Mol Psychiatry.* 2002;7:524,617–625.

40. Braun AR, Stoetter B, Randolph C, et al. The functional neuroanatomy of Tourette's Syndrome: An FDG-PET study. I. Regional changes in cerebral glucose metabolism differentiating patients and controls. *Neuropsychopharmacology* 1993;9:277–291.

41. Moriarty J, Costa DC, Schmitz B, et al. Brain perfusion abnormalities in Gilles de la Tourette's Syndrome. *Br J Psychiatry.* 1995;167:249–254.

42. Sieg KG, Buckingham D, Gaffney GR, et al. Tc-99m HMPAO SPECT brain imaging of Gilles de la Tourette's syndrome. *Clin Nucl Med.* 1993;18:255.

43. Riddle MA, Rasmusson AM, Woods SW, et al. SPECT imaging of cerebral bloodflow in Tourette syndrome. *Adv Neurol.* 1992;58:207–211.

44. Eidelberg D, Moeller JR, Antonini A, et al. The metabolic anatomy of Tourette's syndrome. *Neurology* 1997;48:927–934.

45. Baxter LR, Schwartz JM, Bergman, et al. Caudate glucose metabolic rate changes with both drug and behavior therapy for obsessive-compulsive disorder. *Arch Gen Psychiatry.* 1992;49:681–689.

46. Peterson BS, Skudlarski P, Anderson AW, et al. A functional magnetic resonance imaging study of tic suppression in Tourette syndrome. *Arch Gen Psychiatry.* 1998;55:326–333.

47. Rauch SL, Jenike MA, Alpert NM, et al. Regional cerebral blood flow measured during symptom provocation in obsessive-compulsive disorder using oxygen 15-labeled carbon dioxide and positron emission tomography. *Arch Gen Psychiatry.* 1994;51:62–70.

48. Bliss J. Sensory experiences of Gilles de la Tourette syndrome. *Arch Gen Psychiatry.* 1980;37:1343–1347.

49. Cohen DJ, Leckman JF. Sensory phenomena associated with Gilles de la Tourette's syndrome. *J Clin Psychiatry.* 1992;5:319–323.

50. Leckman JF, Walker DE, Goodman WK, et al. "Just right" perceptions associated with compulsive behavior in Tourette's syndrome. *Am J Psychiatry.* 1994;151:675–680.

51. Leckman JF, Walker DE, Cohen DJ. Premonitory urges in Tourette's syndrome. *Am J Psychiatry.* 1993;150:98–102.

52. Miguel EC, de Rosario-Campos MC, Prado HS, et al. Sensory phenomena in obsessive-compulsive disorder and Tourette's disorder. *J Clin Psychiatry.* 2000;61:150–156.

53. Miguel EC, Baer L, Coffey BJ, et al. Phenomenological differences appearing with repetitive behaviours in obsessive-compulsive disorder and Gilles de la Tourette's syndrome. *Br J Psychiatry.* 1997;170:140–145.

54. Hollenbeck P. A Jangling journey: life with Tourette's syndrome. *Cerebrum* 2004;5:47–60.

55. Swerdlow NR. Cortico-striatal substrates of cognitive, motor and sensory gating: speculations and implications for psychological function and dysfunction. In: J Panksepp, ed. *Advances in Biological Psychiatry.* vol. 2. Greenwich: JAI Press. 1996; 179–208.

56. Swerdlow NR, Geyer MA, Braff DL. Neural circuit regulation of prepulse inhibition of startle in the rat: current knowledge and future challenges. *Psychopharmacology* 2001;156:194–215.

57. Frost WN, Tian LM, Hoppe TA, et al. A cellular mechanism for prepulse inhibition. *Neuron* 2003;40:991–1001.

58. Graham F. The more or less startling effects of weak prestimuli. *Psychophysiology* 1975;12:238–248.

59. Braff D, Stone C, Callaway E, et al. Prestimulus effects on human startle reflex in normals and schizophrenics. *Psychophysiology* 1978;15:339–343.

60. Braff DL, Geyer MA, Swerdlow NR. Human studies of prepulse inhibition of startle: normal subjects, patient groups, and pharmacological studies. *Psychopharmacology* 2001;156:234–258.

61. Swerdlow NR, Paulsen J, Braff DL, et al. Impaired prepulse inhibition of acoustic and tactile startle in patients with Huntington's disease. *J Neurol Neurosurg Psychiatry.* 1995;58:192–200.

62. Valls-Sole J, Munoz JE, Valldeoriola F. Abnormalities of prepulse inhibition do not depend on blink reflex excitability: a study in Parkinson's disease and Huntington's disease. *Clin Neurophysiol.* 2004;115:1527–1536.

63. Swerdlow NR, Benbow CH, Zisook S, et al. A preliminary assessment of sensori-motor gating in patients with obsessive compulsive disorder (OCD). *Biol Psychiatry.* 1993;33:298–301.

64. Schall U, Schon A, Zerbin D, et al. Event-related potentials during an auditory discrimination with prepulse inhibition in patients with schizophrenia, obsessive-compulsive disorder and healthy subjects. *Int J Neurosci.* 1996;84:15–33.

65. Ornitz EM, Hanna GL, de Traversay J. Prestimulation-induced startle modulation in attention-deficit hyperactivity disorder and nocturnal enuresis. *Psychophysiology* 1992;29:437–451.

66. Gomez-Wong E, Marti MJ, Tolosa E, et al. Sensory modulation of the blink reflex in patients with blepharospasm. *Arch Neurol.* 1998;55:1233–1237.

67. Castellanos FX, Fine EJ, Kaysen DL, et al. Sensorimotor gating in boys with Tourette's Syndrome and ADHD: Preliminary results. *Biol Psychiatry.* 1996; 39:33–41.

68. Swerdlow NR, Karban B, Ploum Y, et al. Tactile prepuff inhibition of startle in children with Tourette syndrome: in search of an "fMRI-friendly" startle paradigm. *Biol Psychiatry.* 2001;50:578–585.

69. Swerdlow NR, Koob GF. Dopamine, schizophrenia, mania and depression: toward a unified hypothesis of cortico-striato-pallido-thalamic function. *Behav Brain Sci.* 1987;10:197–245.

70. Smith SJ, Lees AJ. Abnormalities of the blink reflex in Gilles de la Tourette syndrome. *J Neurol Neurosurg Psychiatry.* 1989;52:895–898.

71. Swerdlow NR, Shoemaker J, Stephany N, et al. Prestimulus effects on startle magnitude: sensory or motor? *Behav Neurosci.* 2002;116:672–681.

72. Ziemann U, Paulus W, Rothenberger A. Decreased motor inhibition in Tourette's disorder: evidence from transcranial magnetic stimulation. *Am J Psychiatry.* 1997;154:1277–1284.

73. Swerdlow NR, Braff DL, Taaid N, et al. Assessing the validity of an animal model of sensorimotor gating deficits in schizophrenic patients. *Arch Gen Psychiatry.* 1994;51:139–154.

74. Davis M. Neurochemical modulation of sensory-motor reactivity: acoustic and tactile startle reflexes. *Neurosci Biobehav Rev.* 1980;4:241–263.

75. Swerdlow NR, Braff DL, Geyer MA. Animal models of deficient sensorimotor gating: what we know, what we think we know, and what we hope to know soon. *Behav Pharmacol.* 2000;111:185–204.

76. Blumenthal TD, Elden A, Flaten MA. A comparison of several methods used to quantify prepulse inhibition of eyeblink responding. *Psychophysiology* 2004;41:326–332.

77. Swerdlow NR, Talledo JA, Braff DL. Startle modulation in Caucasian- and Asian-Americans: a prelude to genetic/endophenotypic studies across the "Pacific Rim." *Psychiatr Genet.* 2004. In press.

78. Swerdlow NR, Monroe SM, Hartston HJ, et al. Men are more inhibited than women by weak prepulses. *Biol Psychiatry.* 1993;34:253–261.

79. Swerdlow NR, Hartman PL, Auerbach PP. Changes in sensorimotor inhibition across the menstrual cycle: implications for neuropsychiatric disorders. *Biol Psychiatry.* 1997;41:452–460.

80. Jovanovic T, Szilagyi S, Chakravorty S, et al. Menstrual cycle phase effects on prepulse inhibition of acoustic startle. *Psychophysiology* 2004;41:401–406.

81. Rahman Q, Kumari V, Wilson GD. Sexual orientation-related differences in prepulse inhibition of the human startle response. *Behav Neurosci.* 2003;117:1096–1102.

82. Swerdlow NR, Zisook D, Taaid N. Serouel (ICI 204, 636) restores prepulse inhibition of acoustic startle in apomorphine-treated rats: similarities to clozapine. *Psychopharmacology* 1994;114:675–678.

83. Swerdlow NR, Geyer MA. Using an animal model of deficient sensorimotor gating to study the pathophysiology and new treatments of schizophrenia. *Schizophenia Bulletin* 1998;24:285–302.

84. Suemaru K, Yasuda K, Umeda K, et al. Nicotine blocks apomorphine-induced disruption of prepulse inhibition of the acoustic startle in rats: possible involvement of central nicotinic alpha7 receptors. *Br J Pharmacol.* 2004;142:843–850.

85. Kumari V, Cotter PA, Checkley SA, et al. Effect of acute subcutaneous nicotine on prepulse inhibition of the acoustic startle reflex in healthy male non-smokers. *Psychopharmacology* 1997;132:389–395.

86. Kumari V, Checkley SA, Gray JA. Effect of cigarette smoking on prepulse inhibition of the acoustic startle reflex in healthy male smokers. *Psychopharmacology* 1996;128:54–60.

87. Curzon P, Kim DJ, Decker MW. Effect of nicotine, lobeline, and mecamylamine on sensory gating in the rat. *Pharmacol Biochem Behav.* 1994;49:877–882.

88. Swerdlow NR, Platten A, Shoemaker J, et al. Effects of pergolide on sensorimotor gating of the startle reflex in rats. *Psychopharmacology* 2001;158:230–240.

89. Bohmelt AH, Schell AM, Dawson ME. Attentional modulation of short- and long-lead-interval modification of the acoustic startle eyeblink response: comparing auditory and visual prestimuli. *Int J Psychophysiol.* 1999;32:239–250.

90. Gilbert DL, Dure L, Sethuraman G, et al. Tic reduction with pergolide in a randomized controlled trial in children. *Neurology* 2003;60:606–611.

91. Black KJ, Mink JW. Response to levodopa challenge in Tourette syndrome. *Mov Disord.* 2000;15:1194–1198.

92. Geyer M, Krebs-Thomson K, Braff D, et al. Pharmacological studies of prepulse inhibition models of sensorimotor gating deficits in schizophrenia: a decade in review. *Psychopharmacology* 2001;156:117–154.

93. Carasso BS, Bakshi VP, Geyer MA. Disruption in prepulse inhibition after alpha-1 adrenoceptor stimulation in rats. *Neuropharmacology* 1998;37:401–404.

94. Swerdlow NR, Bongiovanni MJ, Tochen L, et al. Separable noradrenergic and dopaminergic regulation of prepulse inhibition in rats: implications for predictive

validity and Tourette syndrome. *Biol Psychiatry.* 2005; 57:39S.

95. Ernst M, Zametkin AJ, Jons PH, et al. High presynaptic dopaminergic activity in children with Tourette's disorder. *J Am Acad Child Adolesc Psychiatry.* 1999;38: 86–94.

96. Wan FJ, Swerdlow NR. Sensorimotor gating in rats is regulated by different dopamine-glutamate interactions in the nucleus accumbens core and shell subregions. *Brain Res.* 1996;722:168–176.

97. Zhang J, Forkstam C, Engel JA, et al. Role of dopamine in prepulse inhibition of acoustic startle. *Psychopharmacology* 2000;149:181–188.

98. Peterson B, Riddle MA, Cohen DJ, et al. Reduced basal ganglia volumes in Tourette's syndrome using three-dimensional reconstruction techniques from magnetic resonance images. *Neurology* 1993;43:941–949.

99. Kodsi M, Swerdlow NR. Prepulse inhibition in the rat is regulated by ventral and caudodorsal striato pallidal circuitry. *Behav Neurosci.* 1995;109:912–928.

100. Kodsi MH, Swerdlow NR. Reduced prepulse inhibition after electrolytic lesions of nucleus accumbens subregions in the rat. *Brain Res.* 1997;773:45–52.

101. Kodsi MH, Swerdlow NR. Mitochondrial toxin 3-nitropropionic acid produces startle reflex abnormalities and striatal damage in rats that model some features of Huntington's disease. *Neurosci Lett.* 1997;231:1–5.

102. Borrell J, Vela JM, Arevalo-Martin A, et al. Prenatal immune challenge disrupts sensorimotor gating in adult rats. Implications for the etiopathogenesis of schizophrenia. *Neuropsychopharmacology* 2002;26: 204–215.

103. Daenen EW, Wolterink G, Van Der Heyden JA, et al. Neonatal lesions in the amygdala or ventral hippocampus disrupt prepulse inhibition of the acoustic startle response; implications for an animal model of neurodevelopmental disorders like schizophrenia. *Eur Neuropsychopharmacol.* 2003;13:187–197.

104. Lipska BK, Swerdlow NR, Geyer MA, et al. Neonatal excitotoxic hippocampal damage in rats causes postpubertal changes in prepulse inhibition of startle and its disruption by apomorphine. *Psychopharmacology* 1995;122:35–43.

105. Shi L, Fatemi SH, Sidwell RW, et al. Maternal influenza infection causes marked behavioral and pharmacological changes in the offspring. *J Neurosci.* 2003;23:297–302.

106. Tohmi M, Tsuda N, Watanabe Y, et al. Perinatal inflammatory cytokine challenge results in distinct neurobehavioral alterations in rats: implication in psychiatric disorders of developmental origin. *Neurosci Res.* 2004;50:67–75.

107. Engel JA, Zhang J, Bergstrom T, et al. Neonatal herpes simplex virus type 1 brain infection affects the development of sensorimotor gating in rats. *Brain Res.* 2000;863:233–240.

108. Watanabe Y, Hashimoto S, Kakita A, et al. Neonatal impact of leukemia inhibitory factor on neurobehavioral development in rats. *Neurosci Res.* 2004;48: 345–353.

109. Schneider T, Przewlocki R. Behavioral alterations in rats prenatally exposed to valproic acid: animal model of autism. *Neuropsychopharmacology* 2004. In press.

110. Burne TH, Feron F, Brown J, et al. Combined prenatal and chronic postnatal vitamin D deficiency in rats impairs prepulse inhibition of acoustic startle. *Physiol Behav.* 2004;81:651–655.

111. Palmer AA, Printz DJ, Butler PD, et al. Prenatal protein deprivation in rats induces changes in prepulse inhibition and NMDA receptor binding. *Brain Res.* 2004;996:193–201.

112. Elmer GI, Sydnor J, Guard H, et al. Altered prepulse inhibition in rats treated prenatally with the antimitotic Ara-C: an animal model for sensorimotor gating deficits in schizophrenia. *Psychopharmacology* (Berlin) 2004. In press.

113. Wang C, McInnis J, Ross-Sanchez M, et al. Long-term behavioral and neurodegenerative effects of perinatal phencyclidine administration: implications for schizophrenia. *Neuroscience* 2001;107:535–550.

114. Ellenbroek BA, Cools AR. Early maternal deprivation and prepulse inhibition: the role of the postdeprivation environment. *Pharmacol Biochem Behav.* 2002;73: 177–184.

115. Cilia J, Reavill C, Hagan JJ, et al. Long-term evaluation of isolation-rearing induced prepulse inhibition deficits in rats. *Psychopharmacology* (Berlin) 2001; 156:327–337.

116. Martinez ZA, Halim ND, Oostwegel JL, et al. Ontogeny of phencyclidine and apomorphine-induced startle gating deficits in rats. *Pharmacol Biochem Behav.* 2000;65:449–457.

117. Anokhin AP, Heath AC, Myers E, et al. Genetic influences on prepulse inhibition of startle reflex in humans. *Neurosci Lett.* 2003;353:45–48.

118. Carter RJ, Lione LA, Humby T, et al. Characterization of progressive motor deficits in mice transgenic for the human Huntington's disease mutation. *J Neurosci.* 1999;19:3248–3257.

119. Francis DD, Szegda K, Campbell G, et al. Epigenetic sources of behavioral differences in mice. *Nat Neurosci.* 2003;6:445–446.

120. Braff DL, Freedman R. The importance of endophenotypes in studies of the genetics of schizophrenia. In: Davis KL, Charney D, Coyle JT, et al, eds. *Neuropsychopharmacology: The Fifth Generation of Progress.* Baltimore: Lippincott, Williams & Wilkins. 2002; 703–716.

121. Willott JF, Tanner L, O'Steen J, et al. Acoustic startle and prepulse inhibition in 40 inbred strains of mice. *Behav Neurosci.* 2003;117:716–727.

122. Palmer AA, Dulawa SC, Mottiwala AA, et al. Prepulse startle deficit in the Brown Norway rat: a potential genetic model. *Behav Neurosci.* 2000;114:374–388.

123. Swerdlow NR, Shoemaker JM, Crain S, et al. Sensitivity to drug effects on prepulse inhibition in inbred and outbred rat strains. *Pharmacol Biochem Behav.* 2004;77:291–302.

124. Amar S, Jones BC, Nadri C, et al. Genetic correlational analysis of glycogen synthase kinase-3 beta and prepulse inhibition in inbred mice. *Genes Brain Behav.* 2004;3:178–180.

125. Palmer AA, Breen LL, Flodman P, et al. Identification of quantitative trait loci for prepulse inhibition in rats. *Psychopharmacology* (Berlin) 2003;165:270–279.

126. Joober R, Zarate JM, Rouleau GA, et al. Provisional mapping of quantitative trait loci modulating the acoustic startle response and prepulse inhibition of acoustic startle. *Neuropsychopharmacology* 2002; 27:765–781.

127. Tsai G, Ralph-Williams RJ, Martina M, et al. Gene knockout of glycine transporter 1: characterization of the behavioral phenotype. *Proc Natl Acad Sci USA.* 2004;101:8485–8490.

128. Mishima K, Tanoue A, Tsuda M, et al. Characteristics of behavioral abnormalities in alpha1d adrenoceptors deficient mice. *Behav Brain Res.* 2004;152:365–373.

129. Heldt SA, Green A, Ressler KJ. Prepulse inhibition deficits in GAD65 knockout mice and the effect of antipsychotic treatment. *Neuropsychopharmacology* 2004. In press.

130. Mukai J, Liu H, Burt RA, et al. Evidence that the gene encoding ZDHHC8 contributes to the risk of schizophrenia. *Nat Genet.* 2004;36:725–731.

131. The Tourette Syndrome Association International Consortium for Genetics. A complete genome screen in sib pairs affected by Gilles de la Tourette syndrome. *Am J Hum Genet.* 1999;65:1428–1436.

132. Swerdlow NR, Sutherland AN. Using animal models to develop therapeutics for Tourette syndrome. *Pharmacol Ther.* 2005;108:281–293.

7

Neurobiology of Basal Ganglia and Tourette Syndrome: Basal Ganglia Circuits and Thalamocortical Outputs

Jonathan W. Mink

Department of Neurology, Neurobiology and Anatomy, Pediatrics, University of Rochester and Department of Child Neurology, Golisano Children's Hospital at Strong Memorial, Rochester, New York

Tourette syndrome (TS) is defined by the presence of tics: stereotyped, repetitive involuntary movements; however, many individuals with TS also have symptoms of inattention, impulsivity, obsessive thinking, and compulsive behaviors. Thus, the disorder is typically a constellation of motor and non-motor symptoms. The fundamental pathophysiology of TS is not known, but there is now general agreement that it probably involved dysfunction of basal ganglia and frontal cortical circuits (1,2). The basal ganglia are usually viewed as a component of the motor system. However, there is substantial evidence that the basal ganglia interact with all of frontal cortex and with the limbic system. Thus, the basal ganglia have a role in cognitive and emotional function in addition to their role in motor control. Indeed, diseases of the basal ganglia often cause a combination of movement, affective, and cognitive disorders. Thus, dysfunction of basal ganglia-thalamo-cortical circuits may account for both motor and non-motor symptoms of TS.

Popular models of basal ganglia functional anatomy in movement disorders suggests that involuntary movements are associated with decreased inhibitory output from the basal ganglia with resulting excessive activity in frontal cortical areas (3,4). This model has also been invoked to provide a theoretical anatomic framework for understanding obsessive-compulsive disorder, depression, and other psychiatric disorders. With recent modifications, a more general model of basal ganglia function and dysfunction has been proposed (5–7). According to this model, the basal ganglia act to facilitate desired behaviors and inhibit potentially competing or unwanted behaviors to prevent them from interfering with the desired behavior. Recent advances have made it possible to suggest how specific neural mechanisms may relate to specific clinical manifestations of TS. The three major groups of symptoms associated with TS (tics, obsessive-compulsive behaviors, and attention deficit hyperactivity disorder) have impaired inhibition of unwanted behaviors as a common feature.

BASAL GANGLIA ORGANIZATION

The basal ganglia include the striatum (caudate, putamen, nucleus accumbens), the subthalamic nucleus (STN), the globus pallidus (internal segment [GPi], external segment [GPe], ventral pallidum [VP]), and the substantia nigra (pars compacta and pars reticulata). The striatum and STN receive the majority of inputs from outside of the basal ganglia. Most of those inputs come from cerebral cortex, but thalamic nuclei also provide strong inputs to striatum. The bulk of the outputs from the basal ganglia arise from the globus pallidus internal segment, VP, and substantia nigra pars reticulata (SNpr). These outputs are inhibitory to thalamic nuclei that in turn project to frontal lobe.

The striatum receives the bulk of extrinsic input to the basal ganglia. The striatum receives excitatory input from virtually all of cerebral cortex (8). In addition, the ventral striatum (nucleus accumbens and rostroventral extensions of caudate and putamen) receive inputs from hippocampus and amygdala (9,10). The cortical input uses glutamate as its neurotransmitter and terminates largely on the heads of the dendritic spines of medium spiny neurons (11,12). The projection from the cerebral cortex to striatum has a roughly topographic organization. The large dendritic fields of medium spiny neurons (13) allow them to receive input from adjacent projections, which arise from different areas of cortex (14). Inputs to striatum from several functionally related cortical areas overlap and a single cortical area projects divergently to multiple striatal zones (14,15). Thus, there is a multiply convergent and divergent organization within a broader framework of functionally different parallel circuits. This organization provides an anatomical framework for the integration and transformation of cortical information in the striatum (16).

Medium spiny striatal neurons receive a number of other inputs, including gamma-butyric acid (GABA) input from small interneurons (17), a large input from dopamine-containing neurons in the substantia nigra pars compacta (SNpc) (18), and a more sparse input from the serotonin-containing neurons in the dorsal and median raphe nuclei (19). The dopamine and serotonin inputs are of particular interest because of the role of medications that influence these neurotransmitters in the treatment of TS and associated symptoms.

The dopamine input to the striatum terminates largely on the shafts of the dendritic spines of medium spiny neurons where it is in a position to modulate transmission from the cerebral cortex to the striatum (12). Five types of G protein-coupled dopamine receptors have been described (dopamine receptors 1 [D1] through 5 [D5]) (20). These have been grouped into two families based on their linkage to adenylcyclase activity and response to agonists. The D1 family includes D1 and D5 receptors, and the D2 family includes D2, D3, and D4 receptors. D1 receptors are thought to stimulate adenylcyclase activity and may potentiate the effect of cortical input to striatal neurons,

whereas D2 receptors are thought to inhibit adenylcyclase activity and may decrease the effect of cortical input to striatal neurons (21). More recent data indicate that the effect of dopamine on striatal medium spiny neurons is dependent on the membrane potential of the target neurons (22). The role of dopamine in learning and reward is discussed in further detail later in this chapter.

Medium spiny striatal neurons contain the inhibitory neurotransmitter GABA (23) and are inhibitory to their targets. In addition, they have peptide neurotransmitters that are co-localized with GABA (24,25). Based on the type of neurotransmitters and the predominant type of dopamine receptor they contain, the medium spiny neurons can be divided into two populations. One population contains GABA, dynorphin, and substance P and primarily expresses D1 receptors. These neurons project to the basal ganglia output nuclei, GPi, VP, and SNpr (3,26,27). The second population contains GABA and enkephalin and primarily expresses D2 receptors. These neurons project to the external segment of the GPe (3,26,27).

Although there are no apparent regional differences in the striatum based on cell type, an intricate internal organization has been revealed with special stains. When the striatum is stained for acetylcholinesterase (AChE), there is a patchy distribution of lightly staining regions within more heavily stained regions (28). The AChE-poor patches have been called *striosomes* and the AChE-rich areas have been called the *extrastriosomal matrix*. The matrix forms the bulk of the striatal volume and receives input from most areas of cerebral cortex. Within the matrix are clusters of neurons with similar inputs that have been termed *matrisomes* (16). The bulk of the output from cells in the matrix is to both segments of the GP, VP, and to SNpr. The striosomes receive input from prefrontal cortex and send output to SNpc (29). Immunohistochemical techniques have demonstrated that many substances such as substance P, dynorphin, and enkephalin have a patchy distribution that may be partly or wholly in register with the striosomes (30). The striosome-matrix organization suggests a level of functional segregation within the striatum that may be important in understanding the variety of symptoms in TS.

The STN receives an excitatory, glutamatergic input from many areas of frontal lobes with especially large inputs from motor areas of cortex (31–33). The STN also receives an inhibitory GABA input from GPe (34). The output from the STN is glutamatergic and excitatory to the basal ganglia output nuclei, GPi, VP, and SNpr (35,36). STN also sends an excitatory projection back to GPe (37). There is a somatopic organization in STN (38,39) and a relative topographic separation of "motor" and "cognitive" inputs to STN (40).

The primary basal ganglia output arises from GPi, a GPi-like component of VP, and SNpr. As described previously, GPi and SNpr receive excitatory input from STN and inhibitory input from striatum. They also receive an inhibitory input from GPe. The output from GPi, VP, and SNpr is inhibitory and uses GABA as its neurotransmitter (41). The primary output is directed to thalamic nuclei that project to the frontal lobes: the ventrolateral, ventroanterior, and mediodorsal nuclei. The thalamic targets of GPi, VP, and SNpr project, in turn, to frontal lobe, with the strongest output going to motor areas.

The basal ganglia motor output has a somatotopic organization such that the body below the neck is largely represented in GPi and the head and eyes are largely represented in SNpr (39,42,43). The separate representation of different body parts is maintained throughout the basal ganglia. Within the representation of an individual body part, it also appears that there is segregation of outputs to different motor areas of cortex and that an individual GPi neuron sends output via thalamus to just one area of cortex (44,45). Thus, GPi neurons that project via thalamus to motor cortex are adjacent to, but separate from, those that project to premotor cortex or supplementary motor area. GPi neurons that project via thalamus to prefrontal cortex are also separate from those projecting to motor areas and from VP neurons projecting via thalamus to orbitofrontal cortex. The anatomic segregation of basal ganglia-thalamocortical outputs suggests functional segregation, too (43,45). Functional segregation of basal ganglia-thalamocortical circuits has important implications for understanding the anatomical basis for different aspects of TS.

The GPe, and the GPe-like part of VP, may be viewed as intrinsic nuclei of the basal ganglia. Like GPi and SNpr, GPe receives an inhibitory projection from the striatum and an excitatory one from STN. Unlike GPi, the striatal projection to GPe contains GABA and enkephalin but not substance P (3,27). The output of GPe is quite different from the output of GPi. The output is GABAergic and inhibitory and the majority of the output projects to STN. The connections from striatum to GPe, from GPe to STN, and from STN to GPi form the "indirect" striatopallidal pathway to GPi (46). In addition, there is a monosynaptic GABAergic inhibitory output from GPe directly to GPi and to SNpr (47) and a GABAergic projection back to striatum (48). Thus, GPe neurons are in a position to provide feedback inhibition to neurons in striatum and STN and feedforward inhibition to neurons in GPi and SNpr. This circuitry suggests that GPe may act to oppose, limit, or focus the effect of the striatal and STN projections to GPi and SNpr as well as focus activity in these output nuclei.

Dopamine input to the striatum arises from SNpc and the ventral tegmental area (VTA). SNpc projects to most of the striatum; VTA projects to the ventral striatum. The SNpc and VTA are made up of large dopamine-containing cells. SNpc receives input from the striatum, specifically from the striosomes (25). This input is GABAergic and inhibitory. The SNpc and VTA dopamine neurons project to all of caudate and putamen in a topographic manner (49,50). However, the nigral dopamine neurons receive inputs from one striatal circuit and project back to the same and to adjacent circuits (50). Thus, they appear to be in a position to modulate activity across functionally different circuits.

Although the basal ganglia intrinsic circuitry is complex, the overall picture is of two primary pathways through the basal ganglia from cerebral cortex with the output directed via thalamus at the frontal lobes. These pathways consist of two disynaptic pathways from cortex to the basal ganglia output. In addition, there are several multi-synaptic pathways involving GPe. The two disynaptic pathways are from cortex through A) striatum and B) STN to the basal ganglia outputs. These pathways have important anatomical and functional differences. First, the cortical input to STN comes only

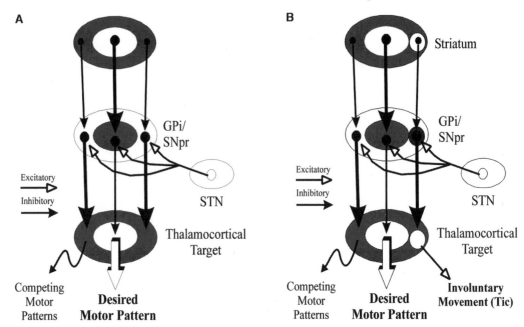

Fig. 7-1. A: Schematic illustration of normal functional organization of the basal ganglia output. Excitatory projections are indicated with *open arrows*; inhibitory projections are indicated with *filled arrows*. Relative magnitude of activity is represented by line thickness. **B:** Schematic illustration of hypothetical reorganization of basal ganglia output in tic disorders. When a discrete set of striatal neurons becomes active inappropriately (*right of figure*) this leads to aberrant inhibition of a discrete set of globus pallidus (internus) neurons. The abnormally inhibited globus pallidus (internus) neurons disinhibit thalamocortical mechanisms involved in a specific unwanted, competing motor pattern resulting in a stereotyped involuntary movement (tic). (Modified from Mink JW. Basal ganglia dysfunction in Tourette's syndrome: a new hypothesis. *Pediatr Neurol.* 2001;25:190–198.)

from frontal lobe whereas the input to striatum arises from virtually all areas of cerebral cortex. Second, the output from STN is excitatory, whereas the output from striatum is inhibitory. Third, the excitatory route through STN is faster than the inhibitory route through striatum (51–53). Finally, the STN projection to GPi is divergent and the striatal projection is more focused (54). Thus, the two disynaptic pathways from cerebral cortex to the basal ganglia output nuclei, GPi and SNpr, provide fast, widespread, divergent excitation through STN and slower, focused, inhibition through striatum. This organization provides an anatomical basis for focused inhibition and surround excitation of neurons in GPi and SNpr (Fig. 7-1A). Because the output of GPi and SNpr is inhibitory, this results in focused facilitation and surround inhibition of basal ganglia thalamocortical targets.

INHIBITION OF COMPETING MOTOR PATTERNS

The authors of this chapter have developed a scheme of normal basal ganglia motor function based on the results of anatomical, physiological, and lesion studies (5,55,56). This scheme is relevant to understanding the neurobiology and pathophysiology of TS (2). In this scheme, the tonically active inhibitory output of the basal ganglia acts as a "brake" on motor pattern generators (MPGs) in the cerebral cortex. When a movement is initiated by a particular MPG, basal ganglia output neurons projecting to competing MPGs increase their firing rate, thereby increasing inhibition and applying a brake on those generators. Other basal ganglia output neurons projecting to the generators involved in the desired movement decrease their discharge, thereby removing tonic inhibition and releasing the "brake" from the desired motor patterns. Thus, the intended movement is enabled and competing movements are prevented from interfering with the desired movement.

The anatomic arrangement of STN and striatal inputs to GPi and SNpr form the basis for a functional center-surround organization as shown in Figure 7-1A. When a voluntary movement is initiated by cortical mechanisms, a separate signal is sent to STN, exciting it. STN projects in a widespread pattern and excites GPi. The increased GPi activity causes inhibition of thalamocortical motor mechanisms. In parallel to the pathway through STN, signals are sent from all areas of cerebral cortex to striatum. The cortical inputs are transformed by the striatal integrative circuitry to a focused, context-dependent output that inhibits specific neurons in GPi. The inhibitory striatal input to GPi is slower, but more powerful, than the excitatory STN input. The resulting focally decreased activity in GPi selectively disinhibits the desired thalamocortical MPGs. Indirect pathways from striatum to GPi (striatum → GPe GPi and striatum → GPe → STN → GPi) result in further focusing of the output. The net result of basal ganglia activity during a voluntary movement is the inhibition of competing motor patterns and focused facilitation of selected voluntary movement pattern generators.

A CIRCUIT-BASED HYPOTHESIS FOR THE PATHOPHYSIOLOGY OF TICS

If a scheme of basal ganglia function is to explain the pathophysiology of tics, it must account for the stereotyped repetitive nature of tics. A pattern of stereotyped motor output can result from a focal population of striatal neurons becoming active. If they become abnormally active and cause unwanted inhibition of a group of basal ganglia output neurons, an unwanted competing motor pattern can be triggered. If a specific set of striatal neurons becomes overactive in discrete repeated episodes, the result would be a repeated, stereotyped, unwanted movement (i.e., a tic). This is illustrated schematically in Figure 7-1B. Multiple tics would result from

abnormal excessive activity of multiple discrete sets of striatal neurons. It has been hypothesized that each tic would correspond to activity of a discrete set of striatal neurons (2).

The discrete sets of striatal neurons in which over-activity can cause tics, may correspond to the striatal matrisomes (16). Matrisomes are thought to be zones of functional homogeneity in an otherwise heterogeneous striatum. If these clusters of neurons become active at inappropriate times, unwanted stereotyped movements would be produced. Microstimulation in the putamen of awake monkeys elicits stereotyped movements of individual body parts (57). At some sites, movement of multiple adjacent body parts is elicited. Increasing the stimulation current can increase the number of contracting muscles, but in a stereotyped pattern for each site. These data indicate that repeated activation of discrete sets of striatal neurons can produce repeated stereotyped movements. The motor output resulting from such activation is stereotyped for each zone (matrisome) and thus could be the substrate for the stereotyped repetitive movements that tics represent. Although no data exist as to what determines the temporal pattern of spontaneous activity in matrisomal neurons, it is tempting to speculate that the intrinsic membrane properties or afferent activity patterns lead to the temporal pattern of tics that is seen clinically (58).

DOPAMINE IN THE BASAL GANGLIA AND TICS

It is widely believed that abnormalities of dopamine neurotransmission have a primary role in the pathophysiology of TS. The "dopamine hypothesis" arises in part from the clinical observation that blockade of dopamine receptors decreases tics and potentiation of dopamine transmission with stimulant medications may elicit tics or increase their severity (59). However, measures of dopamine receptors, presynaptic content, or function in pathological or functional imaging studies have produced conflicting results (as discussed in Chapters 14 and 16). Despite the conflicting data and limitations of the studies summarized previously, the dopamine hypothesis of TS remains important. There may be significant abnormalities of dopamine-mediated function even in the absence of primary abnormalities of dopamine neurons or post-synaptic receptor binding.

The dopamine input of the basal ganglia largely arises from SNpc. As noted above, the action of dopamine on striatal neurons depends on the type of dopamine receptor involved. It is generally agreed that D1 receptors stimulate and D2 receptors inhibit adenylcyclase activity. There is also evidence that dopamine transmission influences the conductance of sodium, potassium, and calcium ions (21), but it appears that these effects are primarily local and have little influence on the membrane potential of the entire cell. Both D1 and D2 receptors are located on medium spiny striatal cells. Some evidence suggests that D1 receptors are preferentially located on cells that project to GPi or SNpr and that D2 receptors are located on cells that project to GPe (26). However, there is evidence that some medium spiny cells contain both D1 and D2 receptors (21). In addition to the postsynaptic localization, D2 receptors are also present presynaptically on corticostriatal terminals and on other dopaminergic terminals (autoreceptors) (60).

The conventional view has been that dopamine acts at D1 receptors to facilitate the activity of post-synaptic neurons and at D2 receptors to inhibit post-synaptic neurons (3,4,26). Indeed, this is a fundamental concept for currently popular models of basal ganglia pathophysiology (3,4). However, it has been shown recently that the effect of dopamine on medium spiny striatal neurons may depend critically on the membrane potential of the medium spiny cell at the time of dopamine release (22,61). The effect of a D1 agonist on the firing rate of medium spiny neurons was studied at both depolarized and hyperpolarized membrane potentials. Normally, the membrane potential of medium spiny neurons fluctuates between two stable resting states: relatively hyperpolarized (approximately –80 mV) and relatively depolarized (approximately –55 mV) (62). In the experiments of Hernandez-Lopez et al. (22) evoked discharge was inhibited by D1 agonists at hyperpolarized membrane potentials, but was facilitated by D1 agonists at more depolarized resting potentials. This effect appears to be mediated by L-type Ca2+ conductance. Thus, D1 receptor activation can either inhibit or enhance evoked activity, depending on the level of membrane depolarization.

In addition to short-term facilitation or inhibition of striatal activity, there is evidence that dopamine can modulate corticostriatal transmission by mechanisms of long-term depression (LTD) and long-term potentiation (LTP) (63–65). The mechanisms of LTD and LTP are thought to rely on time-dependent changes in intra-cellular calcium and second messenger systems. Through these mechanisms, dopamine strengthens or weakens the efficacy of corticostriatal synapses and can thus mediate reinforcement of specific discharge patterns. LTP and LTD are thought to be fundamental to many neural mechanisms of learning and may underlie the hypothesized role of the basal ganglia in habit learning (66,67).

There is increasing evidence for a role of the basal ganglia in procedural learning. Much of the research has focused on the learning of tasks or of sequential behavior. There is increasing evidence for a role of the basal ganglia in procedural learning that leads to the formation of habits and the performance of behavioral routines once they are learned (66). Tonically active striatal neurons and SNpc dopamine neurons fire in relation to behaviorally significant events (68,69). The activity patterns of these neurons change as the task becomes learned and when novel stimuli or events are introduced. Other striatal neurons also change activity in relation in relation to learning. In rats performing a T-maze task, striatal neurons changed activity patterns as the task became learned and more automatic (66). In monkeys performing a discrimination learning task, striatal neurons changed activity as the animal learned new associations between stimuli and reward (70). Functional imaging studies have also shown basal ganglia activity correlated with the learning of new tasks. Striatal lesions or focal striatal dopamine depletion impairs the learning of new movement sequences (71). These findings together support a role for the basal ganglia in certain types of procedural learning.

The state-dependent effect of dopamine and the role of dopamine in LTP and LTD have potential importance to the pathophysiology of TS. Abnormalities in these mechanisms could result in aberrant action of dopamine that might be corrected by dopamine antagonists [or agonists (72)] despite normal dopamine content and transmitter–receptor interaction. Two aspects of dopamine neurotransmission discussed above are appealing candidates in the pathophysiology of tics. If a set of striatal neurons spent excessive periods of time in the depolarized resting state, the effect of dopamine via D1 receptors would be facilitatory and thus would make these cells more likely to fire in response to weak cortical inputs. This aberrant firing would elicit a tic in the manner proposed previously (Fig. 7-1B). Thus, abnormalities in the regulation of the resting potential states of striatal neurons may cause abnormal response to dopamine without a fundamental abnormality of dopamine transmission per se. Changes in the probability of the membrane potential being in the depolarized state over time could underlie the clinical observed temporal fluctuations in tics. Alternatively, abnormally weak LTD or strong LTP of discrete sets of striatal neurons could cause excessive activity resulting in abnormal stereotyped movements as described above. Because LTP and LTD are mediated by dopamine in the striatum, this is another means by which apparently abnormal responses to dopamine may be seen without a fundamental abnormality of dopamine neurotransmission. Despite the emphasis on dopamine, it is also possible that other mechanisms including glutamate-mediated transmission and intracellular signal transduction could lead to abnormal LTP or LTD.

EXTENSION OF THE HYPOTHESIS TO NON-MOTOR MANIFESTATIONS OF TOURETTE SYNDROME

The scheme of basal ganglia function described above was developed specifically for the motor circuits of the basal ganglia-thalamocortical

system (5). However, it is likely that the fundamental principles of function in the somatomotor, oculomotor, limbic, and cognitive basal ganglia circuits are similar. If the basic scheme of facilitation and inhibition of competing movements is extended to encompass more complex behaviors and thoughts, many features of TS can be explained as a failure to inhibit unwanted behaviors and thoughts due to abnormal basal ganglia output patterns.

The segregation of basal ganglia outputs to the frontal lobes via thalamus described previously may provide the anatomical substrate for production of simple tics, complex tics, and compulsions. Abnormal activation of motor cortex via basal ganglia-thalamocortical circuits would be expected to cause relatively simple motor patterns like those seen in simple tics. Abnormal activation of premotor, supplementary motor, and cingulate motor areas would be expected to cause more elaborate motor patterns like those seen in complex tics. Abnormal activation of orbitofrontal cortex would be expected to cause even more elaborate motor patterns seen as compulsions. The premonitory symptoms would likewise be associated with abnormal activity of these areas. Thus, abnormal activation of motor areas may be associated with specific or non-specific sensations and activation of orbitofrontal areas may be associated with obsessions. Finally, abnormal disinhibition of dorsolateral prefrontal mechanisms may be associated with attention deficits. The proposed relationship between different basal ganglia circuits and the different symptoms associated with TS is hypothetical. However, with advances in functional imaging methodology there is an opportunity to test it directly in individual with different manifestations of TS.

SUMMARY

In summary, the scheme of basal ganglia function presented here, in conjunction with known features of anatomical organization and dopamine neurotransmission provides a hypothesis for the pathophysiology of tics (2). According to the hypothesis, clusters of striatal neurons (matrisomes) become abnormally active in inappropriate contexts leading to inhibition of GPi or SNpr neurons that would normally be active to suppress unwanted movements. The inhibition of these GPi or SNpr neurons would then disinhibit thalamocortical circuits, leading to the production of tics. Activity-dependent dopamine effects would inappropriately reinforce these activity patterns leading to stereotyped repetition. Over time, exactly which striatal neuronal clusters are overactive may change under various influences so that the produced movements will also change over time. This hypothesis is testable directly, but requires a valid animal model of tics or higher resolution functional imaging techniques. Continuing work on basic basal ganglia physiology, pathophysiology, and functional imaging in TS is advancing our knowledge of neural circuit abnormalities in TS, but much more work is still needed.

ACKNOWLEDGMENTS

Supported by the Tourette Syndrome Association.

REFERENCES

1. Leckman J, Cohen D. *Tourette's Syndrome—Tics, Obsessions, Compulsions: Developmental Psychopathology and Clinical Care*. New York: John Wiley & Sons; 1999.
2. Mink JW. Basal ganglia dysfunction in Tourette's syndrome: a new hypothesis. *Pediatr Neurol*. 2001;25:190–198.
3. Albin RL, Young AB, Penney JB. The functional anatomy of basal ganglia disorders. *Trends Neurosci*. 1989;12:366–375.
4. DeLong MR. Primate models of movement disorders of basal ganglia origin. *Trends Neurosci*. 1990;13: 281–285.
5. Mink JW. The basal ganglia: focused selection and inhibition of competing motor programs. *Prog Neurobiol*. 1996;50:381–425.
6. Redgrave P, Prescott T, Gurney K. The basal ganglia: a vertebrate solution to the selection problem? *Neuroscience* 1999;89:1009–1023.
7. Mink J. The basal ganglia and involuntary movements: impaired inhibition of competing motor patterns. *Arch Neurol*. 2003;60:1365–1368.
8. Kemp JM, Powell TPS. The corticostriate projection in the monkey. *Brain* 1970;93:525–546.
9. Russchen F, Bakst I, Amaral D, et al. The amygdalostriatal projections in the monkey. An anterograde tracing study. *Brain Res*. 1985;329:241–257.
10. Fudge J, Kunishio K, Walsh C, et al. Amygdaloid projections to ventromedial striatal subterritories in the primate. *Neuroscience* 2002;110:257–275.
11. Cherubini E, Herrling PL, Lanfumey L, et al. Excitatory amino acids in synaptic excitation of rat striatal neurones in vitro. *J Physiol*. 1988;400:677–690.
12. Bouyer JJ, Park DH, Joh TH, et al. Chemical and structural analysis of the relation between cortical inputs and tyrosine hydroxylase-containing terminals in rat neostriatum. *Brain Res*. 1984;302:267–275.
13. Wilson CJ, Groves PM. Fine structure and synaptic connections of the common spiny neuron of the rat neostriatum: A study employing intracellular injection of horseradish peroxidase. *J Comp Neurol*. 1980; 194: 599–614.
14. Selemon LD, Goldman-Rakic PS. Longitudinal topography and interdigitation of corticostriatal projections in the rhesus monkey. *J Neurosci*. 1985;5:776–794.
15. Flaherty AW, Graybiel AM. Corticostriatal transformations in the primate somatosensory system. Projections from physiologically mapped body-part representations. *J Neurophysiol*. 1991;66:1249–1263.
16. Graybiel AM, Aosaki T, Flaherty AW, et al. The basal ganglia and adaptive motor control. *Science* 1994; 265: 1826–1831.
17. Bolam JP, Hanley JJ, Booth PA, et al. Synaptic organization of the basal ganglia. *J Anat*. 2000;196:527–542.
18. Carpenter MB. Anatomy of the corpus striatum and brain stem integrating systems. In: Brooks VB, ed. *Handbook of Physiology: The Nervous System*. Bethesda: American Physiological Society; 1981:947–995.
19. Lavoie B, Parent A. Immunohistochemical study of the serotoninergic innervation of the basal ganglia in the squirrel monkey. *J Comp Neurol*. 1990;299:1–16.
20. Sibley DR, Monsma FJ. Molecular biology of dopamine receptors. *Trends Pharm Sci*. 1992;13:61–69.
21. Surmeier DJ, Reiner A, Levine MS, et al. Are neostriatal dopamine receptors co-localized? *Trends Neurosci*. 1993;16:299–305.
22. Hernandez-Lopez S, Bargas J, Surmeier DJ, et al. D1 receptor activation enhances evoked discharge in neostriatal medium spiny neurons by modulating an L-type Ca2+ conductance. *J Neurosci*. 1997;17:3334–3342.
23. Ribak CE, Vaughn JE, Roberts E. The GABA neurons and their axon terminals in rat corpus striatum as demonstrated by GAD immunocytochemistry. *J Comp Neurol*. 1979;187:261–283.
24. Penny GR, Afsharpour S, Kitai ST. The glutamate decarboxylase-, leucine enkephalin-, methionine enkephalin- and substance P-immunoreactive neurons in the neostriatum of the rat and cat: evidence for partial population overlap. *Neuroscience* 1986;17: 1011–1045.
25. Graybiel AM. Neurotransmitters and neuromodulators in the basal ganglia. *Trends Neurosci*. 1990;13: 244–254.
26. Gerfen CR, Engber TM, Mahan LC, et al. D1 and D2 dopamine receptor-regulated gene expression of striatonigral and striatopallidal neurons. *Science* 1990; 250:1429–1432.
27. Gerfen CR, Young WS III. Distribution of striatonigral and striatopallidal peptidergic neurons in both patch and matrix compartments: an in situ hybridization histochemistry and fluorescent retrograde tracing study. *Brain Res*. 1988;460:161–167.
28. Graybiel AM, Ragsdale CW. Histochemically distinct compartments in the striatum of human, monkey and cat demonstrated by acetylcholinesterase staining. *Proc Natl Acad Sci*. 1978;75:5723–5726.
29. Gerfen CR. The neostriatal mosaic: Multiple levels of compartmental organization in the basal ganglia. *Ann Rev Neurosci*. 1992;15:285–320.

30. Graybiel AM, Ragsdale CW, Yoneika ES, et al. An immunohistochemical study of enkephalins and other neuropeptides in the striatum of the cat with evidence that the opiate peptides are arranged to form mosaic patterns in register with striosomal compartments visible with acetylcholinesterase staining. *Neuroscience* 1981;6:377–397.

31. Rouzaire-Dubois B, Scarnati E. Pharmacological study of the cortical-induced excitation of subthalamic nucleus neurons in the rat: evidence for amino acids as putative neurotransmitters. *Neuroscience* 1987;21:429–440.

32. Fujimoto K, Kita H. Response characteristics of subthalamic neurons to the stimulation of the sensorimotor cortex in the rat. *Brain Res.* 1993;609:185–192.

33. Hartmann-von Monakow K, Akert K, Kunzle H. Projections of the precentral motor cortex and other cortical areas of the frontal lobe to the subthalamic nucleus in the monkey. *Exp Brain Res.* 1978;33:395–403.

34. Kita H, Chang HT, Kitai ST. Pallidal inputs to subthalamus: intracellular analysis. *Brain Res.* 1983;264:255–265.

35. Rinvik E, Ottersen OP. Terminals of subthalamonigral fibres are enriched with glutamate-like immunoreactivity: an electron microscopic, immunogold analysis in the cat. *J Chem Neuroanat.* 1993;6:19–30.

36. Brotchie JM, Crossman AR. D-[3H]Aspartate and [14C]GABA uptake in the basal ganglia of rats following lesions in the subthalamic region suggest a role for excitatory amino acid but not GABA-mediated transmission in subthalamic nucleus efferents. *Exp Neurol.* 1991;113:171–181.

37. Parent A, Smith Y, Filion M, et al. Distinct afferents to internal and external pallidal segments in the squirrel monkey. *Neurosci Lett.* 1989;96:140–144.

38. Nambu A, Takada M, Inase M, et al. Dual somatotopical representations in the primate subthalamic nucleus: evidence for ordered but reversed body-map transformations from the primary motor cortex and the supplementary motor area. *J Neurosci.* 1996;16:2671–2683.

39. DeLong MR, Crutcher MD, Georgopoulos AP. Primate globus pallidus and subthalamic nucleus: functional organization. *J Neurophysiol.* 1985;53:530–543.

40. Maurice N, Deniau J, Glowinski J, et al. Relationships between the prefrontal cortex and the basal ganglia in the rat: physiology of the cortico-subthalamic circuits. *J Neurosci.* 1998;18:9539–9546.

41. Penney JB, Young AB. GABA as the pallidothalamic neurotransmitter: implications for basal ganglia function. *Brain Res.* 1981;207:195–199.

42. Georgopoulos AP, DeLong MR, Crutcher MD. Relation between parameters of step-tracking movements and single cell discharge in the globus pallidus and subthalamic nucleus of the behaving monkey. *J Neurosci.* 1983;3:1586–1598.

43. Alexander GE, DeLong MR, Strick PL. Parallel organization of functionally segregated circuits linking basal ganglia and cortex. *Ann Rev Neurosci.* 1986;9: 357–381.

44. Middleton FA, Strick PL. Anatomical evidence for cerebellar and basal ganglia involvement in higher cognitive function. *Science* 1994;266:458–461.

45. Hoover JE, Strick PL. Multiple output channels in the basal ganglia. *Science* 1993;259:819–821.

46. Alexander GE, Crutcher MD. Functional architecture of basal ganglia circuits: neural substrates of parallel processing. *Trends Neurosci.* 1990;13:266–271.

47. Bolam JP, Smith Y. The striatum and the globus pallidus send convergent synaptic inputs onto single cells in the entopeduncular nucleus of the rat: a double anterograde labelling study combined with postembedding immunocytochemistry for GABA. *J Comp Neurol.* 1992; 321:456–476.

48. Bevan MD, Booth PA, Eaton SA, et al. Selective innervation of neostriatal interneurons by a subclass of neuron in the globus pallidus of the rat. *J Neurosci.* 1998;18:9438–9452.

49. Hedreen JC, DeLong MR. Organization of striatopallidal, striatonigral, and nigrostriatal projections in the macaque. *J Comp Neurol.* 1991;304:569–595.

50. Haber SN, Fudge JL, McFarland NR. Striatonigrostriatal pathways in primates form an ascending spiral from the shell to the dorsolateral striatum. *J Neurosci.* 2000;20:2369–2382.

51. Kita H. Responses of globus pallidus neurons to cortical stimulation: intracellular study in the rat. *Brain Res.* 1992;589:84–90.

52. Maurice N, Deniau J, Glowinski J, et al. Relationships between the prefrontal cortex and the basal ganglia in the rat: physiology of the cortico-nigral circuits. *J Neurosci.* 1999;19:4674–4681.

53. Nambu A, Tokuno H, Hamada I, et al. Excitatory cortical inputs to pallidal neurons via the subthalamic nucleus in the monkey. *J Neurophysiol.* 2000;84: 289–300.

54. Parent A, Hazrati L-N. Anatomical aspects of information processing in primate basal ganglia. *Trends Neurosci.* 1993;16:111–116.

55. Mink JW, Thach WT. Basal ganglia intrinsic circuits and their role in behavior. *Curr Opin Neurobiol.* 1993; 3:950–957.

56. Thach WT, Mink JW, Goodkin HP, et al. Combining versus gating motor programs: differential roles for cerebellum and basal ganglia. In: Mano N, Hamada I, DeLong MR, eds. *Role of the Cerebellum and Basal Ganglia in Voluntary Movement.* Amsterdam: Elsevier Science Publishers; 1993: 235–245.

57. Alexander GE, DeLong MR. Microstimulation of the primate striatum. II. Somatotopic organization of striatal microexcitable zones and their relation to neuronal response properties. *J Neurophysiol.* 1985;53:1417–1430.

58. Peterson B, Leckman J. The temporal dynamics of tics in Gilles de la Tourette syndrome. *Biol Psychiatry.* 1998;44:1337–1348.

59. Singer HS. Neurobiological issues in Tourette syndrome. *Brain Dev.* 1994;16:353–364.

60. Kalsner S, Westfall TC. Presynaptic receptors and the question of autoregulation of neurotransmitter release. *Ann NY Acad Sci.* 1990;604:652–655.

61. Nicola S, Surmeier J, Malenka R. Dopaminergic modulation of neuronal excitability in the striatum and nucleus accumbens. *Ann Rev Neurosci.* 2000;23: 185–215.

62. Wilson CJ, Kawaguchi Y. The origins of two-state spontaneous membrane potential fluctuations of neostriatal spiny neurons. *J Neurosci.* 1996;16:2397–2410.

63. Groves PM, Garcia-Munoz M, Linder JC, et al. Elements of the intrinsic organization and information processing in the neostriatum. In: Houk JC, Davis JL, Beiser DG, eds. *Models of Information Processing in the Basal Ganglia.* Cambridge: MIT Press; 1995:51–96.

64. Wickens J, Kotter R. Cellular models of reinforcement. In: Houk JC, Davis JL, Beiser DG, eds. *Models of Information Processing in the Basal Ganglia*. Cambridge: MIT Press; 1995:187–214.

65. Centonze D, Gubellini P, Picconi B, et al. Unilateral dopamine denervation blocks corticostriatal LTP. *J Neurophysiol*. 1999;82:3575–3579.

66. Jog M, Kubota Y, Connolly C, et al. Building neural representations of habits. *Science* 1999;286: 1745–1749.

67. Knowlton B, Mangels J, Squire L. A neostriatal habit learning system in humans. *Science* 1996;273:1399–1402.

68. Aosaki T, Kimura M, Graybiel AM. Temporal and spatial characteristics of tonically active neurons of the primate's striatum. *J Neurophysiol*. 1995;73: 1234–1252.

69. Schultz W, Romo R, Ljungberg T, et al. Reward-related signals carried by dopamine neurons. In: Houk JC, Davis JL, Beiser DG, eds. *Models of Information Processing in the Basal Ganglia*. Cambridge: MIT Press; 1995:233–249.

70. Tremblay L, Hollerman J, Schultz W. Modifications of reward expectation-related neuronal activity during learning in primate striatum. *J Neurophysiol*. 1998;80:964–977.

71. Matsumoto N, Hanakawa T, Maki S, et al. Role of nigrostriatal dopamine system in learning to perform sequential motor tasks in a predictive manner. *J Neurophysiol*. 1999;82:978–998.

72. Gilbert D, Sethuraman G, Sine L, et al. Tourette's syndrome improvement with pergolide in a randomized, double-blind, crossover trial. *Neurology* 2000;54: 1310–1315.

8

Neurobiology of Basal Ganglia and Tourette Syndrome: Striatal and Dopamine Function

Roger L. Albin

Department of Neurology, University of Michigan School of Medicine, and Geriatrics Research, Education, and Clinical Center, Ann Arbor, Veteran's Affairs Medical Affairs, Ann Arbor, Michigan.

Understanding and treatment of Tourette syndrome (TS) has been hampered by insufficient knowledge regarding the neurobiology of TS. Unlike many neurologic disorders in which postmortem examinations provide crucial clues to the anatomic locus of pathology and pathophysiology of clinical features, the very modest amount of pathologic data from TS subjects has been unrewarding. Inferences derived from clinical observations, imaging research, and basic neurobiology studies, however, are coalescing around the concept that TS results from dysfunction within the basal ganglia and may be specifically associated with abnormalities in the ventral striatum.

EVIDENCE FOR VENTRAL STRIATAL DYSFUNCTION IN TOURETTE SYNDROME

The starting point for any discussion of the neurobiology of TS is the basic clinical phenomenology and clinical pharmacology of TS (1–3). The characteristic tics are repetitive, stereotyped movements, varying considerably in complexity. Although tics may involve almost any body part, there is a strong tendency for tics to involve the face and head. Both within individuals and within families, there is a strong association of tics and obsessive-compulsive behaviors (OCBs). Tics are commonly preceded by a compulsive urge so it is often impossible to distinguish complex tics from compulsive behavior. There may be a spectrum of tic-OCB phenomena with simple motor tics at one end of the spectrum and obsessions at the other end of the spectrum. There is also a suggested overlap between TS and attention deficit hyperactivity disorder (ADHD). Another key feature of TS is the natural history of tic expression. Tics begin typically in the first decade of life, peak between 10 to 14 years, and moderate or even remit with attainment of adulthood. The natural history of TS suggests an abnormality of brain development.

Probably the most fruitful clinical clue regarding the natural history of TS is its clinical pharmacology. Tics are most reliably suppressed by dopamine antagonists. OCBs are improved by treatment with selective serotonin reuptake inhibitors. These facts suggest involvement of central nervous system systems in which dopamine and serotonin play important roles. Dopamine and serotonin systems have a number of common features. Both arise from discrete groups of brainstem neurons; the substantia nigra pars compacta (SNpc)-ventral tegmental area (VTA) complex for dopamine, and the raphe nuclei for serotonin. Both these groups of nuclei give rise to wide-ranging projections that innervate multiple regions of the central nervous system. The principle of parsimony suggests that key areas involved in the pathophysiology of TS would receive both significant dopaminergic and serotonergic innervation. This consideration suggests two candidate regions within the forebrain; the ventral striatum and the SNc-VTA itself. All components of the striatal complex receive massive dopaminergic innervation from the SNc-VTA complex.

The striatum receives a significant serotonergic innervation that is enriched within the ventral striatum (4,5). The dorsal raphe also innervates dopamine neurons in the midbrain, identifying another possible locus of abnormalities in TS.

Some imaging data supports the inference that the ventral striatum is abnormal in TS. Some magnetic resonance imaging morphometric data (as discussed in Chapter 11) suggests the existence of differences in striatal morphology between TS and control subjects. A clever functional imaging study of TS subjects in which subjects were studied while actively suppressing tics revealed significant areas of altered brain activity in several forebrain regions with significant activation in the right ventral striatum (6). Positron emission tomography study of striatal monoaminergic terminals with the type 2 vesicular monoamine transporter (VMAT2) ligand [^{11}C]dihydrotetrabenazine (DTBZ) indicates increased density of DTBZ binding sites within the ventral striatum, particularly the right ventral striatum (7). VMAT2 ligands such as DTBZ bind to synaptic vesicles within monoaminergic—dopamine, serotonin, norepinephrine, histamine—nerve terminals. In the striatum, VMAT2 binding is dominated by nigrostriatal dopaminergic terminals (8). The finding of increased ventral striatal VMAT2 binding suggests increased density of dopaminergic terminals within TS ventral striatum, though increased innervation by other monoaminergic neurons, such as serotonergic raphe neurons, is possible. The notion that TS is characterized by increased ventral striatal dopaminergic innervation is consistent with recent data about the development of the human nigrostriatal dopaminergic system. Haycock et al. (9) reported recently that striatal levels of dopamine and other dopaminergic markers increase gradually from birth to until about 9 years of age and gradually fall to adult levels. Haycock et al. (9) suggest that nigrostriatal innervation becomes "overelaborated" in the preadolescent years with the formation of a relatively high number of synapses and then undergoes developmental regression with the onset of adolescence. This hypothesis is consistent with a good deal of what we know about brain development in the first two decades of life. The

proposed "overelaboration" and regression of dopaminergic innervation parallels the natural history of TS nicely and leads to the suggestion that TS could involve aberrant timing of the development of the nigrostriatal projection during childhood.

Clinical observations in other diseases and parallel developments in other fields are consistent with the idea that the ventral striatum could be implicated in TS. Tics occur commonly in diseases with known striatal pathology such as Huntington disease. The phenomenon of compulsion has some features that overlap with the uncontrollable drug seeking and drug craving behavior that is a prominent component of addiction. A large body of experimental and clinical data implicate alterations of VTA-ventral striatal dopaminergic neurotransmission as crucial factors in the development of addiction (10,11).

A final piece of evidence regarding the probable role of the striatum in TS comes from the very interesting literature describing an important striatal role in the regulation of stereotyped behavioral sequences. Ethological and behavioral neuroscience studies have defined a number of naturally occurring stereotyped and often complex behaviors in a number of mammals. Berridge et al. (12–18) have studied an interesting example of such behaviors in rodents; control of grooming chains. In many rodent species, grooming is a relatively complex and stereotyped sequence (chain) of individual and repetitive motor acts. Components of this sequence can be elicited in decerebrate preparations and a small region in the dorsal striatum is crucial for controlling the appropriate sequencing and expression of grooming chains. The presence of grooming behaviors in decerebrate preparations and the occurrence of grooming chains in many rodent species suggests that this behavior is at least partially "hard-wired" within the central nervous system. Grooming chains are profoundly modified by dopaminergic agents. Grooming chains apparently play a role in conspecific social interactions and may be under selective pressure. Grooming chains may be a paradigmatic example of relatively "hard-wired" behavioral sequences whose performance is regulated by the striatum. A wide variety of other stereotyped and sometimes complex behaviors can be elicited by pharmacologic manipulation of small regions of the striatum, including the ventral striatum. Particularly intriguing is the observation of stereotyped facial movements elicited by focal injections of opioid agonists within small regions of the ventral striatum. Berridge et al. (15) point out that stereotyped movements of this type are seen in a wide variety of mammalian species, including primates, again suggesting that they may be relatively hard-wired. A key role for facial and head movements in humans and other primates is social communication. The likely explanation for the perceived disruptive character of even moderate tics is that they interfere with the continuous and largely subliminal character of social communication carried by facial expression and head movements. It is plausible that the ventral striatum is an important node for regulating the expression of socially significant, stereotyped movements, precisely the sort of actions that tics distort.

DOPAMINERGIC SIGNALING WITHIN THE STRIATUM

The available evidence highlights the importance of the ventral striatum and dopaminergic neurotransmission in the genesis of tics. Dopaminergic signaling within the striatum has a complex character. The relatively small number of midbrain dopaminergic neurons innervate virtually all striatal neurons. The great majority of striatal neurons are medium spiny projection neurons and dopaminergic neurons synapse on medium spiny neurons in a "triadic" arrangement with glutamatergic afferents from the neocortex, amygdala, and the hippocampal formation (19). The glutamatergic afferents terminate in synapses in the heads of spines while dopaminergic afferent terminals form closely adjacent synapses on the necks of spines. Because the nigrostriatal afferents arise from the small population of dopaminergic midbrain neurons and presumably exhibit wide divergence with single dopaminergic neurons innervating multiple striatal neurons, it is likely that dopaminergic neurotransmission conveys some type of general signal(s) to striatal

neurons (as discussed later in text). The glutamatergic cortical afferents are arranged in a topographic manner (reviewed in Chapter 7) and probably subserve specialized functions through broadly parallel circuits. It is likely that a major role for striatal dopamine is to modulate glutamatergic corticostriate neurotransmission, including the functional strength of these synapses (20). The close apposition of glutamatergic and dopaminergic terminals creates multiple opportunities for cross modulation of glutamatergic and dopaminergic neurotransmission. Although axoaxonic synapses between corticostriate and nigrostriatal terminals are not present, there is evidence that presynaptic glutamate and dopamine heteroreceptors modulate dopamine and glutamate release, respectively (21). It is likely that dopaminergic terminals participate in "volume" neurotransmission in which dopamine diffusing from the synaptic cleft can interact with surrounding dopamine receptors on other neurons.

It is very likely that there are postsynaptic interactions as well. The close apposition of glutamatergic and dopaminergic synapses provides the opportunity for dopamine activated signal transduction mechanisms to modify glutamatergic neurotransmission at several points. Svenningsson et al. have dissected a primary mechanism of dopamine receptor signaling, modulation of the activity of the 32 kD dopamine and cyclic adenosine monophosphate (cAMP) regulated phosphoprotein (DARPP-32) (22). Dopamine receptors modulate adenylylcyclase activity and activation of protein kinase A (PKA). The phosphorylation state of DARPP-32 is regulated by PKA. Phosphorylated DARPP-32 is an inhibitor of protein phosphatase 1 (PP1), a multifunctional phosphatase that is an important regulator of the phosphorylation state of numerous important proteins, including glutamate and gamma-butyric acid receptors, ion channels, and transcriptional regulators. The adenylylcyclase-PKA-DARPP-32 cascade is probably not the only signal transduction mechanism for dopamine receptors. The pleiotropic effects of dopamine receptor activation probably cause multiple effects on striatal neuron function ranging from short-term electrophysiologic effects to persistent changes in gene expression. Although the complexity of dopamine signal transduction precludes any easy identification of particular molecular events with clinical phenomena, it presents a large number of targets for potential therapies.

Dopamine interacts with five different G-protein coupled receptor subtypes, dopamine receptors 1 to 5 (D1 to D5). D1 and D2 receptors are expressed at uniquely high levels by medium spiny neurons, probably in a relatively segregated pattern (as reviewed in Chapter 7), and D3 receptors are expressed at high levels within the ventral striatum. There are probably also populations of D2 presynaptic receptors on corticostriate and dopaminergic terminals.

Considerably less is known about serotonin signaling within the striatum. It is likely also to have a formidably complex character. Serotonergic terminals synapse on the shafts of medium spiny neuron dendrites, often closely adjacent to gamma-aminobutyric amino acidergic terminals and sometimes adjacent to dopaminergic terminals (23–25). There is a remarkable plethora of serotonin receptors, including both multiple subtypes of G-protein coupled receptors and ionotropic receptors, several of which are expressed within the striatum. Much less is known about the subcellular localization and actions of striatal serotonin receptors. Some experimental evidence and theoretical treatments suggest that serotonergic systems may oppose the action of dopaminergic systems within the basal ganglia (26).

THE ORGAN OF HABIT

Although the specific molecular mechanisms underlying striatal functions remain unclear, there has been considerable progress in understanding the function of striatum/basal ganglia in broader terms and in associating specific components of the basal ganglia and even neurochemical systems within the basal ganglia with specific behavioral functions. For many years, speculations about the functions of the basal ganglia tended to be discussed in relatively general terms often employing vague terminology and difficult to define concepts.

More recently, experimental work from several fields and theoretical analyses are producing convergence in thinking about the function(s) of the basal ganglia. It is clear now that the striatum plays a crucial role in certain well-defined forms of learning and memory (27,28). Different terms have been used for these forms of learning and memory but habit is a reasonable shorthand for these types of basal ganglia based functions. The basal ganglia are viewed increasingly as responsible, at least in part, for learning and recalling incrementally acquired stimulus-response associations epitomized by the classical paradigms of Pavlovian and instrumental conditioning. These forms of learning and memory are contrasted with more "cognitive" forms of learning and "declarative" memory, which are associated with circuits involving the hippocampal formation. A growing body of literature including both animal experiments and human studies support this conclusion.

The experiments of Knowlton et al. (29), using subjects with Parkinson disease (PD) or classic amnesia, are a good example of this burgeoning literature. This group compared the performance of non-demented PD subjects with that of amnesic subjects on a pair of learning/memory tasks. The amnesic subjects had incurred their memory deficits from injuries to the hippocampal formation or linked structures. One task was a probabilistic learning task that relied on incremental learning of specific stimulus-response associations and for which a conscious memorization strategy was impossible. The second task was a conventional test of declarative memory. PD subjects performed very poorly on the probabilistic learning task and normally on the declarative memory task. The performance of the amnesic subjects was precisely reversed; their performance on the probabilistic learning task was nearly normal and their performance on the declarative memory task was dreadful. This "double dissociation" of memory/learning functions mirrors results in a large number of animal lesion experiments.

Some electrophysiologic work correlates well with the idea of the striatum as the organ of habit. An interesting recent study is that of Blazquez et al. (30). This group used extracellular recording methods in awake monkeys undergoing simple aversive conditioning. They recorded the activity of tonically active neurons (TANs) within the dorsal striatum. TANs are very likely the large cholinergic interneurons whose axons ramify widely within the striatum and synapse on medium spiny projection neurons. The wide divergence of cholinergic innervation suggests that TANs may play some role in coordinating the behavior of wide range of medium spiny neurons. The firing behavior of TANs was modified by several training conditions and the population response behavior of the TANs correlated strongly with the likelihood that a stimulus would lead to a behavioral response. TAN firing behavior coincided with and did not precede motor responses in these paradigms, precluding the possibility that TANs provide a premotor signal. TANs may encode information about response probability and deliver this information to wide range of striatal neurons, a feature that would be essential for a system mediating instrumental conditioning. This interpretation is consistent with the proposed role of the striatum in incremental learning of stimulus-response associations.

Whereas experimental paradigms tend to focus on simpler, discrete, and easily manipulated learning/memory paradigms, it is likely that these mechanisms underlying learning/memory of stimulus-response associations can be elaborated to subserve complex behavioral repertoires. Graybiel (31) has emphasized that the basal ganglia could combine or "chunk" individual stimulus-response associations into more complex sequences for execution as "units." This suggestion is consonant with the literature on striatal regulation of stereotyped behavioral sequences (as noted previously) and is an intuitively attractive correlate of phenomena like complex tics or compulsions. The idea that brain regions can combine individual stimulus-response associations into more complex assemblages has been embodied in a group of formal computational models of learning termed temporal difference models. Results

from a recent functional magnetic resonance imaging study of a more complex second order pain learning task are consistent with predictions of temporal difference models and identify altered neuronal activity within the ventral striatum as a probable key locus for this type of sequential learning (32).

THE ROLE OF DOPAMINE SIGNALING

Recent investigations suggest that dopamine signaling plays a specific role within the general context of habit formation. Most of this work has been driven by the desire to gain better understanding of substance abuse and focuses on the role of dopamine in positively reinforced behaviors. The background of this work is the realization of the importance of the VTA-ventral-striatal projection in initiating and maintaining addiction. Some of the most influential work in this area has been accomplished by the laboratory of Wolfram Schultz (33,34). Briefly, several groups documented that midbrain dopaminergic neurons exhibit phasic firing in response to reward presentation. Others, however, obtained contradictory findings. Schultz's group reconciled these results by establishing a complex relationship between rewards and the phasic firing behavior of dopaminergic neurons. The basic result is that phasic firing in response to reward signals not reward per se but rather information about the difference between reward and the expectation of reward. Phasic dopamine neuron firing is elicited by unexpected presentation of a reward, as occurs during the initial training phase of a visual stimulus-response paradigm. Once the association is learned, reward no longer elicits the phasic response. Omission of the reward, however, results in diminished firing. In a series of systematic and clever experiments, Schultz et al. (33,34) established clearly the relationship between phasic dopamine neuron responses and reward prediction errors. This work ties in nicely some formal models of learning, including the temporal difference models mentioned previously.

Others have offered alternative interpretations of these results. The criticism is not so much that the reward prediction error is incorrect as that it might be incomplete. Redgrave et al. (35), for example, suggested that these results could be interpreted in the context of formal models of attentional processing. The concept that dopamine neuron signaling is participating in processes like allocation of attention has received some support from recent and very interesting results from Schultz's laboratory. Fiorillo et al. (36) reported data in which they modified their basic visual stimulus-reward association task to include a probabilistic component. They documented phasic dopamine neuron responses consistent with their conception of dopaminergic encoding of a reward prediction signal. In addition, they made the unexpected discovery of slower increases in tonic dopamine neuron activity correlated with uncertainty of reward. This correlation may indicate a general role for dopaminergic signaling in conveying information about reward uncertainty and is linked to formal learning theories in which attentional mechanisms are central to acquiring new information (36,37). This interpretation is consistent with rodent lesion studies supporting a role for the ventral striatum in regulating attention (38).

Another attractive hypothesis is that phasic dopamine signaling is related to attaching motivational significance or "salience" to specific stimuli (10,39,40). This idea can be generalized formally to incorporate Schultz's ideas about reward prediction and pushed past the emphasis on reward to describe a general role for the VTA-ventral striatal pathway in assessing a variety of stimuli, including relatively neutral and aversive stimuli (41). This conclusion is supported by animal lesion and human functional magnetic resonance imaging studies supporting a role for the ventral striatum in evaluating the "salience" of a broad range of stimuli (42,43). The general idea that the VTA-ventral striatal system has a key function for assessing the motivational significance of stimuli is a plausible correlate of some of the clinical phenomenology of TS and OCBs and has nice parallels with the idea of the "self under siege" (as discussed in Chapter 1).

VENTRAL STRIATAL CRITIC AND DORSAL STRIATAL ACTOR

Some work suggests specialization of different components of the striatal complex for different aspects of habit formation. Most of the literature on the role of the striatum in learning and memory focuses on the dorsal striatum. Work on assessment of stimuli "salience" concentrates on the ventral striatum. To some extent this recapitulates the widely diffused idea of broad parallel circuits running through the basal ganglia. Sensorimotor circuits run through the putamen, more "cognitive" circuits via the caudate, and limbic circuits through the ventral striatum. Zink et al. (43) presented functional magnetic resonance imaging data indicating activation of ventral striatal regions in response to salient but non-rewarding stimuli. When these stimuli were relevant for performance of a behavioral response, there was also activation of caudate regions. This result is consistent with some kind of specialization of function within the striatal complex. Some formal models of rewarded stimulus-response learning have posited the existence of a two-component process; a "critic" that develops predictions about future reward and an "actor" responsible for maintaining information about outcomes that are used to select action. The idea that the ventral striatum is involved in reward prediction suggests that the critic function can be assigned to the ventral striatum while the role of the dorsal striatum in habit formation suggests that it is the actor. Results of recent functional magnetic resonance imaging experiments are consistent with these predictions (44). The critic and actor would presumably have to have some way for information to transit from critic to actor. An attractive possibility would be Haber's ascending spiral of dopaminergic interconnections between the ventral and dorsal striatum (45,46).

CONCLUSION

Convergent data suggest that the ventral striatum is a locus of abnormality in TS. A broad range of neurobiological work is beginning to cast light on the function of the basal ganglia in ways that can be plausibly connected to the clinical phenomenology of TS. This work emphasizes the role of the striatum in the formation of habits and specifically in relatively complex and socially relevant behavioral sequences. Dopaminergic neurotransmission plays a key role in the learning and memnonic functions of the basal ganglia. Dopamine signaling is likely to participate in assignment of "salience" to stimuli, in encoding information about reward uncertainty, and perhaps in communication between different compartments of the striatal complex. Further work on the basic neurobiology of the striatum will cast further light on the pathogenesis and pathophysiology of tics, OCBs, and attentional deficits.

ACKNOWLEDGMENTS

Supported by NS15655 and a Merit Review Grant.

REFERENCES

1. Jankovic J. Tourette's syndrome. *New Engl J Med.* 2001;345:1184–1192.
2. Leckman JF. Tourette's syndrome. *Lancet* 2002;360: 1577–1586.
3. Robertson MM. Tourette syndrome, associated conditions and the complexities of treatment. *Brain* 2000;123 Pt 3:425–462.
4. Azmitia EC, Segal M. An autoradiographic analysis of the differential ascending projections of the dorsal and median raphe nuclei in the rat. *J Comp Neurol.* 1978; 179:641–667.
5. Gurevich EV, Joyce JN. Comparison of [3H]paroxetine and [3H]cyanoimipramine for quantitative measurement of serotonin transporter sites in human brain. *Neuropsychopharmacology* 1996;14:309–323.
6. Peterson BS, Skudlarski P, Anderson AW, et al. A functional magnetic resonance imaging study of tic suppression in Tourette syndrome. *Arch General Psychiatry.* 1998;55:326–333.
7. Albin RL, Koeppe RA, Bohnen NI, et al. Increased ventral striatal monoaminergic innervation in Tourette syndrome. *Neurology* 2003;61:310–315.
8. Vander Borght TM, Sima AA, Kilbourn MR, et al. [3H]methoxytetrabenazine: a high specific activity ligand for estimating monoaminergic neuronal integrity. *Neuroscience* 1995;68:955–962.
9. Haycock JW, Becker L, Ang L, et al. Marked disparity between age-related changes in dopamine and other presynaptic dopaminergic markers in human striatum. *J Neurochem.* 2003;87:574–585.
10. Robinson TE, Berridge KC. Addiction. *Ann Rev Psychology.* 2003;54:25–53.
11. Kelley AE, Berridge KC. The neuroscience of natural rewards: relevance to addictive drugs. *J Neurosci.* 2002;22:3306–3311.
12. Berridge KC. Progressive degradation of serial grooming chains by descending decerebration. *Behavioural Brain Res.* 1989;33:241–253.
13. Cromwell HC, Berridge KC. Implementation of action sequences by a neostriatal site: a lesion mapping study of grooming syntax. *J Neurosci.* 1996;16:3444–3458.
14. Aldridge JW, Berridge KC. Coding of serial order by neostriatal neurons: a "natural action" approach to movement sequence. *J Neurosci.* 1998;18:2777–2787.
15. Berridge KC, Aldridge JW. Super-stereotypy I: enhancement of a complex movement sequence by systemic dopamine D1 agonists. *Synapse* 2000;37:194–204.
16. Bursten SN, Berridge KC, Owings DH. Do California ground squirrels (Spermophilus beecheyi) use ritualized syntactic cephalocaudal grooming as an agonistic signal? *J Comp Psychology.* 2000;114:281–290.
17. Steiner JE, Glaser D, Hawilo ME, et al. Comparative expression of hedonic impact: affective reactions to taste by human infants and other primates. *Neurosci Biobehavioral Rev.* 2001;25:53–74.
18. Reynolds SM, Berridge KC. Fear and feeding in the nucleus accumbens shell: rostrocaudal segregation of GABA-elicited defensive behavior versus eating behavior. *J Neurosci.* 2001;21:3261–3270.
19. Bolam JP, Hanley JJ, Booth PA, et al. Synaptic organisation of the basal ganglia. *J Anatomy.* 2000;196: 527–542.
20. Horvitz JC. Dopamine gating of glutamatergic sensorimotor and incentive motivational input signals to the striatum. *Behavioural Brain Res.* 2002;137:65–74.
21. Bamford NS, Zhang H, Schmitz Y, et al. Heterosynaptic dopamine neurotransmission selects sets of corticostriatal terminals. *Neuron* 2004;42:653–663.
22. Svenningsson P, Nishi A, Fisone G, et al. DARPP-32: an integrator of neurotransmission. *Ann Rev Pharmacol Toxicol.* 2004;44:269–296.
23. Van Bockstaele EJ, Chan J, Pickel VM. Pre- and postsynaptic sites for serotonin modulation of GABA-containing neurons in the shell region of the rat nucleus accumbens. *J Comp Neurol.* 1996;371:116–128.
24. Van Bockstaele EJ, Pickel VM. Ultrastructure of serotonin-immunoreactive terminals in the core and shell of the rat nucleus accumbens: cellular substrates for interactions with catecholamine afferents. *J Comp Neurol.* 1993;334:603–617.
25. Van Bockstaele EJ, Cestari DM, Pickel VM. Synaptic structure and connectivity of serotonin terminals in the ventral tegmental area: potential sites for modulation of mesolimbic dopamine neurons. *Brain Res.* 1994;647:307–322.
26. Daw ND, Kakade S, Dayan P. Opponent interactions between serotonin and dopamine. *Neural Networks* 2002;15:603–616.
27. Packard MG, Knowlton BJ. Learning and memory functions of the basal ganglia. *Annu Rev Neurosci.* 2002;25:563–593.
28. White NM, McDonald RJ. Theoretical review. Multiple parallel memory systems in the brain of the rat. *Neurobiol Learn Mem.* 2002;77:125–184.
29. Knowlton BJ, Mangels JA, Squire LR. A neostriatal habit learning system in humans. *Science* 1996;273: 1399–1402.

30. Blazquez PM, Fujii N, Kojima J, et al. A network representation of response probability in the striatum. *Neuron* 2002;33:973–982.

31. Graybiel AM. The basal ganglia and chunking of action repertoires. *Neurobiol Learn Mem* 1998;70:119–136.

32. Seymour B, O'Doherty JP, Dayan P, et al. Temporal difference models describe higher-order learning in humans. *Nature* 2004;429:664–667.

33. Schultz W. Getting formal with dopamine and reward. *Neuron* 2002;36:241–263.

34. Schultz W, Tremblay L, Hollerman JR. Changes in behavior-related neuronal activity in the striatum during learning. *Trends Neurosci.* 2003;26:321–328.

35. Redgrave P, Prescott TJ, Gurney K. Is the short-latency dopamine response too short to signal reward error? *Trends Neurosci.* 1999;22:146–151.

36. Fiorillo CD, Tobler PN, Schultz W. Discrete coding of reward probability and uncertainty by dopamine neurons. *Science* 2003;299:1898–1902.

37. Fiorillo CD. The uncertain nature of dopamine. *Mol Psychiatry.* 2004;9:122–123

38. Cardinal RN, Pennicott DR, Sugathapala CL, et al. Impulsive choice induced in rats by lesions of the nucleus accumbens core. *Science* 2001;292:2499–2501.

39. Berridge KC, Robinson TE. Parsing reward. *Trends Neurosci.* 2003;26:507–513.

40. Wise RA. Dopamine, learning and motivation. *Nat Rev Neurosci.* 2004;5:483–494.

41. McClure SM, Daw ND, Montague PR. A computational substrate for incentive salience. *Trends Neurosci.* 2003;26:423–428.

42. Schoenbaum G, Setlow B. Lesions of nucleus accumbens disrupt learning about aversive outcomes. *J Neurosci.* 2003;23:9833–9841.

43. Zink CF, Pagnoni G, Martin ME, et al. Human striatal response to salient nonrewarding stimuli. *J Neurosci.* 2003;23:8092–8097.

44. O'Doherty J, Dayan P, Schultz J, et al. Dissociable roles of ventral and dorsal striatum in instrumental conditioning. *Science* 2004;304:452–454.

45. Groenewegen HJ, van den Heuvel OA, Cath DC, et al. Does an imbalance between the dorsal and ventral striatopallidal systems play a role in Tourette's syndrome? A neuronal circuit approach. *Brain Dev.* 2003:25:S3–S14.

46. Haber SN, Fudge JL, McFarland NR. Striatonigrostriatal pathways in primates form an ascending spiral from the shell to the dorsolateral striatum. *J Neurosci.* 2000;20:2369–2382.

9

Motor Cortex Inhibitory Function in Tourette Syndrome, Attention Deficit Disorder, and Obsessive Compulsive Disorder: Studies Using Transcranial Magnetic Stimulation

Donald L. Gilbert

Department of Neurology, Cincinnati Children's Hospital Medical Center, Cincinnati, Ohio

Dysregulation of activity in the cortical-subcortical circuits connecting the cerebral cortex to the striatum, globus pallidus, thalamus, and back to the cortex (1-3) (Fig. 9-1) may contribute to symptoms of tics in Tourette syndrome (TS), as well as symptoms of obsessive compulsive disorder (OCD) and attention deficit hyperactivity disorder (ADHD) (4-7). Electrophysiologic evidence from primate studies suggests that abnormalities in the basal ganglia result in disinhibition of excitatory neurons in the ventral thalamus, which in turn produces hyperexcitability, or disinhibition, of cortical motor areas, associated with the occurrence of involuntary movements (8). A substantial body of neuroimaging literature also supports the involvement of the basal ganglia in TS (9,10). Nigro-striatal dopaminergic dysfunction may also play a prominent role in TS. Although results have been inconsistent, radioligand imaging studies in adults suggest that excessive tonic or pulsatile striatal dopamine may be present in some individuals with TS (11,12).

USE OF TRANSCRANIAL MAGNETIC STIMULATION TO STUDY PROPERTIES OF THE CORTICAL NODE OF CORTICAL-SUBCORTICAL CIRCUITS

Transcranial magnetic stimulation (TMS) can be used to study the motor cortex node of cortical-subcortical circuits. This technology involves the use of a handheld magnetic coil attached to a capacitor that functions as a high current pulse generator. The operator designates the amount of energy as the percent of the total energy the capacitor can store (1% to 100%). The operator then triggers release of the energy pulse (up to approximately 500 J of energy in 0.1 ms) into the coil either manually (via a foot pedal) or digitally (via computer program). This release produces a magnetic field pulse with strength of up to approximately 2 T, comparable with fields produced by clinical magnetic resonance imaging scanners. When placed on the scalp, the coil's magnetic pulse induces current in underlying brain. The induced current is far less than that produced by electroconvulsive therapy (13) and is generally well tolerated, even in awake children (14,15).

TMS pulses over motor cortex activate pyramidal motor neurons transsynaptically, producing motor evoked potentials (MEPs) in corresponding muscles. Properties of the MEPs can be measured noninvasively using surface electrodes, amplifiers, and electrophysiology software. Changes in the stimulation thresholds, latencies, and amplitudes of these MEPs during development (16,17), in the presence of various neurologic conditions (18–20), and with pharmacologic interventions (21) have yielded important neurobiologic insights.

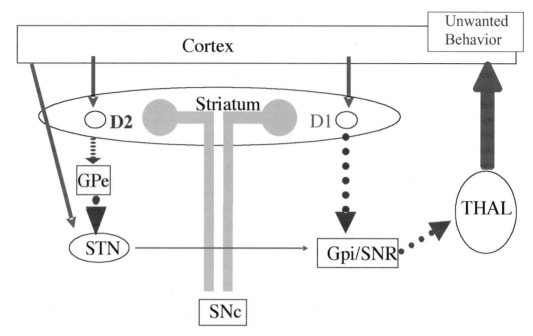

Fig. 9-1. Schematic of cortical-subcortical circuits. Dysregulated striatal function may lead to disinhibted thalamocortical output and unwanted behaviors. *Solid line arrows* are excitatory, glutamatergic projections. *Dotted arrows* are inhibitory, gamma-butyric acid-ergic projections. Projection with circular end is dopaminergic from substantia nigra to striatum. D1, excitatory dopamine receptors; D2, inhibitory dopamine receptors; GPi/GPe, internal and external globus pallidus; SNpc, substantia nigra pars compacta; STN, subthalamic nucleus; Thal, thalamus.

This review focuses on two measures of motor cortex inhibitory function that have been studied using TMS in TS, ADHD, and OCD. The first, *short interval intracortical inhibition* (SICI), is a paired-pulse measure. The first pulse, a subthreshold (below the intensity required to produce a MEP) "conditioning" stimulus, activates the intracortical inhibitory mechanism. After an interstimulus interval of 2 to 5 ms, the second pulse, a suprathreshold "test" stimulus, transsynaptically depolarizes pyramidal output cells (Fig. 9-2). At this interstimulus interval, the paired-pulse-evoked MEP amplitude is typically smaller (inhibited) relative to the single-pulse-evoked MEP amplitude (22). SICI is calculated as the *ratio* of the paired pulse evoked (conditioned) MEP amplitude to the single pulse evoked ("unconditioned") MEP amplitude. The ratio is usually less than 1. When SICI is diminished (motor cortex is disinhibited), the MEP amplitude ratio is higher, approaching or even

exceeding 1 in some cases (23,24). This phenomenon is believed to be mediated by cortical inhibitory interneurons and the gamma-butyric acid A receptors on cortical output cells but may also be affected by subcortical inputs to cortical interneurons and pyramidal cells (21).

The second measure of cortical inhibitory function, the cortical silent period (CSP), is the period of suppression seen in the electromyogram of a voluntarily contracting muscle, following an MEP evoked by TMS (Fig. 9-3). Its basis is less well understood, but its duration is also related to the degree of evokable cortical inhibition (25).

Diminished SICI or a shorter CSP could be surrogate markers for both cortical and subcortical pathological processes. In hyperkinetic disorders due to striatal dysfunction, there may be increased excitatory, glutamatergic output from the disinhibited thalamus to motor cortex. The overexcited motor cortex might be less susceptible to inhibition by cortical interneurons,

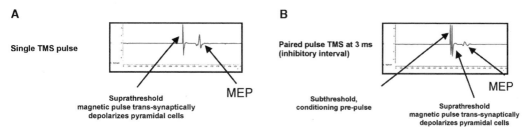

Fig. 9-2. Surface electromyogram tracings after single unconditioned (2a) and 3-msec interstimulus interval conditioned paired pulse (2b) transcranial magnetic stimulations. After the magnetic pulse(s), and a latency that varies with distance and conduction velocity, a motor evoked potential occurs in the target muscle. Although there is significant trial to trial variation (not shown), on average the amplitude of the motor evoked potential after the conditioned pulse (2b) is smaller than that after the single test pulse (2a). The SICI is the conditioned (2b) over the unconditioned (2a) motor evoked potential amplitudes, expressed as a percent or ratio.

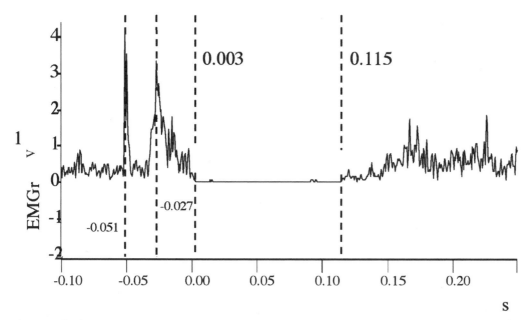

Fig. 9-3. Surface electromyogram tracing in actively contracting muscle shows the cortical silent period. There are four vertical cursors, from left to right: the TMS pulse artifact, the MEP in the target muscle, the cortical silent period onset, and cortical silent period offset. Here the cortical silent period duration based on manually-placed cursors is 112 msec. Cortical silent period onset and offset can also be calculated mathematically (47).

resulting in larger conditioned/unconditioned MEP amplitude ratios (less SICI), or shorter CSPs. Alternatively, in disorders due to dysfunctional cortical inhibitory interneurons, there may be deficient inhibitory capacity within cortex. Dysfunctional intracortical neuronal circuits might be less able to inhibit motor cortex.

Motor Cortex Physiology in Tourette Syndrome

Several studies of cortical inhibition in patients with tic disorders have assessed SICI and the CSP using case-comparison designs. A study comparing adults with TS to healthy controls found reduced SICI (conditioned paired-pulse/

unconditioned single pulse amplitude ratios were larger) in TS (26). There was a trend toward less SICI in a TS subgroup with distal tics. In addition, the CSP measured after pulses that were 10% and 40% above the active motor threshold, was significantly shorter in TS, particularly in the subgroup with distal tics. The presence of ADHD and OCD did not account for significant variance in SICI or CSP.

Two follow-up studies comparing healthy children to children age 10 to 16 years with tic disorders, with ADHD excluded or analyzed as a separate categorical variable, failed to identify reduced SICI in children with tics (27,28). The CSP, measured after a pulse that was 40% above the active motor threshold, was significantly shorter in children with tic disorders.

Motor Cortex Physiology in Obsessive Compulsive Disorder

Using similar experimental paradigms, TMS has been used to compare a cohort of 16 adults with OCD, including five with a history of motor tics, to 11 healthy adults screened extensively for psychopathology (29). In this study, SICI was significantly reduced in subjects with OCD. Subgroup analysis showed the presence of tics was associated with even greater reduction in SICI. However, no correlation was identified between the severity of OCD and reduction in SICI. There were no significant group differences in the length of the cortical silent period after a pulse at 20% above the active motor threshold.

A subsequent study was performed to determine whether altered SICI might be related more generally to anxiety rather than specifically to OCD (30). In this study, 46 healthy volunteers were given the Revised NEO Personality Inventory (NEO-PI-R) personality inventory (31). The results on the neuroticism index, a stable measure of trait-level anxiety and other negative emotions, correlated robustly with SICI (r = 0.48; P <0.001), particularly in the men (r = 0.63; P <0.001).

Motor Cortex Physiology in Attention Deficit Hyperactivity Disorder

In one case-control study, SICI and CSP were compared in children with ADHD ($N = 18$) and healthy controls ($N = 18$) (32). SICI was significantly reduced in the ADHD children, but there was no difference found in CSP, measured after a pulse at 40% above the active motor threshold. Retesting the ADHD children after a single, 10-mg dose of methylphenidate showed increased SICI, although still significantly different from the control group. A subsequent study comparing children with ADHD only ($N = 16$), ADHD plus tics ($N = 16$), tics only ($N = 16$), and no tics or ADHD ($N = 16$) (28) showed that SICI was significantly reduced only in the ADHD groups. CSP was significantly shorter only in the tic disorder groups. Of note, ADHD has also been assessed with several other TMS techniques which measure conduction times and probably reflect dysmaturation of white matter, particularly transcallosal pathways (18,33).

REGRESSION ANALYSIS STUDY OF TICS, ATTENTION DEFICIT HYPERACTIVITY DISORDER, OBSESSIVE COMPULSIVE DISORDER SYMPTOMS, AND CORTICAL INHIBITION IN A TOURETTE SYNDROME COHORT

To clarify inconsistencies in the reported relationships between cortical inhibition and Tic Disorder, ADHD, and OCD diagnoses in children and adults, the author of this chapter recruited a cohort of 35 patients age 8 to 47 years with TS and a broad spectrum of tic, ADHD, and OCD symptoms (34). Tic, ADHD, and OCD symptoms were graded blindly and independently using standard clinical rating scales (35-37). SICI and CSP were measured with TMS techniques similar to those in the case control studies. Correlation and regression analyses were used to estimate the strength of the relationships between current symptom severity and measures of cortical inhibition.

In a univariate analysis, motor tic severity correlated with larger MEP amplitude ratios (r = 0.43, $P = 0.02$); patients with more severe motor tics had less SICI. Post hoc analysis suggested that the motor tic frequency subscale accounted for the most tic-related variance in SICI. However, a more robust univariate correlation was found between larger MEP amplitude ratios (less SICI) and higher ADHD scores

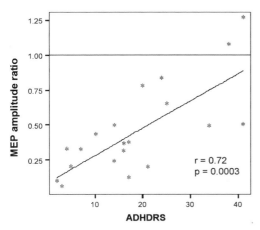

Fig. 9-4. Scatterplot of the attention deficit hyperactivity disorder rating scale (ADHDRS) scores versus 3-msec MEP amplitude ratio (short interval intracortical inhibition) in subjects not taking neuroleptics. Patients with more severe attention deficit hyperactivity disorder symptoms had significantly larger conditioned/unconditioned motor evoked potentials amplitude ratios (less short interval intracortical inhibition). (From Gilbert DL, Bansal AS, Sethuraman G, et al. Association of cortical disinhibition with tic, ADHD, and OCD severity in Tourette syndrome. *Mov Dis.* 2004;19:416-425. Reprinted with permission of Wiley Liss Inc., a subsidiary of John Wiley & Sons, Inc.)

(r = 0.53; P = 0.003), particularly among subjects not taking dopamine 2 (D2)-receptor blocking agents (r = 0.72; P = 0.003) (Fig. 9-4). There was no significant univariate correlation between OCD severity and SICI.

Regression modeling of SICI was performed using the SAS software (The SAS Institute, Inc., Cary, NC). The model was constructed using all demographic (including age) and clinical rating scale variables, with selection of the best fit variables using the maximal r^2 improvement method. This showed that the only significant factors were ADHD and motor tic severity. The severity of ADHD symptoms and motor tics were significantly and independently associated with reduced SICI (r^2 = 0.50; F(2,27) = 13.7; P <0.001), particularly in subjects not taking neuroleptics (r^2 = 0.68; F(2,17) = 17.8; P <0.0001). *Post hoc* analysis suggested that, within ADHD rating scale scores, hyperactivity, rather than inattention, accounted for most of the ADHD-related variance in SICI.

Within this cohort, the range of CSP duration values, measured after a pulse at 30% above the active motor threshold, was consistent with the range reported in the prior case-control studies of patients with tic disorders. However, the study did not identify any clinical or demographic factors that accounted for variance in CSP. In particular, the study found no correlation between tic severity and CSP duration.

Finally, segregating the cohort into four nonoverlapping groups, group means of SICI (MEP amplitude ratios) were: TS only 0.27 (95% CI 0.17–0.41); TS plus OCD 0.28 (95% CI 0.08–1.06); TS plus OCD plus ADHD 0.48 (95% CI 0.28–0.83); TS plus ADHD 0.70 (95% CI 0.47–1.03). SICI differed significantly between these diagnostic groups (one way analysis of variance, F(3,26) = 3.09; P = 0.04). In *post hoc* analysis, after correction for multiple comparisons, the TS plus ADHD group had significantly less SICI (P = 0.05).

The biological validity of dichotomizing ADHD and OCD into present versus not-present in this TS sample is debatable because hyperactivity, impulsivity, inattentiveness, obsessiveness, and compulsiveness were present to some degree in most TS patients. Thus assigning the cut-off value to scale scores in order to make a diagnosis may be arbitrary from the standpoint of research into surrogate markers of neurobehavioral phenotypes. The stronger association between SICI and current ADHD symptoms may be an indication that, compared with tics, hyperactive/impulsive behaviors are anatomically or temporally more closely linked with cortical inhibitory function. A recent quantitative magnetic resonance imaging study implicated more frontal-cortical involvement in ADHD than in TS (38). If TS is viewed as an episodic disorder (39) possibly related more to phasic than tonic neurotransmitter levels it may be the case that SICI fluctuates in TS and is more normal "between tics" (12). Further studies using TMS in TS may need to assess patients during periods of frequent tics.

The reported strong correlation in a study of healthy adult volunteers between anxiety-related neuroticism scores on the NEO-PI-R personality inventory (30) and SICI is intriguing in light of our findings that, within a TS cohort, SICI

TABLE 9-1. *Measures of inhibitory function in motor cortex in children and adults with Tic disorders, attention deficit hyperactivity disorder, and obsessive compulsive disorder*

Study Sample	Subjects, N	Age	SICI (ratio)	S (NS)	CSP in msec	S (NS)	Reference
TD + ADHD + OCD	20	A	0.64	**TD** (ADHD) (OCD)	127	**TD** (ADHD) (OCD)	Ziemann 1997 (45); SICI 1-4 msec; CSP at AMT + 40%
Control	21		0.41		166		
OCD + TD	5	A	~0.88	**OCD**	116	(OCD)	Greenberg 2000 (46);
OCD	11		~0.70	**TD**			SICI at 3 msec; CSP at
Control	11		0.33		103		AMT + 20%
TD + OCD	21	C	0.61	(TD) (OCD)	150	**TD** (OCD)	Moll 1999 (27); SICI at 2-4 msec; CSP at AMT +40%
Control	25		0.57		176		
ADHD	18	C	0.97	**ADHD**	163	(ADHD)	Moll 2000 (32); SICI at 2-5 msec; CSP at AMT + 40%
Control	18		0.66		160		
ADHD + TD	16	C	0.88	**ADHD** (TD)	137	**TD** (ADHD)	Moll 2001 (28); SICI at 2-5 msec; CSP at AMT + 40%
TD	16		0.71		138		
ADHD	16		0.87		172		
Control	16		0.70		163		
TD + ADHD	6	M	0.70	**ADHD**	88	(ADHD)	Gilbert 2004 (34); SICI
TD + ADHD + OCD	8		0.48	(TD)	79	(TD)	at 3 msec; CSP at AMT + 30%
TD + OCD	5		0.28	(OCD)	68	(OCD)	
TD	11		0.27		88		
				Regression analysis			
Factor			*SICI* r^2		*CSP* r^2		
ADHD	30	M	0.25	**ADHD**	-	(ADHD)	
Motor tic			0.22	**Motor tic**	-	(Motor tic)	
(OCD)			-	(OCD)	-	(OCD)	

As shown in reference column, studies differed in interstimulus intervals used to measure short interval cortical inhibition and pulse intensity used to measure cortical silent period. Other differences which may affect TMS measures include intensity of the conditioning pulse for short interval cortical inhibition, coil type, target intrinsic hand muscle, co-morbid diagnoses, and use of medications, particularly neuroleptics. Relationships that were statistically significant are in **bold**. Those which were evaluated and not found significant are in (regular type). N = number of subjects. A, adult; ADHD; attention deficit hyperactivity disorder; C, children; CSP, cortical silent period; M, mixed children and adult; NS, not statistically significant; OCD, obsessive compulsive disorder; S, statistically significant; SICI, short interval cortical inhibition; TD, tic disorders; AMT, active motor threshold.

correlated most strongly with ADHD severity, less strongly with tics, and not at all with OCD severity. Another small study using this inventory in adults found higher scores on the neuroticism index in adults with ADD (40). This suggests disturbances in cortical inhibitory function may underlie both common maladaptive personality traits and ADHD behaviors. Careful, representative sample selection and screening for psychopathology, even in "normal controls," is critical in order to clarify the relationships between cortical inhibitory function and neurobehavioral phenotypes. In postmenarchal females, stage of the menstrual cycle may also account for some variation (41).

CONCLUSIONS

The balance of inhibition and excitation in motor cortex appears to be altered in patients with TS, ADHD, and OCD. Although the neurophysiologic function of subcortical structures cannot be assessed noninvasively, TMS is a well-tolerated, noninvasive technique that can be used to quantify fundamental neurophysiologic properties relating to inhibitory function at the cortical node of the cortical-subcortical circuits, in children and adults (Table 9-1). Two measures, SICI and CSP, appear to differentiate patients with tics, OCD, and ADHD from matched controls. CSP appears generally to be shorter in tic disorders in children and adults, particularly in adults with distal tics, although the study failed to find any correlation between CSP duration and any aspect of tic severity. SICI appears most strongly associated with the presence of ADHD symptoms, in case control and correlational design studies.

There are a number of limitations that must be considered in interpreting the studies summarized in this review. First, as in neuroimaging studies, the quantitative differences between affected and unaffected persons are significant in terms of group means, but there is substantial variation within groups and overlap between groups. Thus a particular CSP duration or SICI MEP amplitude ratio is not diagnostic of the presence of TS, OCD, or ADHD. The overlap in quantitative physiologic or imaging variables between those affected and unaffected by neurobehavioral disorders is not surprising, given the high prevalence of some degree of many of these behaviors in the general population, and the inherent difficulties of rating behavior with subjective scales. Second, all studies to date have involved fairly small samples-of-convenience, thus there exists the possibility of confounding due to unmeasured factors. However, the corroboration of the case-control results in ADHD (28,32) with the robust correlation the study identified between ADHD symptom severity and SICI (34) makes confounding less likely. Third, there are some differences in laboratory techniques between studies. For example, interstimulus intervals used to measure SICI and the pulse strength used for measuring CSP varied between reported studies. The increasing availability of normative data (42,43) and of data on the effects of differing TMS techniques on the variability of neurophysiologic measures (44) has been helpful.

Finally, although TMS pulses evoke cortical neuronal potentials, one cannot determine whether inhibitory abnormalities result from intracortical pathology or subcortical pathology projecting to motor cortex. Fundamentally, it is unknown at the cellular level which populations of neurons are activated by TMS in various paradigms. Achieving additional insights may require combining genetic or neuroimaging data with neurophysiologic measures in a larger, carefully characterized cohort.

ACKNOWLEDGMENTS

This research was supported by a generous grant from the Tourette Syndrome Association, by NINDS K23 NS41920. The author thanks Jie Zhang for expert technical assistance.

REFERENCES

1. Singer HS. Current issues in Tourette syndrome. *Mov Disord.* 2000;15:1051–1063.
2. Penney JB Jr, Young AB. Speculations on the functional anatomy of basal ganglia disorders. *Annu Rev Neurosci.* 1983;6:73–94.
3. Alexander GE, DeLong MR, Strick PL. Parallel organization of functionally segregated circuits linking basal ganglia and cortex. *Annu Rev Neurosci.* 1986;9:357–381.
4. Mink JW. Basal ganglia dysfunction in Tourette's syndrome: a new hypothesis. *Pediatr Neurol.* 2001;25: 190–198.
5. Singer HS. Neurobiology of Tourette syndrome. *Neurol Clin.* 1997;15:357–379.
6. Saxena S, Brody AL, Maidment KM, et al. Localized orbitofrontal and subcortical metabolic changes and predictors of response to paroxetine treatment in obsessive–compulsive disorder. *Neuropsychopharmacology* 1999;21:683–693.
7. Durston S, Tottenham NT, Thomas KM, et al. Differential patterns of striatal activation in young children with and without ADHD. *Biol Psychiatry.* 2003;53: 871–878.
8. Alexander GE, DeLong MR. Microstimulation of the primate neostriatum. II. Somatotopic organization of striatal microexcitable zones and their relation to neuronal response properties. *J Neurophysiol.* 1985;53:1417–1430.
9. Peterson BS, Thomas P, Kane MJ, et al. Basal ganglia volumes in patients with Gilles de la Tourette syndrome. *Arch GenPsychiatry.* 2003;60:415–424.
10. Peterson BS, Skudlarski P, Anderson AW, et al. A functional magnetic resonance imaging study of tic suppression in Tourette syndrome. *Arch Gen Psychiatry.* 1998;55:326–333.
11. Albin RL, Koeppe RA, Bohnen NI, et al. Increased ventral striatal monoaminergic innervation in Tourette syndrome. *Neurology;* 2003;61:310–315.
12. Singer HS, Szymanski S, Giuliano J, et al. Elevated intrasynaptic dopamine release in Tourette's syndrome measured by PET. *Am J Psychiatry.* 2002;159: 1329–1336.
13. Post RM, Speer AM, Weiss SR, et al. Seizure models: anticonvulsant effects of ECT and rTMS. *Prog Neuropsychopharmacol Biol Psychiatry.* 2000;24:1251–1273.
14. Garvey MA, Kaczynski KJ, Becker DA, et al. Subjective reactions of children to single–pulse transcranial magnetic stimulation. *J Child Neurol.* 2001;16:891–894.
15. Gilbert DL, Garvey MA, Bansal AS, et al. Should transcranial magnetic stimulation research in children be considered minimal risk? *Clin Neurophysiol.* 2004;115: 1730–1739.

16. Muller K, Homberg V, Lenard HG. Magnetic stimulation of motor cortex and nerve roots in children. Maturation of cortico–motoneuronal projections. *Electroencephalogr Clin Neurophysiol.* 1991;81:63–70.

17. Eyre JA, Taylor JP, Villagra F, et al. Evidence of activity–dependent withdrawal of corticospinal projections during human development. *Neurology* 2001;57:1543–1554.

18. Ucles P, Lorente S, Rosa F. Neurophysiological methods testing the psychoneural basis of attention deficit hyperactivity disorder. *Childs Nerv Syst.* 1996;12:215–217.

19. Muller K, Homberg V, Aulich A, et al. Magnetoelectrical stimulation of motor cortex in children with motor disturbances. *Electroencephalogr Clin Neurophysiol.* 1992;85:86–94.

20. Brown P, Ridding MC, Werhahn KJ, et al. Abnormalities of the balance between inhibition and excitation in the motor cortex of patients with cortical myoclonus. *Brain* 1996;119:309–317.

21. Ziemann U, Tergau F, Wischer S, et al. Pharmacological control of facilitatory I–wave interaction in the human motor cortex. A paired transcranial magnetic stimulation study. *Electroencephalogr Clin Neurophysiol.* 1998;109:321–330.

22. Kujirai T, Caramia MD, Rothwell JC, et al. Corticocortical inhibition in human motor cortex. *J Physiol.* 1993; 471:501–519.

23. Nakamura H, Kitagawa H, Kawaguchi Y, et al. Intracortical facilitation and inhibition after transcranial magnetic stimulation in conscious humans. *J Physiol.* 1997;498:817–823.

24. Di Lazzaro V, Restuccia D, Oliviero A, et al. Magnetic transcranial stimulation at intensities below active motor threshold activates intracortical inhibitory circuits. *Exp Brain Res.* 1998;119:265–268.

25. Werhahn KJ, Kunesch E, Noachtar S, et al. Differential effects on motorcortical inhibition induced by blockade of GABA uptake in humans. *J Physiol.* 1999;517: 591–597.

26. Ziemann U, Paulus W, Rothenberger A. Decreased motor inhibition in Tourette's disorder: evidence from transcranial magnetic stimulation. *Am J Psychiatry.* 1997;154:1277–1284.

27. Moll GH, Wischer S, Heinrich H, et al. Deficient motor control in children with tic disorder: evidence from transcranial magnetic stimulation. *Neurosci Lett.* 1999; 272:37–40.

28. Moll GH, Heinrich H, Trott G, et al. Children with comorbid attention–deficit–hyperactivity disorder and tic disorder: Evidence for additive inhibitory deficits within the motor system. *Ann Neurol.* 2001; 49:393–396.

29. Greenberg BD, Ziemann U, Cora–Locatelli G, et al. Altered cortical excitability in obsessive–compulsive disorder. *Neurology* 2000;54:142–147.

30. Wassermann EM, Greenberg BD, Nguyen MB, et al. Motor cortex excitability correlates with an anxiety-related personality trait. *Biol Psychiatry.* 2001;50: 377–382.

31. Costa PT, McCrae RR. *Revised NEO Personality Inventory (NEO–PI–R) and NEO Five–Factor Inventory (NEO–FFI) Professional Manual.* Odessa, FL: Psychological Assessment Resources; 1992.

32. Moll GH, Heinrich H, Trott G, et al. Deficient intracortical inhibition in drug–naive children with attention–deficit hyperactivity disorder is enhanced by methylphenidate. *Neurosci Lett.* 2000;284:121–125.

33. Buchmann J, Wolters A, Haessler F, et al. Disturbed transcallosally mediated motor inhibition in children with attention deficit hyperactivity disorder (ADHD). *Clin Neurophysiol.* 2003;114:2036–2042.

34. Gilbert DL, Bansal AS, Sethuraman G, et al. Association of cortical disinhibition with tic, ADHD, and OCD severity in Tourette syndrome. *Mov Disord.* 2004;19: 416–425.

35. Leckman JF, Riddle MA, Hardin MT, et al. The Yale Global Tic Severity Scale: initial testing of a clinician–rated scale of tic severity. *J Am Acad Child Adolesc Psychiatry;* 1989;28:566–573.

36. DuPaul GJ, Power TJ, Anastopoulos AD, et al. *ADHD Rating Scale–IV: Checklist, norms, and clinical interpretations.* New York: Guilford Press; 1998.

37. Scahill L, Riddle MA, McSwiggin–Hardin M, et al. Children's Yale–Brown Obsessive Compulsive Scale: reliability and validity. *J Am Acad Child Adolesc Psychiatry.* 1997;36:844–852.

38. Kates WR, Frederikse M, Mostofsky SH, et al. MRI parcellation of the frontal lobe in boys with attention deficit hyperactivity disorder or Tourette syndrome. *Psychiatry Research;* 2002;116:63–81.

39. Peterson BS, Leckman JF. The temporal dynamics of tics in Gilles de la Tourette syndrome. *Biol Psychiatry.* 1998;44:1337–1348.

40. Ranseen JD, Campbell DA, Baer RA. NEO PI–R profiles of adults with attention deficit disorder. *Assessment* 1998;5:19–24.

41. Smith MJ, Adams LF, Schmidt PJ, et al. Effects of ovarian hormones on human cortical excitability. *Ann Neurol.* 2002;51:599–603.

42. Wassermann EM. Variation in the response to transcranial magnetic brain stimulation in the general population. *Clin Neurophysiol.* 2002;113:1165–1171.

43. Garvey MA, Ziemann U, Bartko JJ, et al. Cortical correlates of neuromotor development in healthy children. *Clin Neurophysiol.* 2003;114:1662–1670.

44. Orth M, Snijders AH, Rothwell JC, et al. The variability of intracortical inhibition and facilitation. *Clin Neurophysiol.* 2003;114:2362–2369.

45. Ziemann U, Paulus W, Rothenberger A. Decreased motor inhibition in Tourette's disorder: evidence from transcranial magnetic stimulation. *Am J Psychiatry.* 1997;154:1277–1284.

46. Greenberg BD, Ziemann U, Cora–Locatelli G, et al. Altered cortical excitability in obsessive–compulsive disorder. *Neurology.* 2000;54:142–147.

47. Garvey MA, Ziemann U, Becker DA, et al. New graphical method to measure silent periods evoked by transcranial magnetic stimulation. *Clin Neurophysiol.* 2001;112:1451–1460.

10

Functional Neuroimaging of Tourette Syndrome: Advances and Future Directions

Tracy Butler[1], Emily Stern[2], and David Silbersweig[3]

1,3Division of Neuropsychiatry, New York Presbyterian Hospital, Department of Psychiatry, Weill Medical College of Cornell University; 2Weill Medical College of Cornell University, Departments of Psychiatry and Neurology

Functional neuroimaging provides an in vivo, noninvasive index of systems-level localized brain activity that can be used to probe neurocircuitry of interest in disorders such as Tourette syndrome (TS). There is much evidence from functional neuroimaging as well as other lines of research suggesting that the pathophysiology of TS involves dysfunction of specific cortical-subcortical neurocircuitry known to mediate motor and emotional/motivational behaviors.

Imaging modalities discussed here include single photon emitted computed tomography (SPECT), positron emission tomography (PET) using tracers reflective of metabolic activity or blood flow; and functional magnetic resonance imaging (fMRI). These modalities as well as related neuroimaging methods and complementary neurophysiological techniques, are part of a translational spectrum of research approaches from animal/basic science research to clinical studies, aimed at elucidating the precise nature and location of this dysfunctional neurocircuitry in TS, with the ultimate goal of informing development of appropriate, targeted therapy.

FUNCTIONAL NEUROIMAGING TECHNIQUES

The broad purpose of functional neuroimaging is to assess neuronal function in specific brain regions. Because noninvasive, direct assessment of neuronal activity is not currently possible, available techniques rely upon various indirect measures of neuronal activity, each of which has its own benefits and limitations. Neuronal activity is closely, though imperfectly coupled to each of these measures via brain metabolic and vascular autoregulation. Measures commonly used in humans include glucose uptake ([FDG] PET); blood flow (SPECT, $H_2^{15}O$ PET; arterial spin labeling fMRI); and blood oxygenation level dependent (BOLD) fMRI. Techniques that have been applied to the study of TS are briefly described.

Single Photon Emitted Computed Tomography

SPECT imaging utilizes an injected gamma-emitting radionuclide, commonly technetium^{99} (Tc99). Because creation of gamma-emitting radioisotopes does not require a cyclotron, SPECT is more widely available than other functional neuroimaging techniques. Although SPECT ligands have been used in TS to examine the density of specific neuroreceptors, this review focuses on SPECT studies of blood flow using Tc99-hexamethylpropylene-amine-oxime or Tc99-ethylcysteinate dimer, both of which provide a "snapshot" of cerebral perfusion during the 30 seconds to 1 minute following injection.

Positron Emission Tomography

PET utilizes positron-emitting radioisotopes, which can be created only with the use of a cyclotron, limiting the availability of this technique. When an emitted positron collides with an electron, two gamma particles are created. Through coincidence detection of these two gamma particles, the location in the brain of the original positron can be accurately determined, providing better spatial resolution with PET than is possible with SPECT. FDG PET studies produce an image reflecting brain activity integrated over approximately 30 minutes. As with SPECT, PET ligands have been used to investigate neuroreceptor binding in TS, although this review focuses on PET blood flow and metabolism studies.

$H_2{}^{15}O$ is a diffusible tracer that measures blood flow. Its 2-minute half-life allows repeated injections during a study session, which makes it possible to examine changes in blood flow pattern in response to specific experimental conditions or subject activities. By measuring blood concentration of radiotracer, quantitative measures of regional blood flow can be obtained using PET, which can facilitate comparisons between different subject groups.

Functional Magnetic Resonance Imaging

fMRI, like structural MRI, detects signal based on differences in the chemical environment of protons in either the brain itself or in flowing blood. The BOLD signal represents the venous decrease in deoxyhemoglobin that accompanies increased blood flow to active brain regions. Another, recently-developed fMRI technique is arterial spin labeling in which signal from blood magnetically labeled in lower slices is detected when it reaches slices of interest in the brain, providing an absolute measure of regional cerebral blood flow (rCBF), analogous to that obtained with quantitative PET techniques (1–3). Quantification of blood flow is not possible with BOLD. The advantages of fMRI include the fact that it is noninvasive and (in most cases) does not require injection of any tracer; it

involves no radiation, making it easily repeatable and more appropriate for children; it provides an extended time series of brain activation data and can therefore be used to study multiple experimental conditions, including event-related paradigms; and it has better temporal and spatial resolution. Limitations of fMRI include its lower signal-to-noise ratio compared to other modalities; its sensitivity to subject movement; the issue of susceptibility artifact in frontal and temporal brain regions; and the fact that the scanner itself is loud and somewhat more physically confining than other image acquisition machines.

NEUROIMAGING ISSUES SPECIFIC TO TOURETTE SYNDROME

In some respects, TS is ideally suited to investigation using functional neuroimaging techniques: it has a prevalence of 5 to 300 cases per 10,000 (4), providing an adequate pool of potential subjects; patients are usually of average or above-average intelligence, and therefore able to consent to research studies and cooperate with investigators' requests; and the key TS symptom—tics—are observable and quantifiable, unlike many neuropsychiatric symptoms, which are accessible only through sometimes-unreliable patient self report. Yet despite greatly increased availability of functional neuroimaging techniques such as fMRI, functional imaging studies of TS have been few. Since publication of a prior review of TS neuroimaging in this series in 2001 (5), fewer than 10 new functional neuroimaging studies of TS could be identified through a search of the scientific literature. This contrasts with a relative explosion in the number of fMRI studies performed on control subjects, or on patients suffering from other neuropsychiatric syndromes such as depression or schizophrenia.

Several unique aspects of TS may account for the paucity of functional neuroimaging studies. The presence of tic-associated head or body movements poses obvious practical difficulties during scanning, especially in fMRI studies. In addition, tics create confounds in experimental design and interpretation, insofar as TS patients, but not control subjects, will often be either ticcing or trying not to tic during any experimental condition.

TS is primarily a disorder in childhood. Although several functional neuroimaging studies in children with TS have been published (6,7), such studies are in general difficult due to the issue of radiation exposure. Even noninvasive, radiation-free techniques such as fMRI pose problems for children in terms of remaining still throughout the experiment in an enclosed space. The developmental trajectory complicates interpretation of functional imaging studies in children, who mature in different domains at very different rates, requiring the use of developmentally appropriate activation paradigms. Functional neuroimaging studies of adult TS patients, while important and easier to perform, may be investigating cases of more severe, persistent or atypical disease (8).

Diagnosing TS is not straightforward despite the increasing availability of validated diagnostic instruments (9). Diagnostic uncertainty and clinical heterogeneity among patients with TS can confound functional neuroimaging results unless careful clinical assessment of subjects is used to identify and quantify TS symptomatology. Furthermore, TS patients differ not only in their manifestations of the disorder, but in the presence or absence of co-morbid/related conditions such as attention deficit hyperactivity disorder (ADHD) and obsessive compulsive disorder (OCD), symptoms of which must be identified and characterized in order to accurately interpret functional neuroimaging findings. Given the range of normal functioning, even normal control subjects probably require rigorous clinical assessment to determine where they fall on a neurobehavioral spectrum.

FUNCTIONAL NEUROIMAGING APPROACHES

Functional imaging approaches can be divided into several main categories, each of which can provide complementary information when studying patients with TS, and each of which

may be more or less appropriate for use with PET, SPECT, and fMRI.

Resting state studies acquire images of brain function while subjects are not engaged in any investigator-specified task. Such studies can demonstrate regional differences in brain function between patients and controls that are present regardless of activity state, and which may or may not be associated with detectable structural alterations. There is evidence for specific "idling" states of activity in different brain regions (10). FDG PET and SPECT are commonly considered resting state studies, although as noted previously, there are important differences between patients with TS and normal control subjects during supposed rest, when TS patients may be actively ticcing or trying to inhibit tics. fMRI can also be used to investigate the resting state, using either arterial spin labeling techniques to provide a quantitative measure of rCBF (1–3), or through post-processing analysis techniques (11), though no resting state fMRI studies of TS have yet been reported.

Activation paradigms involve acquisition of functional images while subjects are presented with specific stimuli or are asked to engage in an investigator-specified cognitive or motor/behavioral task. Task-related brain activity can be ascertained through comparison to brain activity during a baseline or control task (subtraction), a task sharing key features (conjunction) or by examining how brain activity varies with stepwise alterations in experimental variables (correlational or parametric design.) Activation paradigms require sufficient temporal resolution to distinguish brain activity between experimental conditions, as is possible with fMRI and $H_2^{15}O$ PET studies. Typically, experimental tasks and stimuli will be designed to probe brain regions, circuits, or functions of interest, based on clinical symptomatology, neurobiological models, or prior research findings. Activation tasks used in functional neuroimaging studies of TS include hand movements (12,13), voluntary mimicking of tics (14), and voluntary suppression of tics (15). Development of additional tasks that are compatible with neuroimaging and relevant to the pathophysiology of TS is an active area of functional neuroimaging research (16,17).

Activation paradigms can provide critical information about the brain in action, performing specific functions, as occurs in real-world functioning. However, use of activation tasks introduces the potential confound of task performance (e.g., speed, accuracy, strategy, effort, compensation), which may vary systematically between patients and controls. Furthermore, certain assumptions (e.g., that it is valid to subtract control activity from task-related activity, that a task activates relevant neurocircuitry) underlie most activation paradigms. Such factors must be considered when designing or interpreting activation studies.

Symptom capture (or symptom provocation) studies focusing on a key/defining neuropsychiatric symptom represent a naturalistic inroad to the pathophysiology of a disorder with minimal assumptions (18–20). With respect to TS, symptom capture can be applied to tics, which are allowed to occur naturally during functional neuroimaging, with careful attention paid to their precise nature and timing, so brain activity associated with tics can be compared to brain activity during periods when no tics are occurring. Symptom capture paradigms require an imaging modality with good temporal resolution (f MRI or [^{15}OH$_2$]O PET) and careful patient selection to ensure sufficient tics are recorded during the study period, with minimal head movement. Given that TS is a disorder in which manifestations vary tremendously between patients, this approach may be especially well suited for study of individual patients. This approach also allows the neural circuitry associated with the core symptoms to be identified in an unbiased manner.

IMAGE PROCESSING AND ANALYSIS

All neuroimaging modalities require postacquisition image processing and image analysis, to produce an interpretable "picture" (usually a statistical image) indicating localized brain activity. Image processing and analysis may be computationally and mathematically intensive. Not widely appreciated among non-neuroimagers is the fact that the specific processing and analysis techniques used, and the assumptions underlying them, can impact results significantly. Understanding basic aspects of image processing

and analysis can facilitate an understanding of the possibilities, as well as the limitations of functional neuroimaging studies of TS.

Image processing requires multiple steps, which vary in nature and complexity by imaging modality. For example, f MRI requires careful alignment of each scan in the functional series, with mathematical correction for small amounts of head movement. Correction for larger head movements is not usually possible, which limits the utility of f MRI in studying TS patients with neck, head, or sometimes vocal tics. After realignment, functional images are commonly coregistered to high-resolution structural MRI scans to allow precise localization of brain activity. The BOLD signal may be high-pass and/or low-pass filtered to remove various sources of noise. To facilitate group analysis of functional data, individual scans are often morphed to match a template brain, and data may be spatially smoothed to increase the likelihood of intersubject overlap in activation patterns (as well as to facilitate certain statistical analyses.) Analysis of structural data using techniques such as manual tracing of brain regions of interest or voxel-based morphometry can identify structural alterations associated with or underlying functional findings. Each of these processing steps, while important, raises the possibility of pitfalls.

Image analysis depends to a great extent on the modality and the imaging approach, as discussed previously, but can be divided into several broad categories: Studies can focus on a particular brain region of interest (ROI); can assess function across the entire brain using voxel-wise techniques such as statistical parametric mapping (21), necessitating correction for multiple comparisons; or can utilize some combination of ROI and voxel-based approaches. Analysis can be as simple as a t-test to compare image intensity in a given region between patients and controls, or may require sophisticated statistical modeling to extract relevant signal from noise. Multiple linear regression models allow the identification of neural activity associated with specific effects of interest, controlling for potentially confounding variables. Analyses incorporating subject characteristics, scanning parameters and other possibly relevant factors may be useful. Multivariate statistical methods can be used to evaluate relationships among brain regions.

Single Photon Emitted Computed Tomography Studies of Tourette Syndrome

Most functional neuroimaging studies of TS have been SPECT studies, likely because of the wide availability and ease of use of this technique in clinical settings. SPECT studies of TS tend to be less sophisticated and reliable, though the more recent studies have used careful subject selection and characterization and appropriate analysis techniques, providing useful results. In general, most SPECT studies have demonstrated abnormally decreased blood flow in the basal ganglia, and altered symmetry, with greater left-sided dysfunction, though there are important variations in subjects, techniques and results, as listed in Table 10-1.

Fluorodeoxyglucose Positron Emission Tomography Studies of Tourette Syndrome

An early functional neuroimaging study of TS was performed by Chase et al. (42). Twelve drug-free adult TS patients and 12 controls underwent FDG PET scanning. There was a 15% reduction in glucose utilization rates in TS patients relative to controls in horizontal section from 8.4 to 8.8 cm caudal to the vertex, encompassing inferior striatum and frontal, cingulate, and possibly insular cortex. Lack of precise anatomical information is a limitation of this early study. An inverse correlation was found between tic severity and glucose utilization in these regions. This study demonstrated decreased activity in subcortical brain regions including basal ganglia in TS, a finding which has been replicated in multiple subsequent studies.

In an enlightening series of FDG PET studies, Braun et al. (43–45) have furthered an understanding of anatomic regions implicated in TS and their interrelation. In an initial comparison of 16 adult TS patients (who were drug-free for at least 2 weeks) with 16 healthy control subjects (43), they demonstrated decreased normalized metabolic rates in orbitofrontal regions,

insula, parahippocampi, ventral striatum, and midbrain in TS. *Increased* metabolic activity in the supplemental motor area (SMA), lateral premotor area, and primary motor cortex were found in TS compared with controls. These changes discriminated TS patients from controls and were interpreted as indicating an altered relation between emotion/motivation-related regions and motor-related regions. Impairments in subcortical/basal ganglia activity were consistent with most SPECT studies. Increased activity in motor-related regions could have been due to tics, or attempts to suppress tics, at the time of scanning. The authors reported that tics during scanning were rare, but did not quantify their occurrence.

Expanding their cohort of TS patients to 18, a follow-up study correlated patterns of regional cerebral activity with neuropsychologic impairment and degree of neurobehavioral symptoms consisting of OCD, echophenomena, coprolalia, impulsivity, self-injurious behavior, and depression (44). Although the validity of grouping these diverse symptoms together can be questioned, it is nonetheless interesting that increased expression of these behaviors and of neuropsychological dysfunction was associated with *increased* metabolism in orbitofrontal regions (and to lesser extent, putamen). Given that orbitofrontal activity was actually decreased in these same TS patients as compared to healthy controls (43), and orbitofrontal lesions commonly cause behavioral disinhibition (46), the interpretation of these findings was that increased orbitofrontal glucose utilization may represent dysfunctional modulation or compensatory orbitofrontal activity in the most severely behaviorally and cognitively affected TS patients.

Additional analyses on these same 18 TS patients and 16 control subjects aimed to move beyond documenting simple increases or decreases in localized brain activity to examine correlations between brain regions, and how such correlations may differ between TS patients and controls (45,47). A total of 182 ROIs were identified, and the degree of correlation between all ROI pairs was computed and compared between TS patients and controls. A key difference between TS patients and controls was

TABLE 10-1. *Single photon emitted computed tomography studies of Tourette syndrome*

Authors	Year	Subjects	Patient characterization	State assessment	Processing/Analysis	Findings
Hall et al. (22)	1991	Adults and children; 25 TS	NR	"...involuntary movements before, during, and ... after injection"	Visual interpretation	Perfusion deficits in frontal, parietal and temporal cortices, especially head of caudate and mesial temporal
George et al. (23)	1992	Adults; 20 TS, half with OCD; 8 NC	Exam, YBOC, LOI, symptom history	eyes open, "largely quiet... and free of tics"	ROI/visual cortex ratios	↑ R frontal rCBF in TS; no effect of comorbid OCD
Riddle et al. (24)	1992	Adults; 9 TS; 9 NC	NR	"eyes and ears covered"	ROI/whole brain (minus cerebellum) ratios	↓ L putamen/globus pallidus rCBF in TS; tic severity correlated with L thalamic rCBF
Sieg et al. (25)	1993	1 TS (11-year-old child)	NR	NR	Visual interpretation	↓ L BG rCBF
Moriarty et al. (26)	1995	Adults; 50 TS (half with OCD); 20 NC	DSM-III criteria, BDI, Tic severity and OCD questions	"at rest with their eyes open"; shorter scans in pts with disruptive tics	ROI/visual cortex ratios	↓ L caudate, L DLPFC, ACC rCBF in TS; tic severity correlated with L caudate, ACC, L medial temporal hypoperfusion.
Moriarty et al. (27)	1997	20 TS family members, half children: 8 TS, 3 OCD, 1 tics, 1 tic + OCD, 7 unaffected.	DSM-III criteria, NHSTRD	"rest, eyes closed"; visual analog anxiety scale	Qualitative comparison to normal scan database; ROI/cerebellum ratios	↓ striatal, frontal, temporal rCBF in family members of TS pts. with tic or OCD symptoms.
Klieger et al. (28)	1997	Adults; 6 TS; 9 NC;	DSM-III criteria	"eyes open in a quiet, dimly lit room"	ROI/cerebellum ratios	↓ R BG rCBF, ↑BG asymmetry in TS
Lampreave et al. (29)	1998	Children; 15 TS (6–16), 13 rescanned medicated; 13 young adult NC	YGTSS	"eyes open in a quiet, dimly lit room"	ROI/cerebellum ratios; factor analysis	↑ rCBF in b/l orbitofrontal, mesial frontal and temporal regions in TS, improved with neuroleptic treatment

Crespo-Facorro et al. (30)	1999	Adults; 20 OCD; 7 OCD with tics; 16 NC	YBOCS; HAM; MADRS; YGTSS; SCID	Resting, supine, eyes closed; "motor tics were not reported"	ROI/cerebellum ratios	↓ rCBF in R orbitofrontal in OCD pts *without* tics compared with NC; no rCBF differences between OCD pts. with and without TS
Chiu et al. (6)	2001	Children (6–15); 27 TS; 11 CT	TSCG criteria; DSM-III-R criteria for ADHD; LOI; Parent Symptom Questionnaire	NR	Inspection; ROI/cerebellum ratios; asymmetry indices	↓ left temporal; asymmetric frontal and temporal rCBF in TS versus CT
Diler et al. (7)	2002	Children (7–14); 38 TS; 18 NC	DSM-IV criteria; CDI; MOCQ; Goetz scale	Eyes open; no disruptive tics based on Goetz scale (35)	ROI/occipital ratios	↓ L caudate, ACC, R cerebellum, L DLPFC, L orbitofrontal in TS; Vocal tic severity correlated with rCBF in cerebellum, DLPFC

Abbreviations and test names with references: ACC, anterior cingulate cortex; BDI, Beck Depression Inventory (33); BG, basal ganglia; b/l, bilateral; CDI, Children's Depression Inventory (CDI) (Psychological Corporation, 1992); Conner Parent Symptom Questionnaire; CT, chronic tic disorder; DSM-III, *Diagnostic and Statistical Manual of Mental Disorders, 3rd ed.*; DSM-IV, *Diagnostic and Statistical Manual of Mental Disorders, 4th ed.*; DLPFC, dorsolateral prefrontal cortex; Goetz scale (35); HAM, Hamilton Depression Rating Scale (37); L, left; LOI, Leyton Obsessional Inventory (34); MADRS, Montgomery-Asberg Depression Rating Scale (38); MOCQ, Maudsley Obsessive Compulsive Questionnaire (36); NC, normal control subjects; NHSTRD, National Hospital schedule for tics and related disorder (31); NR, not reported; OCD, patients with obsessive compulsive disorder; R, right; ROI, region of interest; rCBF, regional cerebral blood flow; SCID, Structured Clinical Interview for Diagnosis based on DSM (40); TS, patients with Tourette Syndrome; TSCG, Tourette Syndrome Classification Group (41); YBOC, Yale-Brown Obsessive-Compulsive Scale (32); YGTSS, Yale Global Tic Severity Scale (39).

reversal of the functional relationship between ventral striatum and motor and premotor cortices: The correlation was negative in controls, but positive in TS. This abnormal coupling of limbic/paralimbic regions with motor structures in TS was interpreted as suggesting abnormal crosstalk between normally-segregated cortico-striatal-thalamocortical (CSTC) loops for motor and emotional/motivational functioning (48), perhaps related to the effect of an abnormal dopaminergic system. Another possible explanation relates to divergent activity at time of scan: TS patients, but not control subjects, were engaging in or suppressing tics during scanning. Without careful quantification of tic occurrence and/or suppression, it is difficult to know whether this important difference in the relationship between emotion-related brain areas and motor-related areas is a core aspect of TS pathophysiology, or an epiphenomenon of its symptomatology (or both).

This issue is addressed in another FDG PET study (49) using the technique of Scaled Subprofile Model to extract patterns of regional metabolic covariation and determine extent of pattern expression in individual subjects. Ten drug-free TS patients with mild to moderate disease and 10 healthy control subjects were studied. Two basic patterns of brain activity were found: covariance pattern 1 consisted of increased activity in movement-related cortical regions, which had been previously found to be nonspecifically activated in hyperkinetic movement disorders. Covariance pattern 1 was therefore considered an epiphenomenon of movement during scanning. Covariance pattern 2, in contrast, consisting of decreased activity in left caudate, bilateral thalamus, lentiform nuclei, temporal regions and midbrain, correlated with the severity of TS. Although there were no significant differences in the expression of covariance pattern 2 between TS patients and normal controls, these findings are nonetheless suggestive of dysfunctional CSTC loops in TS.

In a case study of one patient with severe TS and OCD, [^{15}O]H$_2$O PET showed caudate and thalamic hypermetabolism which normalized after surgical lesioning of the anterior hypothalamus and inferior anterior cingulate gyrus (limbic leucotomy) (50). Systematic pre treatment and post-treatment functional neuroimaging

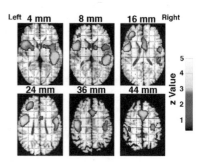

Fig. 10-1. Stereotactic axial sections of brain areas with significantly increased activity during tics (motor and vocal) in six patients with Tourette syndrome. Functional positron emission tomography results (thresholded at $P < .005$, with spatial extent corrected for multiple comparisons at a threshold of $P < .05$) are displayed in color, superimposed on a single structural T1-weighted magnetic resonance imaging scan that has been transformed into the stereotactic coordinate space of Talairach and Tournoux (for anatomical reference). Section numbers refer to the distance (in millimeters) from the anterior commissure–posterior commissure line, with positive numbers being superior to the line.

studies may one day help guide treatment, but at present, it is difficult to draw conclusions from single cases.

A [^{15}O]H$_2$O PET study from our group developed a symptom capture paradigm in which audio/video monitoring detected tics during scanning. Six male TS patients with frequent tics were studied. Information about the exact timing of tics relative to radiotracer delivery to the brain was used to identify brain regions in which activity correlated with tic occurrence. Tic-related increased activity was found in medial and lateral premotor cortex, anterior cingulate cortex, dorsolateral prefrontal cortex, inferior parietal region, putamen, caudate, primary motor cortex, Broca's area, superior temporal gyrus, insula, and claustrum (Fig. 10-1). In one patient example, coprolalic tics were found to correlate with increased rCBF in the left inferior frontal region, whereas motor tics correlated with increased rCBF in sensorimotor cortex, demonstrating somatotopy and the specificity of tic efferent modalities (Figs. 10-1 and 10-2).

In addition, there were specific regions of decreased brain activity associated with tics.

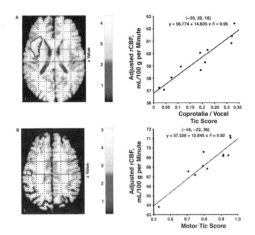

Fig. 10-2. Correlations in a single patient with Tourette syndrome between regional cerebral blood flow (rCBF) and scan scores for coprolalia in the left frontal operculum/inferior frontal gyrus (A), and for motor tics in the left sensorimotor cortex (B). These activated regions (thresholded at P <.001, with spatial extent corrected for multiple comparisons at P <.05) are superimposed in color on axial slices from a stereotactically transformed structural magnetic resonance imaging template. *L* indicates left. (From Stern E, Silbersweig DA, Chee KY, Holmes A, Robertson MM, Trimble M, et al. A functional neuroanatomy of tics in Tourette syndrome. *Arch Gen Psychiatry.* 2000;57:741–748. With permission.)

Activity in right rostral frontal cortex and precuneus decreased significantly during tics. These regions, part of a resting state network (10) mediating the near-constant processing of sensory information (51), are involved in self-awareness and self monitoring. Tic-associated decreased activity in these regions may relate to impairments in executive function and monitoring demonstrated in TS (52,53), and suggest the possibility that transient decreased internal and external awareness may accompany tics. Whether such a momentary state of diminished awareness precedes or follows tics, has any behaviorally detectable features, or is etiologically relevant to tics themselves or to conscious behavioral control, will require further study.

Such findings were the first to identify the neural correlates of tics, and demonstrate the utility of a symptom-oriented approach. They provide evidence for localized, tic-related CSTC circuitry activity, implicating specific cortical and sub-

cortical regions associated with the control and expression of motor and vocal behavior. Tic-related activity in frontal brain regions involved in volitional and executive functioning suggests a substrate for abnormal urges and disordered voluntary control in TS. Although there are complexities, future studies employing this approach can employ a comparison condition of mimicked tics to control for the sensorimotor aspects of the movement itself, with the goal of teasing apart the role of motor, premotor, and executive brain regions in the initiation and/or inhibition of both normal movements and tics in TS.

Functional Magnetic Resonance Imaging Studies of Tourette Syndrome

The first fMRI study of TS used bilateral finger tapping as an activation paradigm in five patients with TS and five normal controls (13). Echoplanar BOLD imaging showed greater number and dispersion of pixels activated by finger tapping in TS patients as compared to controls. This finding was interpreted as indicating altered organization of motor function in TS, though it may also reflect unwitnessed tics disrupting finger tapping, or an effect of suppressed tics.

To address the issue of tic suppression, Peterson et al. (15) studied 22 adult TS patients with echoplanar BOLD imaging under two conditions: volitional tic suppression versus allowing free occurrence of tics. Measures of tic severity (obtained outside the scanner) were correlated with regional fMRI signal change. Results showed that the magnitude of fMRI signal in subcortical regions (basal ganglia/thalamus) during tic inhibition correlated *inversely* with tic severity, whereas signal in cortical regions (prefrontal, parietal, temporal, cingulate) involved in behavioral inhibition correlated poorly with tic severity. The interpretation was that the pathogenesis of tics involves impaired inhibitory modulation of activity in subcortical circuitry. Although all subjects stated that they successfully suppressed all tics during the tic suppression condition, the fact that tics were not actually measured during scanning represents a limitation that can affect the interpretation of results. This finding deserves further exploration using additional paradigms and methodologies, with the aim of elucidating the nature of these cortical-subcortical interactions.

Rauch et al. (17) studied six drug-free TS patients and 12 controls using a motor task designed to specifically probe CSTC circuitry. Their serial reaction-time task, which they have also applied to the study of patients with OCD (54), provides a measure of implicit sequence learning involving motor as well as visuospatial learning elements. During implicit learning, controls, but not TS patients, demonstrated right striatal activation and early thalamic deactivation, suggesting deficient striatal recruitment and striato-thalamic gating in TS, perhaps associated with impaired filtering/suppression of irrelevant sensorimotor input.

In a case study, a 15-year-old male patient with TS underwent fMRI scanning during expression of frequent coprolalic tics and was compared with a healthy control subject mimicking identical tics (14). Tic-related activity was present in the caudate, cingulate, cuneus, left angular gyrus, left inferior parietal lobe and occipital region. These preliminary results obtained using a symptom-capture approach with fMRI require validation using additional subjects and rigorous analysis methods.

A recent fMRI study involved only three TS patients and three controls, but used precise behavioral and electromyographic assessment of grip-load force control during execution of a rhythmical motor task, with additional TS and control subjects assessed outside the scanner. TS patients demonstrated inaccurate specification of precision grip. During scanning, TS patients showed no task-related activation of SMA, which was interpreted as indicating that SMA is active at rest in TS due to the constant premonitory urge to move, which interferes with SMA participation in other motor planning. This study requires replication with larger numbers of subjects, and with other measures to assess the interpretation regarding baseline activity. The initial findings are somewhat at odds with intriguing electrophysiological observations that the premotor or Breitschaft potential—commonly thought to correspond to motor preparatory activity in the general region of the SMA—precedes voluntary movements in both normal subjects and TS patients, but is not present prior to most tics (55,56). Future multimodal functional neuroimaging studies utilizing careful monitoring of tics or other movements, ideally with electromyography, perhaps accompanied by electrophysiologic recordings, could help elucidate the nature and time course of activity in the SMA and its subregions in TS, during voluntary movements and tics.

A recent study applied the innovative technique of pharmacologic fMRI to TS. In eight TS patients performing a working memory task, abnormally increased activity (compared with control subjects) in parietal cortex, medial frontal gyrus, and thalamus was normalized following administration of intravenous levodopa, contributing to an understanding of the role of dopamine in regional brain dysfunction in TS (57).

INTEGRATION OF FINDINGS

Considering all the functional neuroimaging studies of TS reviewed, several convergent findings emerge: TS functional neuroanatomy is characterized by dorsal (premotor, motor) cortical hyperactivity, ventral (basal ganglia) hypoactivity, paralimbic abnormalities, and aberrant connectivity of emotional/motivational and motor systems. There is strong evidence for dysmodulation of CSTC loops, especially motor, resulting in abnormally increased motor output. Considered traditionally, this increased motor output could be due to hyperactivity of the direct pathway (putamen to globus pallidus to substantia nigra pars reticulata) and/or hypoactivity of the indirect pathway (putamen to external globus pallidus to subthalamic nucleus to external globus pallidus or substantia nigra pars reticulata), either of which would result in excess movement via disinhibition of thalamo-cortical motor pathways. Predominant (though variable) functional neuroimaging findings of basal ganglia hypometabolism and hypoperfusion suggest indirect pathway dysfunction. However, tics differ from other sorts of hyperkinetic movement disorders in important ways:

they are intermittent, stereotyped, suppressible, and often complex. This contrasts with hemiballismus caused by subthalamic nucleus stroke, for example, which corresponds to more straightforward indirect pathway dysfunction. The dynamic nature of tics suggests a dynamic, complex dysfunction in CSTC circuitry rather than a static lesion. Conflicting reports from many of the earlier imaging studies discussed previously, including findings of both hypoactivity and hyperactivity in the basal ganglia, may relate to attempts to study TS with insufficient consideration to timing factors, or inadequate spatial or temporal resolution.

It is possible that increased localized activity during tics may be associated with decreased activity in same region when tics are not occurring, perhaps via tonic increased inhibition alternating with phasic escape from inhibition. This would be analogous to clinical nuclear medicine examinations of patients with localization-related epilepsy, which typically show hyperperfusion during a seizure (ictal SPECT) but hypoperfusion or hypometabolism at baseline (FDG PET or interictal SPECT.) Detection and investigation of such temporal fluctuations in TS would require precise behavioral assessments over time in association with an imaging technique with high temporal resolution, and would be difficult to detect using integrated measures of brain activity such as FDG PET. Such fluctuation may account for some divergent SPECT findings, since a patient's activity at the time of injection would be expected to affect imaging results, showing hypoperfusion or hyperperfusion depending on the state of the patient at the time of injection, which is not often recorded.

Recent fine-grained anatomic research has identified a promising model for understanding the pathophysiology of tics in TS, which may help explain some conflicting imaging findings. Matrisomes represent zones of functional homogeneity in the striatum made up of clusters of neurons with similar inputs and outputs. When stimulated, they appear to produce stereotyped movements in primates (58). Intermittent overactivity of specific matrisomes, or sets of matrisomes (rather than of the striatum as a whole)

represents a plausible explanation for tics (59). Given the focality of most tics, such hyperactive matrisomes are likely to correspond to only a small proportion of the striatum, which would be expected to vary in location between TS patients based on their tic phenotype, and may even vary in a given patient over time. Functional investigation of matrisomes in humans may therefore require high-resolution imaging methods such as high-field MRI focused on the basal ganglia, perhaps forgoing the spatial smoothing and normalization processing steps commonly performed to facilitate group image analysis. Such hyperactive matrisomes would be most active only during tics (which, fortunately for most patients, do not occur constantly) and might therefore be very difficult to detect without careful attention to tic timing and use of an imaging method with high temporal resolution.

If one accepts the idea of tics correlating with temporal fluctuations in the activity state of CSTC circuitry, the question arises as to which part of the circuit initiates the abnormal impulse? Although most models concern a role for disordered basal ganglia functioning in TS, it remains uncertain whether basal ganglia dysfunction is primary or secondary. It is possible that the impulse which ultimately leads to a tic arises cortically, perhaps in premotor/executive regions when related to a motor tic, in a sensory region when accompanied by a sensory phenomenon, in a region known to contain mirror neurons (60) when associated with an urge to mimic or touch someone or a "phantom" tic located extracorporally (61), or in a paralimbic region when related to strong emotion. TMS studies demonstrate impaired cortical inhibition in TS (62,63). Unlike other movement disorders associated with basal ganglia degeneration or lesions, TS is characterized by "*un*voluntary" [i.e., suppressible and perceived by patients as willed (64)] rather than true involuntary movements, again suggesting a higher-order, potentially cortically-mediated dysfunction. In support of this idea are findings of extensive premotor activation during tics (20) suggesting that cortical motor and pre-motor activation detected during tic occurrence represents not just the expected neural correlates of the movement itself, but may be associated with the characteristic urge, which may be etiologically relevant to the neurobiology of tics and potential treatment modalities.

TOURETTE SYNDROME AS PART OF SPECTRUM

There is substantial clinical overlap between TS, OCD, and ADHD, with most TS patients meeting criteria for at least one of these two disorders (65,66). Several studies have already demonstrated functional neuroanatomic commonalities between TS and OCD (17,23, 26,30). It may be useful to view TS as part of a spectrum of impulse control disorders having their neurobiologic basis in dysfunction of the CSTC circuitry mediating purposeful behavior (67), with differences in the nature of the aberrant behavior related to the specific CSTC loop affected: relatively simple motor or vocal tics or sensory urges in TS due to "sensorimotor loop" dysfunction (primary and supplementary somatosensory cortex, dorsolateral striatum, globus pallidus, ventrolateral/centromedian/ intralaminar thalamus); more complex motor compulsions or recurrent thoughts in OCD due to "limbic loop" dysfunction (orbitofrontal cortex, ventromedial caudate, globus pallidus, medial dorsal nucleus of the thalamus) (68); and deficits of attention in ADHD due to "association loop" dysfunction (dorsolateral prefrontal cortex, dorsalateral caudate, globus pallidus, ventral anterial nucleus of the thalamus) (69). Dysfunction of CSTC loops mediating eye movement control have recently been demonstrated in TS (70). Increasing evidence that these distinct, parallel CSTC loops actually demonstrate substantial cross-connectivity under normal conditions (71), which may be enhanced in neuropsychiatric disorders such as TS (45) may help explain the overlapping clinical features of TS, OCD, and ADHD. Reconceptualizing these disorders as similar in form but varying in content has implications for diagnostic classification and treatment, and can provide a useful theoretical framework for investigation using neuroimaging and other techniques.

FUTURE DIRECTIONS

Functional neuroimaging in TS remains in its infancy, with much exciting work to be done to continue defining the pathophysiology of TS via multiple means, including paradigm development and integration of varied imaging techniques with one another and with other scientific methods, with the long-term goal of broadening and optimizing treatment options available to patients with TS. In this context, neuroimaging can be combined with genetics and used to identify intermediate phenotypes. Other promising avenues include study of clinically- and genetically-defined subpopulations of TS patients, as well as normal subjects at different stages of development, based on the fact that tics represent a normal occurrence at certain developmental stages (72).

Paradigm Development

Development of activation tasks to probe relevant neurocircuitry can build upon existing conflict and conscious response inhibition tasks (17) as well as more automatic tasks such as pre-pulse inhibition (16) and habit learning (73), both of which have been shown to be abnormal in TS. Frontal-subcortical mechanisms of response inhibition in TS are also being explored, using a go-no-go paradigm (Stewart Mostofsky, 2004, oral communication). Tasks could also be developed that TS patients actually perform better than healthy controls. In addition to their anecdotally-described advantages in speed of thought and action (74), TS patients have been found to be better than controls at making accurate drawing movements with their non-dominant hand (75). Use of similar tasks in functional neuroimaging studies could address, in a novel manner, confounds inherent to unequal performance between patients and controls, and might also provide additional insight into disorders like Parkinson disease in which these functions are impaired, or perhaps contribute to an explanation for the prevalence of TS, which may relate to a one-time evolutionary advantage afforded individuals with certain TS characteristics.

Multimodal Approaches

As discussed previously, every functional neuroimaging method has advantages and disadvantages. Combining different modalities provides the opportunity to benefit from the best aspects of each technique. In particular, combining techniques with excellent spatial resolution (e.g., MRI) with techniques providing excellent temporal resolution (electroencephalography or magnetoencephalography) while technically demanding, may be necessary to understand fully the origin and nature of tics, which almost certainly involve rapid fluctuations in the activity state of CSTC circuitry. Future useful multimodal techniques could include correlation of detailed structural information such as shape/texture (76), cortical thickness (77), or structural connectivity as assessed by diffusion tensor imaging or other assessment of white matter (78), with measures of function, including functional connectivity; radioligand PET or SPECT combined with measures of localized neural activity to explore the role of different neurotransmitters in the genesis of focal dysfunction; use of electromyography and/or evoked potentials to precisely correlate normal and tic-related movement with brain activity; pharmacologic challenge using short-acting agents to alter dopaminergic or other neurotransmitter function (57); and relating genetic information (e.g., dopamine receptor polymorphisms) to specific patterns of brain activity.

Relevance of Functional Neuroimaging to Treatment

Better understanding of the pathophysiology of TS may have implications for treatment using psychologic, pharmacologic, and somatic therapies, including transcranial magnetic stimulation (TMS) (77). Pretreatment and post-treatment functional imaging studies may help guide selection of appropriate medical and/or psychological therapies, perhaps eventually helping to predict the optimal treatment (e.g., anti-dopaminergic agent versus pro-serotonin agent versus habit reversal therapy) to modulate specific nodes in TS-related neurocircuitry.

Functional neuroimaging studies of TS may prove especially useful in guiding the use of neurostimulators, at present most commonly used as treatment for motor symptoms of Parkinson disease (79), but increasingly considered for other diseases, including psychiatric disorders (80). Neurostimulators can be implanted safely in the cortex (81) as well as the subcortex, and are currently under study in TS (82). Although theoretically less appealing due to its irreversibility, neurosurgery aimed at resecting or disconnecting dysfunctional brain regions—already applied to patients with TS, with variable results (83)—could in the future be guided by neuroanatomically precise information derived from functional neuroimaging studies of TS in general and of individual TS patients.

REFERENCES

1. Yang Y, Engelien W, Xu S, et al. Transit time, trailing time, and cerebral blood flow during brain activation: measurement using multislice, pulsed spin-labeling perfusion imaging. *Magn Reson Med*. 2000;44:680–685.
2. Yang Y, Engelien W, Pan H, et al. A CBF-based event-related brain activation paradigm: characterization of impulse-response function and comparison to BOLD. *Neuroimage* 2000;12:287–297.
3. Detre JA, Alsop DC. Perfusion magnetic resonance imaging with continuous arterial spin labeling: methods and clinical applications in the central nervous system. *Eur J Radiol*. 1999;30:115–124.
4. Scahill L, Tanner C, Dure L. The epidemiology of tics and Tourette syndrome in children and adolescents. *Adv Neurol*. 2001;85:261–271.
5. Peterson BS. Neuroimaging studies of Tourette syndrome: a decade of progress. *Adv Neurol*. 2001;85:179–196.
6. Chiu NT, Chang YC, Lee BF, et al. Differences in 99mTc-HMPAO brain SPET perfusion imaging between Tourette's syndrome and chronic tic disorder in children. *Eur J Nucl Med*. 2001;28:183–190.
7. Diler RS, Reyhanli M, Toros F, et al. Tc-99m-ECD SPECT brain imaging in children with Tourette's syndrome. *Yonsei Med J*. 2002;43:403–410.
8. Gerard E, Peterson BS. Developmental processes and brain imaging studies in Tourette syndrome. *J Psychosom Res*. 2003;55:13–22.
9. Goetz CG, Kompoliti K. Rating scales and quantitative assessment of tics. *Adv Neurol*. 2001;85:31–42.
10. Raichle ME, MacLeod AM, Snyder AZ, et al. A default mode of brain function. *Proc Natl Acad Sci USA*. 2001;98:676–682.
11. Greicius MD, Krasnow B, Reiss AL, et al. Functional connectivity in the resting brain: a network analysis of the default mode hypothesis. *Proc Natl Acad Sci USA*. 2003;100:253–258.

12. Serrien DJ, Nirkko AC, Loher TJ, et al. Movement control of manipulative tasks in patients with Gilles de la Tourette syndrome. *Brain* 2002;125:290–300.

13. Biswal B, Ulmer JL, Krippendorf RL, et al. Abnormal cerebral activation associated with a motor task in Tourette syndrome. *AJNR Am J Neuroradiol.* 1998; 19:1509–1512.

14. Gates L, Clarke JR, Stokes A, et al. Neuroanatomy of coprolalia in Tourette syndrome using functional magnetic resonance imaging. *Prog Neuropsychopharmacol Biol Psychiatry.* 2004;28:397–400.

15. Peterson BS, Skudlarski P, Anderson AW, et al. A functional magnetic resonance imaging study of tic suppression in Tourette syndrome. *Arch Gen Psychiatry.* 1998;55:326–333.

16. Swerdlow NR, Karban B, Ploum Y, et al. Tactile pre-puff inhibition of startle in children with Tourette's syndrome: in search of an "fMRI-friendly" startle paradigm. *Biol Psychiatry.* 2001;50:578–585.

17. Rauch SL, Whalen PJ, Curran T, et al. Probing striato-thalamic function in obsessive-compulsive disorder and Tourette syndrome using neuroimaging methods. *Adv Neurol.* 2001;85:207–224.

18. Silbersweig DA, Stern E, Frith C, et al. A functional neuroanatomy of hallucinations in schizophrenia. *Nature* 1995;378:176–179.

19. Silbersweig DA, Stern E. Symptom localization in neuropsychiatry. A functional neuroimaging approach. *Ann N Y Acad Sci.* 1997;835:410–420.

20. Stern E, Silbersweig DA, Chee KY, et al. A functional neuroanatomy of tics in Tourette syndrome. *Arch Gen Psychiatry.* 2000;57:741–748.

21. Frackowiak RS, Price C, Zeki S, et al. *Human Brain Function.* 2nd ed: Elsevier/Academic Press; 2003.

22. Hall M, Costa D, Shields J, et al. Brain perfusion patterns with ^{99}Tc^m-HMPAO/SPET in patients with Gilles de la Tourette Syndrome—Short Report. In: *Nuclear Medicine: The State of the Art of Nuclear Medicine in Europe.* Stuttgart: Schattauer; 1991:243–245.

23. George MS, Trimble MR, Costa DC, et al. Elevated frontal cerebral blood flow in Gilles de la Tourette syndrome: a 99Tcm-HMPAO SPECT study. *Psychiatry Res.* 1992;45:143–151.

24. Riddle MA, Rasmusson AM, Woods SW, et al. SPECT imaging of cerebral blood flow in Tourette syndrome. *Adv Neurol.* 1992;58:207–211.

25. Sieg KG, Buckingham D, Gaffney GR, et al. Tc-99m HMPAO SPECT brain imaging of Gilles de la Tourette's syndrome. *Clin Nucl Med.* 1993;18:255.

26. Moriarty J, Costa DC, Schmitz B, et al. Brain perfusion abnormalities in Gilles de la Tourette's syndrome. *Br J Psychiatry.* 1995;167:249–254.

27. Moriarty J, Eapen V, Costa DC, et al. HMPAO SPET does not distinguish obsessive-compulsive and tic syndromes in families multiply affected with Gilles de la Tourette's syndrome. *Psychol Med.* 1997;27:737–740.

28. Klieger PS, Fett KA, Dimitsopulos T, et al. Asymmetry of basal ganglia perfusion in Tourette's syndrome shown by technetium-99m-HMPAO SPECT. *J Nucl Med.* 1997;38:188–191.

29. Lampreave JL, Molina V, Mardomingo MJ, et al. Technetium-99m-HMPAO in Tourette's syndrome on neuroleptic therapy and after withdrawal. *J Nucl Med.* 1998; 39:624–628.

30. Crespo-Facorro B, Cabranes JA, Lopez-Ibor Alcocer MI, et al. Regional cerebral blood flow in obsessive-compulsive patients with and without a chronic tic disorder. A SPECT study. *Eur Arch Psychiatry Clin Neurosci.* 1999;249:156–161.

31. Eapen V, Pauls DL, Robertson MM. Evidence for autosomal dominant transmission in Tourette's syndrome. United Kingdom cohort study. *Br J Psychiatry.* 1993;162:593–596.

32. Goodman WK, Price LH, Rasmussen SA, et al. The Yale-Brown Obsessive Compulsive Scale. II. Validity. *Arch Gen Psychiatry.* 1989;46:1012–1016.

33. Beck AT, Rial WY, Rickets K. Short form of depression inventory: cross-validation. *Psychological Reports.* 1974; 34:1184–1186.

34. Berg CJ, Rapoport JL, Flament M. The Leyton Obsessional Inventory-Child Version. *J Am Acad Child Psychiatry.* 1986;25:84–91.

35. Goetz CG, Tanner CM, Wilson RS, et al. A rating scale for Gilles de la Tourette's syndrome: description, reliability, and validity data. *Neurology* 1987;37:1542–1544.

36. Hodgson RJ, Rachman S. Obsessional-compulsive complaints. *Behav Res Ther.* 1977;15:389–395.

37. Hamilton M. A rating scale for depression. *J Neurol Neurosurg Psychiatry.* 1960;23:56–62.

38. Montgomery SA, Asberg M. A new depression scale designed to be sensitive to change. *Br J Psychiatry.* 1979;134:382–389.

39. Leckman JF, Riddle MA, Hardin MT, et al. The Yale Global Tic Severity Scale: initial testing of a clinician-rated scale of tic severity. *J Am Acad Child Adolesc Psychiatry* 1989;28:566–73.

40. American Psychiatric Association. *Diagnostic and Statistical Manual of Mental Disorders, 4th ed. (DSM-IV).* Washington, DC, 1994.

41. The Tourette Syndrome Classification Study Group. Definitions and classification of tic disorders. *Arch Neurol.* 1993;50(10):1013–1016.

42. Chase TN, Geoffrey V, Gillespie M, et al. Structural and functional studies of Gilles de la Tourette syndrome. *Rev Neurol* (Paris). 1986;142:851–855.

43. Braun AR, Stoetter B, Randolph C, et al. The functional neuroanatomy of Tourette's syndrome: an FDG-PET study. I. Regional changes in cerebral glucose metabolism differentiating patients and controls. *Neuropsychopharmacology* 1993;9:277–291.

44. Braun AR, Randolph C, Stoetter B, et al. The functional neuroanatomy of Tourette's syndrome: an FDG-PET Study. II: Relationships between regional cerebral metabolism and associated behavioral and cognitive features of the illness. *Neuropsychopharmacology* 1995;13:151–168.

45. Jeffries KJ, Schooler C, Schoenbach C, et al. The functional neuroanatomy of Tourette's syndrome: an FDG PET study III: functional coupling of regional cerebral metabolic rates. *Neuropsychopharmacology* 2002;27: 92–104.

46. Lichter DG, Cummings JL. *Frontal-subcortical circuits in psychiatric and neurological disorders.* New York: Guilford Press; 2001.

47. Stoetter B, Braun AR, Randolph C, et al. Functional neuroanatomy of Tourette syndrome. Limbic-motor interactions studied with FDG PET. *Adv Neurol.* 1992; 58:213–226.

48. Alexander GE, Crutcher MD, DeLong MR. Basal ganglia-thalamocortical circuits: parallel substrates for motor, oculomotor, "prefrontal" and "limbic" functions. *Prog Brain Res.* 1990;85:119–146.

49. Eidelberg D, Moeller JR, Antonini A, et al. The metabolic anatomy of Tourette's syndrome. *Neurology* 1997;48:927–934.

50. Sawle GV, Lees AJ, Hymas NF, et al. The metabolic effects of limbic leucotomy in Gilles de la Tourette syndrome. *J Neurol Neurosurg Psychiatry.* 1993;56:1016–1019.

51. Vogt BA, Finch DM, Olson CR. Functional heterogeneity in cingulate cortex: the anterior executive and posterior evaluative regions. *Cereb Cortex.* 1992;2:435–443.

52. Muller SV, Johannes S, Wieringa B, et al. Disturbed monitoring and response inhibition in patients with Gilles de la Tourette syndrome and co-morbid obsessive compulsive disorder. *Behav Neurol.* 2003;14:29–37.

53. Channon S, Pratt P, Robertson MM. Executive function, memory, and learning in Tourette's syndrome. *Neuropsychology* 2003;17:247–254.

54. Rauch SL, Savage CR, Alpert NM, et al. Probing striatal function in obsessive-compulsive disorder: a PET study of implicit sequence learning. J *Neuropsychiatry Clin Neurosci.* 1997;9:568–573.

55. Karp BI, Porter S, Toro C, et al. Simple motor tics may be preceded by a premotor potential. *J Neurol Neurosurg Psychiatry.* 1996;61:103–106.

56. Obeso JA, Rothwell JC, Marsden CD. Simple tics in Gilles de la Tourette's syndrome are not prefaced by a normal premovement EEG potential. *J Neurol Neurosurg Psychiatry.* 1981;44:735–738.

57. Hershey T, Black KJ, Hartlein JM, et al. Cognitive-pharmacologic functional magnetic resonance imaging in tourette syndrome: a pilot study. *Biol Psychiatry.* 2004;55:916–925.

58. Alexander GE, DeLong MR. Microstimulation of the primate neostriatum. II. Somatotopic organization of striatal microexcitable zones and their relation to neuronal response properties. *J Neurophysiol.* 1985;53:1417–1430.

59. Mink JW. Neurobiology of basal ganglia circuits in Tourette syndrome: faulty inhibition of unwanted motor patterns? *Adv Neurol.* 2001;85:113–122.

60. Rizzolatti G, Craighero L. The mirror-neuron system. *Annu Rev Neurosci.* 2004;27:169–192.

61. Karp BI, Hallett M. Extracorporeal "phantom" tics in Tourette's syndrome. *Neurology* 1996;46:38–40.

62. George MS, Sallee FR, Nahas Z, et al. Transcranial magnetic stimulation (TMS) as a research tool in Tourette syndrome and related disorders. *Adv Neurol.* 2001;85:225–235.

63. Ziemann U, Paulus W, Rothenberger A. Decreased motor inhibition in Tourette's disorder: evidence from transcranial magnetic stimulation. *Am J Psychiatry.* 1997;154:1277–1284.

64. Jankovic J. Tourette syndrome. Phenomenology and classification of tics. *Neurol Clin.* 1997;15:267–275.

65. Steingard R, Dillon-Stout D. Tourette's syndrome and obsessive compulsive disorder. Clinical aspects. *Psychiatr Clin North Am.* 1992;15:849–860.

66. Spencer T, Biederman J, Coffey B, et al. Tourette disorder and ADHD. *Adv Neurol.* 2001;85:57–77.

67. Alexander GE, DeLong MR, Strick PL. Parallel organization of functionally segregated circuits linking basal ganglia and cortex. *Annu Rev Neurosci.* 1986;9:357–381.

68. Saxena S, Bota RG, Brody AL. Brain-behavior relationships in obsessive-compulsive disorder. *Semin Clin Neuropsychiatry.* 2001;6:82–101.

69. Castellanos FX. Neural substrates of attention-deficit hyperactivity disorder. *Adv Neurol.* 2001;85:197–206.

70. Nomura Y, Fukuda H, Terao Y, et al. Abnormalities of voluntary saccades in Gilles de la Tourette's syndrome: pathophysiological consideration. *Brain Dev.* 2003;25 suppl 1:S48–54.

71. Joel D, Weiner I. The organization of the basal ganglia-thalamocortical circuits: open interconnected rather than closed segregated. *Neuroscience* 1994;63:363–379.

72. Kurlan R. Hypothesis II: Tourette's syndrome is part of a clinical spectrum that includes normal brain development. *Arch Neurol.* 1994;51:1145–1150.

73. Marsh R, Alexander GM, Packard MG, et al. Habit learning in Tourette syndrome: a translational neuroscience approach to a developmental psychopathology. *Arch Gen Psychiatry.* 2004;61:1259–1268.

74. Sacks O. A Neurologist's Notebook. *The New Yorker* 2004 August 23:60.

75. Georgiou N, Bradshaw JL, Phillips JG, et al. Functional asymmetries in the movement kinematics of patients with Tourette's syndrome. *J Neurol Neurosurg Psychiatry.* 1997;63:188–195.

76. Castellano G, Bonilla L, Li LM, et al. Texture analysis of medical images. *Clin Radiol.* 2004;59:1061–1069.

77. Fischl B, Dale AM. Measuring the thickness of the human cerebral cortex from magnetic resonance images. *Proc Natl Acad Sci USA.* 2000;97:11050–11055.

78. Plessen KJ, Wentzel-Larsen T, Hugdahl K, et al. Altered interhemispheric connectivity in individuals with Tourette's disorder. *Am J Psychiatry.* 2004;161:2028–2037.

79. Volkmann J. Deep brain stimulation for the treatment of Parkinson's disease. *J Clin Neurophysiol.* 2004;21:6–17.

80. Greenberg BD, Rezai AR. Mechanisms and the current state of deep brain stimulation in neuropsychiatry. *CNS Spectr.* 2003;8:522–526.

81. Vossler D, Doherty M, Goodman R, et al. Early safety experience with a fully implanted intracranial responsive neurostimulator for epilepsy [abstract]. *Epilepsia* 2004;45 suppl 7:1–393.

82. Visser-Vandewalle V, Temel Y, Boon P, et al. Chronic bilateral thalamic stimulation: a new therapeutic approach in intractable Tourette syndrome. Report of three cases. *J Neurosurg.* 2003;99:1094–1100.

83. Temel Y, Visser-Vandewalle V. Surgery in Tourette syndrome. *Mov Disord.* 2004;19:3–14.

11

A Genome-Wide Scan and Fine Mapping in Tourette Syndrome Families

David L. Pauls

*Psychiatric and Neurodevelopmental Genetics Unit, Massachusetts General Hospital,
Harvard Medical School, Boston, Massachusetts*

Gilles de la Tourette's syndrome or Tourette syndrome (TS) is a neuropsychiatric disorder that emerges early in development. For nearly a century after its original description in 1885, TS was considered a rare neuropsychiatric disorder. It received relatively little attention until the late 1960s when interest was renewed largely as a result of the work of Shapiro and others who found many patients responded to haloperidol, a dopamine receptor inhibitor. As a result of this discovery and the active publicity campaign of the Tourette Syndrome Association, scientific research on TS has increased dramatically over the last four decades.

The familial nature of TS and CT has been well documented (1). Furthermore, twin studies implicate genetic factors in the expression of TS. Price et al. (2) and Hyde et al. (3) reported significantly higher concordance rates among monozygotic (MZ) twins compared to dizygotic (DZ) twins when twins with TS, CT, or obsessive compulsive disorder (OCD) were considered as affected. In contrast, the MZ twin data suggest that non-genetic factors also play a role in the manifestation of TS and tics; MZ concordance rates are less than 1.0.

Early complex segregation analyses of family study data provided strong evidence that the mode of transmission was compatible with an autosomal dominant model (4,5). However, subsequent segregation analyses completed by members of the Tourette Syndrome Association International Consortium for Genetics (TSAICG)

(6–8) and others (9) suggest that the mode of inheritance is more complex.

Although the mode of inheritance is not simple, it is clear that TS has a significant genetic basis and that some individuals with TS, CT, and OCD manifest variant expressions of the same genetic susceptibility factors. A number of investigators have documented a wide range of phenotypes that unfold throughout development (6,10–13). A more complete understanding of that genetic basis and of the interactions between relevant genotypes and relevant environmental factors will be vital for understanding this developmental process.

PHENOTYPE AND GENETIC APPROACHES

Until recently, most genetic studies of complex behavioral traits have relied primarily on the analysis of dichotomous diagnostic phenotypes (i.e., affected/not affected). Recently, it has become increasingly apparent that traditional methods for classifying individuals as affected or unaffected are inadequate for genetic studies of complex traits. Gottesman and Gould (14) have summarized the current situation in neuropsychiatric genetics when they state that:

> "Despite the successful characterization of the nucleotide base-pair order that represents the human genome, and although a legion of genetic linkage and association studies have been done, psychiatry has had little success in

definitively identifying 'culprit' genes or gene regions in the development of diseases categorized by using the field's diagnostic classification schemas. The reason there is so much difficulty is undoubtedly—in part—that psychiatry's classification systems describe heterogeneous disorders. In addition to the inherent complexity of psychiatric disorders,…, [it is clear that] the brain is the most complex of all organs.… Furthermore, the brain is subject to complex interactions not just among genes, proteins, cells and circuits of cells but also between individuals and their changing experiences. Therefore, the phenotypic output from the brain i.e., behavior, is not simply a sum of all its parts. *It stands to reason that more optimally reduced measures of neuropsychiatric functioning should be more useful than behavioral 'macros' in studies pursuing the biological and genetic components of psychiatric disorders."*

A number of investigators have employed a variety of methods that address multiple quantitative phenotypic dimensions with the goal of examining distinct components of complex phenotypes. In studies of TS and OCD, principal components analyses have identified elements of TS (15) and OCD (16) that are comprised of symptom clusters that appear to represent unique heritable elements of each complex phenotype (17). Given the co-morbidity that has been observed between TS and OCD a reasonable next step will be to determine if there are unique heritable components of symptoms and/or neuropsychologic functions that span these diagnostic classifications. If such components can be elucidated and if they are heritable, it could lead to a major advance in identifying more precisely the candidate genes that may reside in some of the regions of interest that will be identified in linkage studies.

GENOME SCANNING FOR TOURETTE SYNDROME SUSCEPTIBILITY GENES

Genetic linkage and, more recently, association studies have been recognized as some of the most powerful methods for clarifying the role of genetic factors in the expression of complex disorders like TS. A number of complex disorders have been mapped (e.g., breast cancer, epilepsy). Until recently, no genes for neuropsychiatric illnesses had been localized. However,

in the last several years significant linkages have been reported and replicated for specific reading disability (18–24), autism (see 25, 26 for review), and schizophrenia (27,28). Furthermore, as described later in text, a genome scan has been completed for TS on a large sample of affected sib-pair and multigenerational families. In addition, recent findings in two large families being studied as part of the TSAICG project provide evidence for a locus on chromosome 17q (29).

The localization and characterization of genes important for the expression of the TS phenotype will be a major advance in the understanding of the pathogenesis of this disorder and will also provide a general model for the study of other developmental disorders. Unquestionably, the localization and characterization of these genes will be a major step forward in the understanding of the specific genetic/biological risk factors important for the expression of TS. Furthermore, once genes conferring susceptibility to TS and associated behaviors have been characterized, further work will allow the identification of additional non-genetic factors important for the manifestation or the amelioration of the symptoms of the disorders. As discussed by Kidd (30) the identification of a linked marker will permit the design of much more incisive studies to illuminate the physiological/biochemical etiology of TS by examination of the gene product and its impact on the development of the disorders. In contrast, by controlling for genetic factors, through the genetic case-control research paradigm (30), it will be possible to document more carefully the environmental/non-genetic factors important for the expression of TS and other disorders.

It is only recently that comprehensive genetic studies of complex behavioral traits have become feasible. Several developments have paved the way. In particular, large-scale genome scans have been made possible and affordable by the complete sequencing of the human genome, the ready availability of instrumentation for high-throughput genomic analysis, and the generation of new analytical and bioinformatics tools.

Single nucleotide polymorphisms (SNPs) have now been identified over virtually all segments of the human genome. It is now feasible to follow up genome-wide linkage studies with fine mapping and association studies in which thousands of SNPs can be reliably assayed at relatively low cost. Such fine mapping is currently underway in the sample collected by the TSAICG. The International HapMap Project, and other ongoing efforts to map the distribution of linkage disequilibrium in the genome (31,32) will likely increase the efficiency of association studies that will be synergistic with the linkage studies underway. The identification of positional candidate genes will benefit from the much lower cost of DNA sequencing, which makes extensive resequencing efforts feasible, and from the opportunities now available to conduct comparative genomic analyses between human sequence and that of several closely related species, including chimpanzee and rhesus macaque (33). A variety of strategies have detected previously unrecognized common variants in genome structure (e.g., duplications and inversions), which suggests the possibility that such variation may play a role in susceptibility to complex traits such as TS (34,35). Functional validation of candidate variants will likely be facilitated by a plethora of methodologies for profiling patterns of gene expression.

Recent Progress

At the present time, the TSAICG has collected a sample of 256 sib-pair families yielding 356 independent sib-pairs. A genome scan has been completed on this sib-pair sample and a sample of 23 multigenerational families with at least three family members affected with TS. Genotyping was completed at the Centre National de Genotypage in Evry Cedex France, and data analyses are currently underway.

A total of 2,192 DNA samples were sent to the Centre National de Genotypage, 1,079 from the affected sib-pair sample and 1,113 from the multigenerational family samples. The 23 multigenerational families range in size from a family of 14 individuals with three TS affected members to a family of 244 individuals with

106 TS affected members. Altogether there were 285 individuals with TS in these 23 multigenerational families.

All individuals in all of the sib-pair and multigenerational families were evaluated with an extensive battery of assessments evaluating the full range of neuropsychiatric disorders. Briefly, all individuals were interviewed extensively about lifetime symptoms of TS, OCD, and attention deficit hyperactivity disorder using an interview designed specifically for this sib-pair study. In addition, every person 18 years of age and older was interviewed with either the Structured Clinical Interview for DSM Diagnoses to obtain information regarding any major psychiatric disorders they may have had over their lifetime. The children's version of the Schedule for Affective Disorders and Schizophrenia was used to obtain similar information about children younger than age 18 years.

In the ascertainment of the affected sib-pair families, families were excluded if both parents were affected with TS, or if one parent had TS, CT, or OCD and the other parent also had CT and/or OCD. All diagnoses were made using DSM-IV-TR criteria. As noted, the final sib-pair sample sent to the Centre National de Genotypage for genotyping consisted of 256 families. Both phenotypic and genotypic information was available for both parents in 233 sib-pair families. In the remaining 23 families information was available for only one of the parents. Information was available for 252 mothers and 237 fathers. The average age of the fathers was 44.1 years and the average of the mothers was 42.2 years. Altogether there were 165 daughters and 425 sons in the sib-pair families. The average age of daughters was 14.6 years and the average age for sons was 13.9 years.

While the genotyping was being completed, all available clinical information was reviewed by the clinicians in the TSAICG and best estimate diagnoses assigned. A number of families were excluded after the best estimate process was completed. The primary reason for exclusion was that one of the siblings in the family did not meet full DSM-IV-TR criteria for TS. As a result, only 236 families were included in the initial analyses of the sib-pair sample. The average age and the gender distribution in the families included in the analyses did not differ from that for the total sample genotyped. As noted previously, 1,113 individuals in 23 multigenerational families were included in the genome scan. Only individuals for whom complete phenotypic information was available were included in the sample that was genotyped and all are included in the analyses. The panel of markers genotyped included 408 highly informative DNA markers. The observed average heterozygosity of these markers was 0.78.

In the data analyses that are ongoing, nonparametric linkage analyses are being completed using MAPMAKER/SIBS and GENEHUNTER for the sib-pair families and SIMWALK2 computer applications for the multigenerational families. Non-parametric analyses have the advantage that the specific mode of transmission need not be specified as in parametric analyses. Both single-point and multipoint analyses will be completed. In the single-point analysis the identity-by-descent distribution will be estimated given the marker genotypes for each marker individually. In the multipoint analysis, NPL scores will be computed for more than 4000 different locations relative to the markers (average step size <1 cM). For sib-pair families with more than two affected siblings, all possible pairs were included in the initial analyses and the results will be weighted by a factor equal to 2/n, for which n is the number of affected children in the sibship. Applying this weighting results in a sample that is equivalent to a sample of 327 "independent" sib-pairs.

Because all of the analyses will be nonparametric, Fisher's rule will be used to combine the results from the total sample of sibpair and multigenerational families where analyses of either sample results in an NPL score greater than 1.5. Fisher's rule states that $-2\ln(p_1 * p_2 * * * * p_k)$ is distributed as a chi-square with 2k degrees of freedom where k is the number of samples being combined.

Finally, analyses will be undertaken to determine the extent of heterogeneity among the multigenerational families and to examine whether combing those families with similar patterns of NPL scores and identity-by-descent distributions will identify the subset of families contributing to the score of the total sample of families. Current heterogeneity analyses for linkage require that parametric analyses be completed so that a heterogeneity lod score can be estimated for the proportion of families that appear to be linked to a specific locus. Because all of the analyses to be completed in these families will be nonparametric, a series of analyses similar to those described by Coon et al. (36) will be completed to estimate the heterogeneity in the sample of multigenerational families.

Several other linkage studies of large families have been completed, and there have been some interesting findings. A region on 17q has shown positive linkage results in three multigenerational families. The 17q region is spanned by markers D17S784 and D17S928. Subsequently, this specific region has been extensively examined by Paschou et al (29). The strongest signal was obtained for the most telomeric marker, D17S928. D17S928 is now known to be at 77,846 kb (May 2004 assembly), centromeric to CD7 (a gene encoding a transmembrane protein which is a member of the immunoglobulin superfamily), whereas the "17qter" single tandem repeat polymorphism is at 78,941 kb in intron 38 of Tubulin-Specific Chaperone D (TBCD). TBCD is an interesting gene that is expressed at varying levels in all human tissues examined (e.g., brain, spinal cord, liver, pancreas, kidney, spleen, heart, lung, skeletal muscle, testis, ovary, fetal brain, and fetal liver). Within the brain, TBCD expression was found in all regions tested (e.g., amygdala, corpus callosum, cerebellum, caudate nucleus, hippocampus, substantia nigra, subthalamic nucleus, and thalamus). As noted in Paschou et al., 2004, an unusual pattern of extended linkage disequilibrium has been identified on distal 17q; this is unexpected since on most chromosomes telomeric regions have elevated recombination. More work is needed to understand more fully these findings.

In another linkage study examining one large French Canadian family, strong suggestive linkage was reported for a region on 11q (37). No additional reports have been published regarding this family so it is not known if specific candidate genes are being examined in this region in this family.

Once the analyses of the current linkage data are completed, regions showing strong suggestive evidence for linkage will be followed up with fine mapping using both microsatellite markers and SNPs to narrow the regions of interest. If the regions are narrowed and specific candidate genes are identified in these regions, association studies will be undertaken in a sample of triad families using a family based association design.

As discussed by Altshuler and Altshuler (38) success in the application of these new technologies to complex diseases will require sustained effort by "goal-oriented, multidisciplinary teams." The Tourette Syndrome Association International Consortium on Genetics is such a multidisciplinary team composed of clinicians, geneticists, statistical geneticists and genetic epidemiologists. As described previously, over the last 5 years, with support from NIH grant NS40024 and the TSA, the TSAICG has succeeded in recruiting a large sample of affected sib-pair and multigenerational families and has completed a genome scan on these families. Results from the complete analyses of these data should provide the best evidence to date for genomic regions that harbor susceptibility loci for TS. Findings from the sib-pair sample will be corroborated in some of the multigenerational families and heterogeneity analyses will be conducted to determine if there are genomic regions that provide statistically significant evidence for results for linkage of TS. Finally, these findings will be examined with association studies using a family based association design. When susceptibility genes for TS are found, the focus of the research will shift to work designed to elucidate the function of these genes in the brain. The ultimate goal is to understand the underlying mechanisms important for the manifestation of TS so that more effective interventions can be developed. Knowing which genes increase the risk for TS, should also allow earlier detection of children at risk, so that prevention measures can be employed to minimize the severity of the disorder.

ACKNOWLEDGMENTS

Supported by NIH grant NS40024.

REFERENCES

1. Pauls DL. An update on the genetics of Gilles de la Tourette syndrome. *J Psychosom Res.* 2003;55:7–12.
2. Price RA, Kidd KK, Cohen DJ. A twin study of Tourette syndrome. *Arch Gen Psychiatry.* 1985;42:815–820.
3. Hyde TM, Aaronson BA, Randolph C, et al. Relationship of birth weight to the phenotypic expression of Gilles de la Tourette's syndrome in monozygotic twins. *Neurology* 1992;42, 652–658.
4. Pauls DL, Leckman JF. The inheritance of Gilles de la Tourette's syndrome and associated behaviors: Evidence for autosomal dominant transmission. *N Engl J Med.* 1986;315:993–997.
5. Eapen V, Pauls DL, Robertson MM. Evidence for autosomal dominant transmission in Tourette's Syndrome— United Kingdom Cohort Study. *Br J Psychiatry.* 1993; 162:593–596.
6. Pauls DL, Alsobrook JP II, Almasy L. Genetic and epidemiological analyses of the Yale Tourette's Syndrome Family Study data. *Psychiatr Genet.* 1991;2:28.
7. Hasstedt S, Leppert M, Filloux F, et al. Intermediate inheritance of Tourette syndrome, assuming assortative mating. *Am J Hum Genet.* 1995;57:682–689.
8. Walkup JT, LaBuda MC, Singer HS, et al. Family study and segregation analysis of Tourette syndrome: evidence for a mixed model of inheritance. *Am J Hum Genet.* 1996;59:684–693.
9. Seuchter SA, Hebebrand J, Klug B, et al. Complex segregation analysis of families ascertained through Gilles de la Tourette syndrome. *Genet Epidemiol.* 2000;18:33–47.
10. Pauls DL, Leckman JF, Cohen DJ. The familial relationship between Gilles de la Tourette's Syndrome, attention deficit disorder, learning disabilities, speech disorders and stuttering. *J Am Acad Child Adolesc Psychiatry.* 1993;32:1044–1050.
11. Pauls DL, Leckman JF, Cohen DJ. Evidence against a genetic relationship between Gilles de la Tourette's syndrome and anxiety, depression, panic and phobic disorders. *Br J Psychiatry.* 1994;164:215–221.
12. Eapen V, Robertson MM, Alsobrook JP II, et al. Obsessive compulsive symptoms in Gilles de la Tourette's syndrome and obsessive compulsive disorder: Differences by diagnosis and family history. *Am J Med Genet B Neuropsychiatr Genet.* 1997;74:432–438.
13. Grados MA, Riddle MA, Samuels JF, et al. The familial phenotype of obsessive-compulsive disorder in relation to tic disorders: the Hopkins OCD family study. *Biol Psychiatry.* 2001;50:559–565.
14. Gottesman II, Gould TD. The endophenotype concept in psychiatry: etymology and strategic intentions. *Am J Psychiatry.* 2003;160:636–645.
15. Alsobrook JP II, Pauls DL. A factor analysis of tic symptoms in Gilles de la Tourette syndrome. *Am J Psychiatry.* 2002;159:291–296.
16. Leckman JF, Grice DE, Boardman J, et al. Symptoms of obsessive compulsive disorder. *Am J Psychiatry.* 1997;154:911–917.
17. Leckman J F, Pauls DL, Zhang H, et al. Obsessive-compulsive symptom dimensions in affected sibling

pairs diagnosed with Gilles de la Tourette syndrome. *Am J Med Genet B Neuropsychiatr Genet.* 2003; 116B:60–68.

18. Grigorenko EL, Wood FB, Meyer MS, et al. Susceptibility loci for distinct components of developmental dyslexia on chromosomes 6 and 15. *Am J Hum Genet.* 1997;60:27–39.

19. Grigorenko EL, Wood FB, Meyer MS, et al. The Chromosome 6p influences on different dyslexia-related cognitive processes: Further confirmation. *Am J Hum Genet.* 2000;66:715–723.

20. Fisher SE, Marlow AJ, Lamb J, et al. A quantitative-trait locus on chromosome 6p influences different aspects of developmental dyslexia. *Am J Hum Genet.* 1999;64:146–156.

21. Gayán J, Smith SD, Cherny SS, et al. Quantitative-trait locus for specific language and reading deficits on chromosome 6p. *Am J Hum Genet.* 1999;64:157–164.

22. Kaplan DE, Gayan J, Ahn J, et al. Evidence for linkage and association with reading disability on 6p21.3–22. *Am J Hum Genet.* 2002;70:1287–1298.

23. Turic D, Robinson L, Duke M, et al. Linkage disequilibrium mapping provides further evidence of a gene for reading disability on chromosome 6p21.3-22. *Mole Psychiatry.* 2003;8:176–185.

24. Deffenbacher KE, Kenyon JB, Hoover DM, et al. Refinement of the 6p21.3 quantitative trait locus influencing dyslexia: linkage and association analyses. *Hum Genet.* 2004;115:128–138.

25. Lamb JA, Parr JR, Bailey AJ, et al. Autism: in search of susceptibility genes. *Neuromolecular Medicine.* 2002; 2:11–28

26. Volkmar FR, Pauls D. Autism. *Lancet* 2003;62: 1133–1141.

27. Lewis DA, Glantz LA, Pierri JN, et al. Altered cortical glutamate neurotransmission in schizophrenia: evidence from morphological studies of pyramidal neurons. *Ann N Y Acad Sci.* 2003;1003;102–112.

28. Sklar P, Pato MT, Kirby A, et al. Genome-wide scan in Portuguese Island families identifies 5q31-5q35 as a susceptibility locus for schizophrenia and psychosis. *Mol Psychiatry.* 2004;9:213–18.

29. Paschou P, Feng Y, Pakstis AJ, et al. Indications of linkage and association of Gilles de la Tourette syndrome in two independent family samples: 17q25 is a putative susceptibility region. *Am J Hum Genet.* 2004;75:545–560.

30. Kidd, KK. New genetic strategies for studying psychiatric disorders. In: Sakai T, Tsuboi T (eds). *Genetic Aspects of Human Behavior.* Igaku-Shoin, Tokyo; 1984:325–346.

31. The International HapMap Consortium. The International HapMap Project. *Nature* 2003;426:789–796.

32. Maniatis N, Collins A, Gibson J, et al. Positional cloning by linkage disequilibrium. *Am J Hum Genet.* 2004;74:846–855.

33. Dorus S, Vallender EJ, Evans PD, et al. Accelerated evolution of nervous system genes in the origin of Homo sapiens. *Cell* 2004;119:1027–1040.

34. Mehan MR, Freimer NB, Ophoff RA. A genome-wide survey of segmental duplications that mediate common human genetic variation of chromosomal architecture. *Hum Genomics.* 2004;1:335–344.

35. Sebat J, Lakshmi B, Troge J, et al. Large-scale copy number polymorphism in the human genome. *Science* 2004;305:525–528.

36. Coon H, Myers RH, Borecki IB, et al. Replication of linkage of familial combined hyperlipidenia to chromosome 1q with additional heterogeneous effect of apolipoprotein A-I/C-III/A-IV locus: the NHLBI Family Hear Study. *Arterioscler Thromb Vasc Biol.* 2000;20:2275–2280.

37. Merétte C, Brassard A, Potvin A, et al. Significant linkage for Tourette syndrome in a large French Canadian family. *Am J Hum Genet.* 2000;67(4):1008–1013.

38. Altshuler JS, Altshuler D. Organizational challenges in clinical genomic research. *Nature* 2004;429:478–481.

12

Web-Based Consensus Diagnosis for Genetics Studies of Gilles De La Tourette Syndrome

William M. McMahon, Cornelia L. Illmann, and Meghan M. McGinn

Tourette Research Program, University of Utah, Division of Child and Adolescent Psychiatry, Salt Lake City, Utah

Genetic factors have long been considered important in the syndrome of Gilles de la Tourette (Tourette syndrome [TS]), as first noted in Dr. Tourette's original paper, published in 1885 (1). Ironically, molecular technology and computerized analytic tools are improving so rapidly that the rate-limiting step for TS gene discovery is arguably the collection and diagnosis of families affected with TS. In 1999, the Tourette Syndrome Association International Consortium for Genetics (TSAICG) reported evidence suggestive of loci contributing to risk of TS in a genome scan of 76 multiplex families (2). To follow-up those results, as well as findings by other investigators (3) the TSAICG has collected a second wave of affected families. To address the challenges associated with the larger sample size and to integrate the efforts of expert clinicians across 10 ascertainment sites, a new tool has been developed. This tool is a web-based process for Best Estimate (BE) diagnosis. This chapter describes the web-based BE process and details the resulting benefits and limitations.

THE WEB-BASED BEST ESTIMATE PROCESS

BE consensus diagnosis has been an important tool in psychiatric research for nearly a quarter of a century (4). BE diagnosis "refers to a process in which one or more diagnosticians review all available data on a subject (e.g., direct and informant interviews, clinical records, and psychological and laboratory test results) and use their clinical judgment to derive final diagnoses" (5). For the TSAICG linkage study reported in 1999, three expert clinicians spent 8 days sequestered in a room with boxes of files containing interview and clinical records of probands and family members from 76 multiplex families (nearly 300 total individuals). For each subject, two clinicians independently reviewed all clinical material and then submitted separate diagnoses. The diagnoses were compared and any discrepancies were resolved by inspecting the relevant records and arriving at consensus through discussion. If consensus was not achieved, ambiguous subject records were clarified by the clinician at the subject's site of origin or a third clinician was asked to join the process.

BE diagnoses on the recent second wave of TSAICG families have now been carried out by web-adapting the process used on the first wave of families (described in 2). The first step in the new process was to remove all personal identifiers and scan each file into portable document format (pdf) files in the database. These files contained all available information about the individual, including the self-report booklets, semi-structured interviews, and clinic records when available. Assessment instruments included:

- The Family Self Report Questionnaire for Tics, Obsessive-Compulsiveness, Attentional Difficulties, Impulsivity and Motor Hyperactivity (2)

Tourette Sib-Pair Consortium Best Estimate System

You have reached the main page of the Tourette Sib-Pair Consortium Best Estimate System. You should see the patients you have been assigned to review below. You may click on the logo in the upper right-hand corner at any time to return to this screen. Administrators, click on the 'Administrative' link in the footer to manage the site. In order to log out from the system you <u>must</u> close your browser window.

Patient	Instrument	Status	Other Clinician	
001-004-04	KSADS	Not Started	John Doe	Review
001-009-03	SCIDS	Not Started	John Doe	Review
001-010-01	SCIDS	Not Started	John Doe	Review
001-013-04	KSADS	Not Started	John Doe	Review
001-014-02	SCIDS	Not Started	John Doe	Review
001-020-01	SCIDS	Not Started	John Doe	Review
001-024-01	SCIDS	Not Started	Bill McMahon (william.mcmahon@hsc.utah.edu)	Review
001-025-04	KSADS	Not Started	Bill McMahon (william.mcmahon@hsc.utah.edu)	Review
005-007-01	SCIDS	Not Started	John Doe	Review
005-051-02	SCIDS	Not Started	John Doe	Review

 MASSACHUSETTS GENERAL HOSPITAL

Home | Edit Profile | Administrative

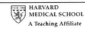 HARVARD MEDICAL SCHOOL A Teaching Affiliate

Fig. 12-1. Clinician home page.

symptom inventory and ordinal severity scales modified from the Yale Global Tic Severity Scale (YGTSS) (6) and the Yale-Brown Obsessive-Compulsive Scale (YBOCS) (7)

- Clinician interview using the YGTSS (6)
- Clinician interview using modified YBOCS (8) or Children's YBOCS (CYBOCS) (9)
- Conners Parent Rating Scale-Revised Long version (CPRS-RL) (10) or Conners Adult Attention Deficit Hyperactivity Disorder (ADHD) Rating Scale (CAARS-RL) (11)
- Diagnostic Confidence Index (12)
- Kiddie Schedule for Affective Disorders and Schizophrenia (KSADS) (13,14) for patients younger than age 18 years
- Structured Clinical Interview for DSM-IIIR (SCID) (15)

The original assessment file materials, usually several hundred paper pages were organized into six categories (TSAICG Self Report, DCI, YGTSS, YBOCS or CYBOCS, SCID or KSADS, Other). The larger assessment instruments, such as the TSAICG Self-Report booklet

containing modified YGTSS and YBOCS were also bookmarked. This created an electronic table of contents with pdf tabs that required only a click to bring up the desired page. Once all of the pdf files for a subject were assembled in the database, the case was assigned to two clinicians for independent BE diagnoses.

The second step was the on-line review of subject materials by expert clinicians. After logging into the password-protected site, each clinician could view his or her individual homepage listing anonymous case numbers (Fig. 12-1).

Besides seeing the list of cases assigned to him or her, the clinician could learn whether the individual was a child or adult (KSADS indicated children, SCID indicated adult), the status of the review, the other assigned clinician and the status of the BE process. From the list of cases, the clinician selected one case and reviewed the corresponding assessment files so that diagnoses could be determined. The clinician directly entered each diagnosis on the coding sheet, by choosing from a list of five mutually exclusive categories: 1–not present

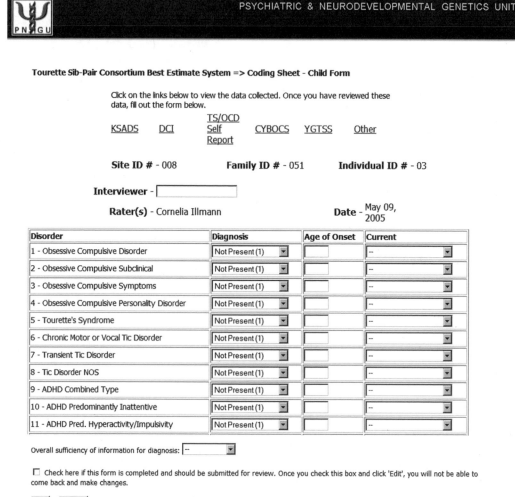

Fig. 12-2. Coding sheet—child form.

(no evidence of the disorder); 2–possible (some characteristics of the disorder, but not a convincing case); 3–probable (meets many, but not all of the required diagnostic criteria); 4–definite (fully meets diagnostic criteria); and 9–unable to code (insufficient information to make a diagnosis). Figure 12-2, Coding Sheet-Child Form, is an image illustrating the data input form that structured the clinician's on-line data entry for diagnosis. Diagnostic criteria from DSM-IV-TR were used to diagnose TS, obsessive-compulsive disorder (OCD) and the three categories of

ADHD. In addition, milder variants of tic disorders and OCD were also coded, giving a total of 11 tic/OCD/ADHD categories. Additional DSM-IV disorders from the SCID or KSADS were also listed online, but they were not completed for this phase of the study and are not shown in Figure 12-2.

Besides entering diagnoses, the clinician was also required to enter the age at onset and whether the disorder was currently occurring or only occurred in the past. Once the diagnostic categories were entered, the clinician rated the overall sufficiency of the information for diagnosis on a four-point ordinal scale (poor, fair, good, or excellent) and checked a box to indicate the coding was complete and ready for consensus comparison. If the clinician could not complete the coding sheet in the first on-line session, whatever was completed could be stored in the database and the case could be re-opened to be completed in any number of subsequent sessions.

Each subject record was independently evaluated by two diagnosticians. Once submitted to the database, the best estimates of the two diagnosticians were immediately compared and feedback was provided by the web-system software. This feedback was emailed to each clinician. When there was disagreement between the two raters, the areas of disagreement were identified in the email notification. The two diagnosticians then reviewed the relevant file with a focus on the specific diagnostic disagreement, and subsequently communicated with each other by telephone or email to arrive at consensus. The final diagnosis was then entered online by one diagnostician and verified by the other. If consensus was not possible, the source of disagreement was identified and subsequent alternative steps were taken. Disagreements resulted from inadequate or ambiguous records, differing interpretations of data, and differing interpretations of decision rules for specific diagnoses. If the disagreement resulted from inadequate or ambiguous subject records, then clarification was requested from the clinician at the site that submitted the case. If the disagreement resulted from interpretation of the clinical data or diagnostic decision rules and consensus between the two clinicians could not be achieved by discussion, then the case was sent to a third diagnostician for both independent diagnosis and consensus discussion with the first two diagnosticians. In some cases, decision rules were discussed and clarified in a conference call with all the clinicians. Table 12-1 gives the decision rules for developed by the expert clinician group for distinguishing between OCD, subclinical OCD, and obsessive compulsive

TABLE 12-1. *Decision matrix for obsessive compulsive categories*

	Time (required)	Distress*	Interference*
Obsessive compulsive disorder	≥1 hr	> Mild	> Mild
Subclinical Obsessive compulsive disorder	<1 hr	Mild	Mild
Obsessive compulsive symptoms	None	None	None

*Either distress or interference is required for obsessive compulsive disorder and subclinical obsessive compulsive disorder.

symptoms. If there was still disagreement, the family would be removed from the sample; however, consensus was achieved on all cases in this sample.

PROJECT ADMINISTRATION

In addition to the web-based process that diagnosticians utilized, the administrators of the project (coordinator, database systems administrators, and principal investigator) used other database tools to assign, monitor, and summarize the work. One of the primary administrative tasks was the addition of new cases. To add a new case, the subject identification number was entered and the adult or child version of the diagnosis coding sheet was selected. After entering the subject identification information, the pdf files of the subject's clinical materials, such as the SCID or YGTSS, were uploaded. A new case could not be stored in the system until at least one instrument was uploaded.

The next step in the administrative process involved the assignment of clinicians. Typically, two clinicians were assigned to each case. To begin to use the system and establish baseline rater agreement, an identical sample of 25 test cases was given to each clinician. For these initial test cases, all of the participating clinicians were assigned to the same cases. Subsequently, new cases were assigned in batches of 10 to rotating pairs of BE clinicians.

PSYCHIATRIC & NEURODEVELOPMENTAL GENETICS UNIT

Tourette Sib-Pair Consortium Best Estimate System => Administrative Home => Diagnoses Reporting

Click on the links below to view the data sources for this individual.

SCIDS   DCI   TS/OCD
Self Report   YBOCS   YGTSS   Other

Below are the diagnoses made by all the clinicians who are doing 'test' or 'clinician' or 'final' diagnoses.

Site ID # - 000   Family ID # - 012   Individual ID # - 01

Data Field	User/Response		
Clinician's Name	Bill McMahon	John Doe	Bill McMahon
Diagnosis Purpose	clinician	clinician	final
Date Created	Apr 27, 2004	Apr 27, 2004	Sep 05, 2004
Date Last Modified	Sep 05, 2004	Jul 22, 2004	Sep 05, 2004
Age At Interview			
Completed	Yes	Yes	Yes
Started	Yes	Yes	Yes
Interviewer			
Sufficiency Of Information	3	3	3
Disorders			
1 - Obsessive Compulsive Disorder	4 Definite	4 Definite	4 Definite
2 - Obsessive Compulsive Subclinical	1 Not Present	1 Not Present	1 Not Present
3 - Obsessive Compulsive Symptoms	1 Not Present	1 Not Present	1 Not Present
4 - Obsessive Compulsive Personality Dis.	1 Not Present	1 Not Present	1 Not Present
5 - Tourette's Syndrome	4 Definite	4 Definite	4 Definite
6 - Chronic Motor or Vocal Tic Disorder	1 Not Present	1 Not Present	1 Not Present
7 - Transient Tic Disorder	1 Not Present	1 Not Present	1 Not Present
8 - Tic Disorder NOS	1 Not Present	1 Not Present	1 Not Present
9 - ADHD Combined Type	1 Not Present	1 Not Present	1 Not Present
10 - ADHD Predominantly Inattentive	1 Not Present	1 Not Present	1 Not Present
11 - ADHD Pred. Hyperactivity/Impulsivity	1 Not Present	1 Not Present	1 Not Present

MASSACHUSETTS
GENERAL HOSPITAL   Home | Edit Profile | Administrative

Fig. 12-3. Administrative home-diagnoses reporting.

Monitoring the progress of the consensus process was accomplished using the "Patient Report by ID" query tool. If a specific identification number of a case was entered, each clinician's completed diagnosis record, as well as the final consensus diagnoses, could be examined. Moreover, another query tool could create a side-by-side comparison of each clinician's initial diagnoses, and the final consensus diagnoses were also available (Fig. 12-3).

The dates that the cases were created in the best estimates system as well as the dates of submission of the clinician diagnoses and final consensus diagnoses were all accessible here. Other administrative tools allowed checking progress by site and by family.

PERFORMANCE OF THE WEB-BASED BEST ESTIMATE SYSTEM

For wave 2 of the TSAICG sib-pair studies, diagnostic materials for 566 individuals (154 sib-pair families) were entered into the database and reviewed by at least two members of the team of eight clinicians. Initial BE efforts focused on TS, chronic motor/vocal tics, transient tic disorder, tic disorder not otherwise specified, OCD, obsessive compulsive subclinical, obsessive compulsive symptoms, ADHD-predominantly inattentive type, ADHD-predominantly hyperactive-impulsive type, and ADHD-combined. (Additional DSM-IV disorders from the SCID or KSADS were not completed for this phase of the study.)

Initial independent BE diagnoses showed good rates of agreement between diagnosticians for DSM-IV-TR TS, 93.5% for all subjects; 92.5% for parents only ($N = 226$ parents); and 94.1% for siblings only ($N = 340$). The slightly higher rate of agreement for sibs compared with parents was expected from the design of the study because the sib-pair linkage study sample was ascertained with the goal of including only families with at least two siblings manifesting TS. Even though personal identifiers were stripped from case files, the fact that a subject was a child potentially biased diagnosticians toward the presence of a disorder, especially TS. However, parent diagnoses were not expected to manifest a disorder to the same degree as siblings. Thus, the rate of agreement for parents only (92.5%) provides a more conservative measure of agreement than the sibling only rate (94.1%). Good agreement was found for parent cases in other tic categories: chronic tic disorder (motor or phonic) 90.7%; transient tic disorder 98.2%; tic disorder not otherwise specified 98.7%. For obsessive compulsive categories agreement rates were not as high as for the tic categories. Agreement rates on parents ($N = 226$) were 89.9% for OCD; 88.5% for subclinical OCD; and 86.8% for OC symptoms. Attention disorder categories were the most difficult, resulting in parent diagnosis agreement rates of 84.1% for ADHD combined, 88.5% for ADHD inattentive, and 90.7% for ADHD.

Hyperactive/Impulsive

Disagreement on BE diagnoses for all diagnostic categories was lower in cases in which assessment records were less complete, legible, or clear. One diagnostic score sheet item required

diagnosticians to rate quality of information for the total subject record on a four-point ordinal scale, with 4 defined as the highest quality. For 566 cases, the average quality of record score was 2.62 (SD = 0.57) and the quality rating was negatively correlated with agreement (r = 0.201; $P < 0.001$).

Although all diagnostic categories were affected by completeness, legibility, and clarity of assessment records, the ADHD categories appeared the most challenging. For the three ADHD categories combined in the total sample, only 78.3% of initial BE diagnoses were concordant. Furthermore, diagnosticians submitted "unable to code" for ADHD categories in 47 cases, compared with 10 for tic categories and 8 for OC categories. Even after the consensus discussions, 30 cases of ADD were given the label "unable to code" as the final diagnosis. This probably reflects multiple challenges regarding ADHD diagnoses. Perhaps the most important is that our assessment focused on tics and OCD, and used well developed diagnostic instruments. For ADHD, assessment instruments were limited to Conners' child and adult rating forms [CPRS-RL (10) and CAARS-RL (11)], parent or self report history of onset before age 7 years, and follow-up brief interviewer questions. No school reports or ratings were available for children. The assessment for adult attention disorders was imperfect because childhood history was limited to self-report and current symptoms were often not corroborated by spouse reports. Diagnosing adult ADHD in our parents of children with TS (and many with OCD additionally) may also have been more challenging because of the increased frequency of TS and OCD in the parents themselves.

ADVANTAGES OF WEB-BASED BEST ESTIMATE

The web-based BE diagnosis process we used for the TSAICG wave 2 sib-pair study provided a number of advantages over the paper-based procedure used for wave 1. First, web-based BE facilitated the distribution of the work load across clinicians, time, and space. In wave 1, three clinicians traveled to one site for a grueling marathon BE session. In wave 2, eight clinicians across three continents worked at times of their choosing and without traveling. The web-based system was accessible wherever clinicians had internet access, meaning that work could be done nearly anywhere and at any time. Besides increasing the overall BE capacity, utilizing clinicians from each site and rotating pairs of consensus partners may also have increased group cohesiveness and problem solving.

A second benefit of the web-based BE database software was the on-line algorithm for scoring agreement and updating progress. The system compared diagnoses of BE pairs and notified the clinicians immediately by email. For cases of agreement, the diagnoses were entered by the system and removed from the clinician assignment list. For disagreements, the clinicians were informed of the specific areas of disagreement. The web-based BE system eliminated much scoring, entering, and list-making that had been done by hand in previous BE work. This both decreased data entry work and increased accuracy. Furthermore, the query tools allowed project administrators to easily track progress by subject, family, site, or clinician.

A third area of advantage of web-based BE resulted from scanning original assessment documents into pdf files for on-line review. This eliminated the need for making and shipping photo copies and decreased the risk of losing or misplacing the original documents. The book-marking feature allowed quick and selective inspection of critical pages in large documents. Clinicians found that they could review large subject files quicker electronically than was possible with paper.

LIMITATIONS OF WEB-BASED BEST ESTIMATE

The primary disadvantages of the TSAICG web-based BE are startup time and cost, learning curve, rigidity, and ghosts in the machine. Development of the web-based BE software has taken many months longer and more money than expected. Besides the software and hardware expenses at the Massachusetts General Hospital, clinicians at each site have had to upgrade connectivity and personal computer hardware. Although clinician users have learned to use the system after a brief orientation, the initial efforts were occasionally frustrating and speed came only with practice. Certain features of the system limited administrative flexibility. For example, editing of a subject record was difficult. If an assessment document was scanned into a subject file, and the original document was illegible or incorrect, then the file could not be edited once a clinician submitted a diagnosis. Finally, start-up errors (ghosts) became evident once the system was in use. For example, clinicians submitted diagnoses for some cases and subsequently learned that there was no record of their work because administrative activities (changing forms) had eliminated the data they had submitted. Clinicians found that keeping their own notes was prudent.

CONCLUSIONS

The web-based BE diagnostic system has increased clinician efficiency by decreasing the need for travel and commitment of extended blocks of time. This adaptation of new technology to facilitate the BE process has required time, money, and collaboration. Some limitations persist but future large-scale studies requiring BE diagnoses will benefit from this web-based system.

ACKNOWLEDGMENTS

The authors express their deep gratitude to the families who have donated their time, energy, hope and DNA to the TSAICG studies. Thanks also to Sue Levi-Pearl and Heather Cowley of TSA; David Pauls; Claire Donehower and Julia O'Rourke of Massachusetts General Hospital; and Tracy Green at the University of Utah.

This work was funded in part by RO1 NS40024 (David Pauls, PI) and funds from the TSA. Clinicians who contributed to the development of the web-based best estimate process include: Danielle Cath, Amsterdam; Yves Dion, Montreal; George Gericke, Pretoria; Marco Grados, Baltimore; Robert King, New Haven; Roger Kurlan, Rochester; James Leckman, New

Haven; William McMahon, Salt Lake City; Carol Mathews, San Diego; Mary Robertson, London; Paul Sandor, Toronto; and John Walkup, Baltimore.

REFERENCES

1. Goetz CG, Klawans HL. Gilles de la Tourette. In: Friedhoff AJ, Chase TN, eds. *Advances in Neurology*, Vol. 35. New York City, NY: Raven Press; 1982:1–16.
2. A complete genome screen in sib pairs affected by Gilles de la Tourette syndrome. The Tourette Syndrome Association International Consortium for Genetics. *Am J Hum Genet*. 1999;65:1428–1436.
3. Merrette C, Brassard A, Potvin A, et al. Significant linkage for Tourette syndrome in a large French Canadian family. *Am J Hum Genet*. 2000;67:1008–1013.
4. Leckman JF, Sholomskas D, Thompson WD, et al. Best estimate of lifetime psychiatric diagnosis: a methodological study. *Arch Gen Psychiatry*. 1982;39:879–883.
5. Klein DN, Ouimette PC, Kelly HS, et al. Test-retest reliability of team consensus best-estimate diagnosis of Axis I and II disorders in a family study. *Am J Psychiatry*. 1994;151:1043–1047.
6. Leckman JF, Riddle MA, Ort SI, et al. The Yale Global Tic Severity Scale: Initial testing of a clinic-rated scale of tic severity. *J Am Acad Child Adolesc Psychiatry*. 1989;28:566–573.
7. Goodman WK, Price LH, Rasmussen SA, et al. The Yale-Brown Obsessive Compulsive Scale II: validity. *Arch Gen Psychiatry*. 1989;46:1012–1016.
8. Goodman WK, Price LH, Rasmussen SA, et al. The Yale-Brown Obsessive Compulsive Scale, I: development, use, and reliability. *Arch Gen Psychiatry*. 1989;46:1006–1011.
9. Scahill L, Riddle MA, McSwiggin-Hardin M, et al. Children's Yale-Brown Obsessive Compulsive Scale: reliability and validity. *J Am Acad Child Adolesc Psychiatry*. 1997;36:844–852.
10. Conners CK. *Conners' Parent Rating Scale—Revised (L)*. Toronto, Canada: Multi-Health Systems, Inc; 1997.
11. Conners CK, Erhardt D, Sparrow EP. *The Conners Adult ADHD Rating Scale (CAARS)*. Toronto, Canada: Multi-Health Systems, Inc; 1998. Conners CK. Erhardt D, Sparrow EP. *CAARS—Self-Report: Long Version*. North Tonawanda, NY: Multi-Health Systems; 1997.
12. Robertson MM, Banerjee S, Kurlan R, et al. The Tourette Syndrome Diagnostic Confidence Index: Development and clinical associations. *Neurology* 1999;59:2108–2112.
13. Chambers WJ, Puig-Antich J, Hirsch M, et al. The assessment of affective disorders in children and adolescents by semistructured interview. Test-retest reliability of the schedule for affective disorders and schizophrenia for school-aged children, present episode version. *Arch Gen Psychiatry*. 1985;42:696–702.
14. Kaufman J, Birmaher B, Brent D, et al. Schedule for Affective Disorders and Schizophrenia for School-Aged Children-Present and Lifetime Version (K-SADS-PL): Initial Reliability and Validity Data. *J Am Acad Child Adolesc Psychiatry*. 1997;36:980–988.
15. First M, Spitzer R, Gibbon M, et al. *Structured Clinical Interview for DSM-IV Axis I Disorders*. Washington, DC: American Psychiatric Press; 1997.

13

Genes and Tourette Syndrome: Scientific, Ethical, and Social Implications

Nancy M. P. King

School of Medicine, University of North Carolina-Chapel Hill, Chapel Hill, NC

The Human Genome Project has not only stimulated society's interest in genes and what they do: it has also spurred thought about the implications of scientific and medical advances. Since the structure of DNA was determined and the genetic paradigm transformed science and medicine, understanding the human genome has always been envisioned both as a means of understanding what it means to be human and as a means of altering much of what seems inevitable about being human: the limitations of human physical nature; the hand that heredity has dealt every individual; illness, aging, and death. Science has now accumulated much information about the human genetic heritage, but researchers still understand very little about the intricate relationships between genes and environment, and the ability to use genetic knowledge to treat disease is in its infancy.

What are the implications of all this unfulfilled promise for genetic disorders such as Tourette syndrome (TS)? As scientists, clinicians, TS patients, families, and advocates work to see that the promise of genetics is fulfilled, it can be very tempting to ignore some of the implications of imperfect knowledge. This essay is an attempt to pose questions and encourage critical reflection, so that society can keep up with science and guide it.

Regarding genes and TS, there are four general things to think about: identifying the TS gene or genes; looking for the gene using modern microarray technologies; instituting screening and testing programs for TS; and the meaning and implications of the results.

GENE FINDING

Despite the great hopes raised by the Human Genome Project, reliably identifying a gene or genes linked to a particular disease or disorder has proven to be difficult, time-consuming, expensive work—especially for complex neurobehavioral disorders such as TS. Affected individuals and their families have to provide DNA that can be examined as part of the search process. In many instances those same families and their advocacy networks have organized themselves and collaborated with investigators to provide specimens and even financial support. Indeed, the Tourette Syndrome Association and its members have engaged in just such an effort. Once one or more TS genes are identified in this way, it will be necessary to envision and develop ways of applying the discovery to the disorder. Some investigators may focus on developing a genetic test with sufficient sensitivity and specificity to provide reliable identification of the gene in at-risk individuals. Other investigators may concentrate on developing potential treatments, such as gene transfer; protein-based or enzyme-based interventions; or targeted pharmacogenetic interventions. And in today's market-oriented environment, all such developments typically also become patentable, potentially profitable products.

The sad history of the development of a genetic test for Canavan disease is an important cautionary tale. After considerable cooperative efforts in the development of an effective test, a patenting dispute rendered the test too expensive to be readily accessible to potentially affected families—the same families who had collaborated so closely in its development. Other disease advocacy groups have since learned from the experience with Canavan disease. They have become quite expert in patent and contract law, and some (pseudoxanthoma elasticum, or PXE, is a well-known example) have created elaborate research and development mechanisms in order to serve their members by maintaining better control of genetic and biotechnological products. Whether such efforts will pay off remains to be seen.

Different pitfalls appear when it comes to developing treatments. Despite great promise and even greater hype during its short 15-year history, gene transfer research has not yet become gene *therapy* for any disease or disorder. Gene therapy for TS seems an unlikely prospect. Meaningful predictions are difficult at present. However, depending on what is learned about the enzymatic and regulatory functions of the TS gene or genes, potential therapies are more likely to be found in enzyme replacement, targeted pharmacology, or even dietary approaches. Thus, finding a TS gene or genes must be recognized as a first step on a long scientific road—*not* as the prelude to a cure. And of course, the process of testing experimental interventions intended as future treatments has its own universe of research ethics challenges.

GENE TROLLING

In the course of developing and using a genetic test, technological advances in finding particular genes can give rise to unusual ethical issues. To give a relatively simple example, the apolipoprotein E gene that is associated with Alzheimer disease was originally identified and described as predictive of heart disease. When the new association with Alzheimer disease appeared, physicians and patients who had sought genetic testing out of concern about the risk of developing one condition had to face discussing the potential to develop a far more upsetting and less treatable condition. Today, when clinicians and scientists go looking for a given gene, they are likely to use microarray technology, which trolls through—and turns up—hundreds of different genes. If DNA is run through a microarray, a TS gene may be found—and almost certainly a large number of other genes will be found, with greater or lesser degrees of medical significance for their owners.

What should a researcher do if the test also finds genes associated with other diseases, disorders, and conditions, including disease susceptibilities and even physical or nonphysical personal traits or characteristics? Does the researcher narrow the test? Does the researcher simply not disclose findings unrelated to the gene sought? Does the researcher tell everything, regardless of what it might mean for individuals and families? Or does the researcher disclose some findings, but not others? As can be plainly seen once the possibilities are listed, there is more than one potentially acceptable answer—but the researcher must think about it, talk about it, and make a conscious and deliberate choice, *before* facing the dilemma in someone's genome.

GENETIC SCREENING AND TESTING

TS is a chronic, non-life-threatening disorder. It has a broad spectrum of symptom severity, with most individuals affected mildly to moderately. Bearing this in mind, once a genetic test for TS has been developed, how exactly should it be used? Should it be used to test at-risk individuals only—and how broadly should "at-risk" be defined? Certainly, asymptomatic members of affected families would be considered to be at risk. In the case of TS, many at-risk individuals would probably be young children. Testing asymptomatic children for a disorder like TS raises many more ethical and social questions than does the testing of adults, who can make their own informed decisions about whether to be tested. Even more complex questions would be raised if members of affected families wanted to use assisted reproductive technologies, and decided to test embryos for TS before implantation, in order to avoid giving birth to offspring with a TS gene.

If a test for TS were available, would screening of the general population for TS be proposed? If screening is attempted, who should be screened? Would screening of newborns be sensible or desirable? As with all genetic screening, false negative and false positive results are possible. What should the counseling process before screening be like? What is an acceptable number of false positive or false negative test results? How should preliminary results be followed up on? If affected newborns are identified through screening, will their parents be pressured to test their siblings—and to have themselves tested?

Of course, if affected newborns are identified at all, they will be identified before it can be known how TS will affect them. That is, genetic screening of newborns for TS, like genetic testing of asymptomatic individuals in affected families, will be "presymptomatic." How should this knowledge of their genetic status be regarded and used by their families, health care providers, and school authorities? What should be done with the knowledge that someone who has no symptoms has a TS gene? Might such individuals—especially children—be scrutinized, stigmatized, even discriminated against, in the absence of symptoms?

Should finding a TS gene, and having the ability to identify it in asymptomatic people, affect how researchers and families think about TS? Could knowledge of the genetic status of asymptomatic people create pressures to devise early interventions for treatment (for example, starting a child on medication before symptoms appear, as is currently being advocated for children at risk for schizophrenia)? In the absence of genuinely effective treatments, early identification of affected individuals could help spur research into more effective treatments or symptom-preventing interventions—perhaps making children with genetically identified but presymptomatic TS especially desirable research subjects. Yet because it cannot really be known how an individual with TS is affected by

it before symptoms develop, it seems likely that what it means to have TS could be altered by genetic identification, whether or not it is followed by development of new treatments.

Genetic identification could change the understanding of TS in another way as well. Depending on the nature of the genetic disorder being studied, genetic screening and testing has the potential to identify not only individuals with a particular disorder, but also so-called "carriers," who do not have the disorder themselves but are able to pass it to offspring. Carrier status is a significant issue for some genetic diseases, such as Huntington disease, cystic fibrosis, or sickle cell disease. Carrier status is also often misunderstood—as it was, scandalously, for sickle cell disease in the 1970s—and the term itself can be stigmatizing (*Typhoid Mary,* for example). But in some disorders it is now recognized that carrier status has specific health effects; for example, carrier status in Fragile X syndrome is now called by some a "predisease state". Should carrier status matter in TS? And if it should—or even only if the label is applied—what does it mean to be a carrier of TS?

Most of the many questions just listed deserve much more discussion. Some of them are probably premature, given the current state of knowledge about TS and its genetic component. But they all lead directly to the heart of the matter: What does it mean to have a TS gene?

WHAT DO GENES MEAN?

The excitement about the Human Genome Project can easily elevate genetics to an overly powerful position in society's understanding of humankind and perspective on health and illness. This tendency is known as "genetic essentialism" or "genetic reductionism"—equating all the significance of a characteristic or condition with the gene itself. The oversimplicity of this view of human individuality was initially very tempting to both scientists and the public. However, what researchers have since learned through the Human Genome Project itself has made clear that genetic essentialism is at best radically incomplete, and at worst deeply wrongheaded.

For all its challenges and miseries, TS is a perfect example of how wrong reducing humans to genes can be. Just three reasons why are discussed here, although there are many others.

First, TS certainly has variable penetrance: individuals with TS can be anywhere on an extraordinarily broad spectrum of symptom severity, from barely to extremely affected. In addition, the effects they exhibit can range across an equally broad spectrum and in many combinations, can wax and wane, and can change greatly over time. Individuals with TS may or may not also be diagnosed with other disorders that have an equally broad severity spectrum, such as obsessive compulsive disorder. This suggests that having a TS gene tells researchers and clinicians very little about an individual's experience of having the disorder.

Second, TS is one of the best examples there is of the complex relationship between genes and their expression, nature and nurture, as well as the relationship between biology and society and culture. Having the gene says little by itself because the relationship of the individual to his or her time and place is what defines TS for that person. Many examples of these complex relationships, and of the "socially situated" nature of TS, have been well explored in TS scholarship, including how cultural context may influence the manifestations of TS, and how the nature and severity of symptoms can change in relationship to the individual's immediate circumstances. This point leads directly to the third reason:

TS has an immensely rich "meaning history." An important component of medical education is the effort to systematically remind medical students of the experiences of patients. Although physicians diagnose *diseases*, they enter into relationships with patients who are *people*, who have lives and tell stories. Surely everyone who has received a diagnosis of TS—and everyone who interacts with someone with the diagnosis—has thought about, and struggled to understand, the relationship between the disorder and the person. People with TS—and often those close to them—may experience considerable distress, stigmatization, and discrimination. Coming to terms with TS often means addressing extraordinarily complicated, morally freighted questions about identity, family, and future.

Because TS symptoms can be addressed through a variety of treatments—albeit imperfect ones—but not cured, these questions have lifelong implications. And because people are so much more than their genes, even the most intensive scientific focus on the TS gene is unlikely to shed light on the lived experience and sense of self of the person with TS.

So if looking for genes, and looking at genes, carries clinicians and researchers away from the lived experience of TS, then the best science can only be partially helpful. Instead, if people affected by TS, with their varied experiences and nuanced stories, were to collaborate with genetic scientists, they could make a real contribution by leading the way in reintegrating genes and environment, biology and personhood. This kind of newly "recomplicated" view of genetic disease—which is actually a very old view—is desperately needed right now, because enormous attention is currently being given to bad misunderstandings of behavioral genetics.

Even the best science needs good ethics, and good ethics starts with considering the social and personal context in which scientific progress takes place. Researchers simply need to remember that most of what is known about disorders such as TS is complicated because the relationship between genes and behavior is complicated. Looking to science for simple answers to complicated questions does not work. Instead, it is essential to ask as many questions as possible. This approach usually makes life more complicated, but ultimately far more interesting, and well worth the effort.

14

Preclinical/Clinical Evidence of Central Nervous System Infectious Etiology in PANDAS

Tanya K. Murphy, David S. Husted, and Paula J. Edge

Department of Psychiatry, University of Florida

CENTRAL NERVOUS SYSTEM AUTOIMMUNITY

Autoimmunity is loss of self-tolerance by the immune system. This loss of self-tolerance allows the immune system to target the organism's own tissues. Autoimmunity is present to some degree in all humans, but is usually benign and even, at times, protective (1). Disease is defined by the progression of autoimmunity to a degree that is pathologic to the organism, disrupting function and/or causing symptomatology. Genetic factors and environmental triggers influence this progression from a normal physiologic process to a disease state. In the past decade, a large body of literature has been generated concerning the role that a malfunctioning immune system may serve in the etiology of neuropsychiatric disorders. This chapter will concentrate on emerging support for autoimmunity of tics and other neuropsychiatric disorders with a special focus on group A streptococcus (GAS).

RHEUMATIC FEVER AND PANDAS

In the 40 years following World War II, the rate of rheumatic fever (RF) fell dramatically; many believed the disease virtually nonexistent. Surprisingly, in 1987 there was a resurgence of acute RF in the United States in disparate geographical locations, with most demonstrating either no symptoms or subclinical symptoms of a preceding pharyngitis (2). Unlike pre-World War II outbreaks, these subsequent RF cases had a greater proportion of individuals who developed Sydenham chorea (SC) (3). A major manifestation of RF, SC is believed to be the result of a cross-reaction between antibodies directed against GAS and epitopes on neurons of the basal ganglia (as well as other regions of the central nervous system [CNS]), resulting in disturbances both motoric and behavioral (4,5).

Susan Swedo, a National Institutes of Mental Health researcher, et al. (6) noted a high prevalence of obsessive-compulsive disorder (OCD) symptoms in patients with SC. Subsequently, she and others conducted systematic investigations into the neuropsychiatric aspects of SC, finding that more than 70% of RF patients with SC presented with classic obsessive compulsive disorder (OCD) symptoms, whereas OCD symptoms were absent in RF patients without SC (7–9). Although Swedo's initial focus was on the OCD symptoms in SC patients, tic disorders (including Tourette syndrome [TS]), emotional lability, separation anxiety, inattention, and hyperactivity were also frequently reported in SC patients (7). Around this time, Louise Kiessling also noticed a large increase in incidence of tic disorders coinciding with GAS outbreak in her developmental pediatric practice (10). Reasoning that if RF and SC are secondary to GAS infections, then the higher incidence of OCD and tics also could be GAS related, Swedo et al. coined the term *PANDAS* (*P*ediatric *A*utoimmune *N*europsychiatric *D*isorders *A*ssociated with *S*treptococcal infection).

The current criteria for diagnosing PANDAS are 1) the presence of OCD and/or a tic disorder, 2) childhood onset of symptoms (age 3 years to puberty), 3) an episodic or sawtooth course of symptom severity, 4) an association with GAS infection (a positive throat culture for strep or history of scarlet fever), and 5) evidence of concurrent neurologic abnormalities (motoric hyperactivity or adventitious movements, such as choreiform movements). Factors that determine whether the symptoms of PANDAS remit following an acute episode or progress to a more chronic illness are not yet known. Regardless, the symptoms and characteristic course of PANDAS is often typical of OCD and tics early in the illness.

NEUROLOGIC FACTORS

There is a high co-morbidity among childhood onset OCD, tics, attention deficit hyperactivity disorder (ADHD) and the presence of neurologic soft signs, such as choreiform movements and pronator sign/drift. Recent studies (11,12) have presented evidence that an overall worsening of neurologic performance was concurrent with or followed neuropsychiatric symptoms. The clinical neurologic picture of a child with a presentation of PANDAS can be complicated, given that neurologic soft signs may only present intermittently in a particular child, the clinical significance of these findings is unknown, and no causal relationship has been identified to account for these neurologic performance fluctuations. Additional research is requisite, both to clarify the neurologic issues and to better differentiate choreiform movements from chorea (13), and chorea from tics—a distinction that has troubled physicians for years due to the overlap of movements seen in choreiform disorders and tic disorders (14).

SUPPORT FOR GROUP A STREPTOCOCCUS IN THE PRESENTATION OF PANDAS

Strong support has long existed in the literature in favor of GAS as the inciting agent in the development of RF and its neuropsychiatric expression SC (5). PANDAS may be a subtype of OCD/tic disorder that has a unique pathophysiology distinct from SC, as does post-streptococcal reactive arthritis from RF (15). Thus post-streptococcal reactive arthritis is a case in point; although similar to the arthritis seen in RF, post-streptococcal reactive arthritis does not meet the criteria for RF in that few reports of carditis exist (16,17) and none exist describing CNS involvement. Similarly, PANDAS, by exclusion, does not meet the criteria for carditis and arthritis but shares overlap with RF in the quality of neuropsychiatric symptoms observed. Subtle pathophysiologic differences may exist leading to the clinical presentation of RF, SC, post-streptococcal reactive arthritis, or PANDAS based on serotype, strain, streptococcus group differences, and the genetic/developmental susceptibility of the child.

Swedo et al. (18) has described at least 50 PANDAS cases, many of which had an acute and dramatic onset that was frequently associated with preceding streptococcal pharyngitis (44%). When followed prospectively, 31% of the 144 observed neuropsychiatric exacerbations were associated with documented GAS infection, whereas only 33 episodes (22.9%) had no evidence of an infectious trigger.

Many other associations of GAS with OCD and/or tic disorders have been described in the literature (11,19–26). Observations have been made that attributed tics and/or OCD onset/exacerbation to recent strep or respiratory infection or to categorically elevated GAS titers. For example, a study examining children for first evaluation of tic disorders found a significant increase in anti-streptolysin O titer elevations, with 38% of 150 children with tics having anti-streptolysin O >500 IU/mL compared with 2% of 150 healthy controls (21). When children with tics and OCD were followed prospectively, those with a clinical course consistent with PANDAS showed an association between marked exacerbations of OCD or tic symptoms and an increase in GAS titers (11). Although the relationship of GAS infection to the onset of tics or OCD has been reported, causality has yet to be established. In a retrospective survey of 80 children (5 to 17 years of age) diagnosed with a tic disorder, 53% of patients described acute and severe onset or worsening of their tic symptoms (22). Of those, only 21% reported their abrupt changes occurred within 6 weeks of a preceding streptococcal infection. A prospective study examining associated factors in all cases of new onset OCD and tics will be necessary to provide a better assessment of the role of infections in illness presentation. Children ($N = 12$) who presented to a pediatric practice over a 3-year period with a sudden onset of a neuropsychiatric problem such as OCD, a tic disorder, or late age-onset ADHD and concurrent GAS pharyngitis were described in a case study, although it is unclear how many subjects with new onset OCD, tics, or ADHD presented without a concurrent GAS infection. Interestingly, these children also had a high prevalence of urinary frequency, and the neuropsychiatric symptoms rapidly remitted with antibiotic therapy (27).

GROUP A STREPTOCOCCUS PATHOGENESIS

In the past decade, the incidence and severity of GAS infections has increased significantly, and a greater degree of allelic diversity has been appreciated. To date, 80 serotypes of GAS have been described, with 150 alleles of the M protein, 89 alleles of the streptococcal pyrotoxic exotoxin B, and 269 alleles of the Sic protein known to exist. In fact, 16 of the 44 known GAS proteins have been found to be immunogenic. Table 14-1 shows some of the currently known virulence factors. GAS produces a number of toxic factors, including opacity factor (which is hemolytic), streptolysin O and streptolysin S (both hemolytic and cytotoxic), hyaluronidase (hydrolyzes hyaluronic acid), NAD+ glycohydrolase (which enables tissue invasion), streptokinase (involved in nephritis), and M-like proteins (bind to immunoglobulin and possibly interfere with complement). Some

Table 14-1. *Streptococcus pyogenes possesses many possibilities of pathogenicity*

Virulence factors	Mechanism of virulence
Peptidoglyceen	Activates alternative complement pathway
Lipoteichoic acid	Adhesin
M protein	Adhesin: binds factor H and prevents activation of complement
Fibronectin binding protein	Adhesin: fibrinogen
Collagen binding protein	Adhesin
Hyaluronic acid capsule	Antiphagocytic: highly mucoid strains increased in rheumatic fever and invasive disease
C5a peptidase	Antiphagocytic: decreases neutrophil chemotaxis
Streptococcal complement inhibitory protein	Antiphagocytic: inactivates membrane attack complex of complement
M-like proteins	Bind immunoglobulins and may interfere with complement activation, cross reactive with cardiac proteins
Opacity factor	Fibronectin binding, lipoproteinase
Streptolysin O	Hemolysin: cytotoxic
Streptolysin S	Hemolysin: cytotoxic
Nicotine-adenine-dinucleotidase	Positive invasive strains
Streptokinase	Plasminogenactivator
Pyrotoxic exotoxins (A, B, C)	Potentiate shock, induce fever, act as superantigens

of the suspected virulence factors were not present in earlier strains of GAS (28). This finding is possibly due to the fact the GAS genome randomly reassorts over time, increasing the chance of new virulence factors developing.

Clinical evidence that GAS may be changing is reflected in changes in the clinical manifestations of illnesses caused by GAS. Scarlet fever and necrotizing fasciitis have increased dramatically in incidence in the past few decades (29,30). In the outbreaks of RF in the mid-1980s, a higher representation of certain serotypes and mucoid strains of GAS was noted (31), and a large proportion (75% in one study) of individuals had only mild or no history of prior pharyngitis (32).

The role of bacterial superantigens (also called *exotoxins*) in the pathogenesis of autoimmune disorders, including RF, has recently received increased attention (33,34). Superantigens are molecules that exert a dramatic immunostimulatory response by interacting with the class II major histocompatibility complex and the variable region of the beta chain (Vβ) of the T-cell receptor. This interaction bypasses the typical immune response, causing an oligoclonal expansion of one or more Vβ components. This activation leads to a prodigious production of cytokines, which is thought to be at least partly responsible for the associated toxicity of superantigens (35). The streptococcal pyrotoxic exotoxins (A, B, C), as well as components of the cell (particularly the M protein), are some elements believed to have superantigenic activity (36–38). Some of these proteins, such as streptococcal phopholipase, share homology with the C subunit of textilotoxin, a neurotoxin from the Australian common brown snake (39,40). Many superantigens have been discovered recently; their exact role in GAS virulence is not well elucidated.

Epidemiologic studies show that the same streptococcal strain can cause infection of varying severity in different individuals, suggesting that host factors play an important role in determining the severity and outcome of GAS infections (41,42). Although several studies have demonstrated that aging, underlying chronic diseases, and immunosuppressive states contribute to greater severity of GAS infections, the presence of severe invasive disease in young, healthy individuals suggests that host genetics plays an important role in predisposition to disease severity (43,44). Indeed, patients with a propensity to produce high levels of proinflammatory cytokines in response to GAS products are noted to exhibit severe clinical manifestations (45). A child's risk of a severe response to GAS and/or developing PANDAS is likely due to a combination of his or her genetic predisposition and pathogen/environmental factors.

ESTABLISHING THE GROUNDWORK FOR IMMUNOLOGIC SUBTYPE OF OBSESSIVE COMPULSIVE DISORDER/TIC DISORDER

For a given disease, evidence of an autoimmune etiology has been categorized by Rose and Bona (46) into three different levels of significance: direct, indirect, and circumstantial. For direct evidence of autoimmunity, transmissibility of the characteristic lesions of the disease from human to human or human to animal must be demonstrated. Indirect evidence of autoimmunity consists of re-creation of the human disease in an animal model. Circumstantial evidence of autoimmunity is obtained by listing markers that are descriptive of the disease. Markers that are characteristic of autoimmune diseases include the presence of infiltrating mononuclear cells or antigen-antibody complexes in the affected organ or tissue, the presence of other autoimmune diseases in the same patient, the preferential usage of certain major histocompatibility complex class II alleles, improvement of symptoms with immune modulators, high serum levels of immunoglobulin G autoantibodies, or a positive family history of the same disease or other known autoimmune diseases (46). To date, circumstantial evidence (Table 14-2) is all that exists for demonstrating the autoimmune nature of PANDAS (13). Clearly, it is impossible to biopsy the basal ganglia and definitively demonstrate inflammatory cells; however, the demonstrated efficacy of treatment with immunomodulatory therapy (47), and high serum levels of cross-reacting antibodies (48) suggest the autoimmune nature of PANDAS.

A number of studies have demonstrated the high prevalence of OCD in patients with RF and SC, which led to the PANDAS concept (6,8,9,12). In addition, Slattery et al. (49) demonstrated a significantly higher prevalence of OCD in a cohort of 50 systemic lupus erythematosus patients. OCD was 10 to 15 times more common in this study group compared with those in community-based studies of OCD. Likewise, in an investigation of 230 patients with myasthenia gravis, a significantly higher rate of compulsive behavior was noted relative

Table 14-2. *Circumstantial evidence of autoimmunity in pediatric autoimmune neuropsychiatric disorders associated with streptococcal infection*

Markers suggesting autoimmune disease	Support for autoimmune obsessive compulsive disorder/tic
Presence in the same patient of other known autoimmune diseases	[a]Swedo et al. 1989, 1994 (6,8) [a]Rohr 1992 (50) [a]Miguel et al. 1995 (51) [a]Asbahr et al. 1998 (9) [a]Mercadante et al. 2000 (12) [a]Slattery et al. 2004 (49)
Positive family history for the same disease, or for other autoimmune diseases	Lougee et al. 2000 (53)
Preferential usage of certain major histocompatibility complex class II allele	No support
Improvement of symptom with use of immunosuppressive drugs or immunomodulatory therapy	Perlmutter et al. 1999 (47)
High serum levels of immunoglobulin G autoantibodies	Church, et al. 2003 (48)
Presence of infiltrating mononuclear cells in the affected organ or tissue	No support
Deposition of antigen-antibody complexes in the affected organ or tissue	No support

[a]These studies show presence of increased obsessive compulsive disorder in other autoimmune disorders. No studies have examined the rate of autoimmunity in Tourette syndrome/obsessive compulsive disorder.

to healthy controls (50), whereas Miguel et al. (51) reported a higher prevalence of OCD in patients with multiple sclerosis. A chart review study (52) concluded that adult OCD patients appeared to have an increased rate of immune-related diseases beyond that seen in other psychiatric disorders. Future research concerning the prevalence of OCD in patients with other autoimmune disorders appears warranted.

To date, there has been only one report looking specifically at the family histories of PANDAS patients (53). In this study, researchers examined the first-degree relatives of 54 PANDAS probands evaluating for the presence of tics, OCD, subclinical OCD, or other *Diagnostic and Statistical Manual–Fourth Edition* (DMS-IV) Axis I disorders. The rates of OCD and tic disorders in these first-degree relatives were shown to mirror those previously reported in probands with childhood onset OCD and TS. Major depressive disorder, ADHD, and phobias are other psychiatric disorders that were observed in a number of the family members of PANDAS patients and have been found by clinicians to be commonly co-morbid with cases of OCD and TS.

MARKERS OF AUTOIMMUNE DISEASE

The search for markers of CNS injury in neurologic illnesses has led to findings of increased levels of the CNS proteins S-100 and enolase in both cerebral spinal fluid and serum (54,55). Peripheral levels of S-100 have been found to be elevated in patients with TS relative to age-matched controls, supporting the hypothesis that CNS inflammation is involved in this disorder (56). Pediatric patients (7 to 17 years of age) with TS and/or OCD ($N = 47$) and healthy control subjects ($N = 19$) were prospectively monitored for newly acquired GAS infections as well as nonspecific markers of acute inflammatory responses, (57). Neopterin, a pyrazinopyrimidine compound that serves as a marker of cellular immune system activation, was noted to be higher in patients (22% versus 0%), but no difference was observed in C-reactive protein.

Peripheral markers of CNS disease could result from CNS injury or inflammation with resultant release of protein and escape of the marker via a breached blood-brain barrier, or from overproduction of a protein in the CNS or peripherally. Identification of an immune marker in OCD/TS could aid in determining the patient subtype best suited for immune therapies. The search for a marker for immune mediated OCD/tics started as an extension of studies of a putative peripheral marker of susceptibility to RF. Monoclonal antibodies to D8/17, an alloantigen found on B lymphocytes, was originally isolated from a patient with rheumatic carditis, and since has been found to react with epitopes expressed on expanded populations of B lymphocytes in a majority of patients with documented RF (58,59). Studies involving cross-reactivity experiments using the D8/17 antibody suggest the B cell antigen is homologous to helical coiled-coil molecules such as myosin, tropomyosin, and the M6 protein of GAS. However, whereas strong binding to smooth muscle has been reported, only weak fluorescence in the cytoplasm of cortical and caudate neuronal cells was detected (60). To date, no other work has been reported on D8/17 expression within various areas of the CNS or on the characterization of the putative antigen.

The possibility of an immune mediated pathogenesis of OCD/TS also has generated interest in the potential of monoclonal antibodies D8/17 helping to identify patients at risk for streptococcal-precipitated neuropsychiatric disorders. In flow cytometric studies, a subpopulation of D8/17-positive B cells was not found, but increased binding was observed in neuropsychiatric patients compared to controls (19,61). The potential for D8/17 to serve as marker of immune function at points of neuropsychiatric exacerbation would suggest the possibility of reflecting a state marker instead of trait marker as suggested in the RF literature. However, although OCD/TS patients demonstrated significantly higher levels of D8/17-reactive cells compared with control subjects, there was no consistent pattern of change in D8/17 levels when exacerbation time points were compared with baseline or follow-up time points (57).

To date, due to concerns regarding methodology and reagents (19,62,63), an assay for the alloantigen D8/17 has not been correlated reliably with suspected PANDAS cases, leaving the diagnostic potential of this antibody and its relationship to the pathophysiology of psychiatric disorders doubtful (64,65). Weisz et al. (63) failed to demonstrate an elevated percentage of D8/17-positive B cells in patients with either acute RF or TS. The authors did find, however, a significant increase in CD19-positive B cells in acute RF and TS patients compared with those in normal controls. In this

study, group A streptococcal pharyngitis patients also had an elevated percentage of CD19 B cells. Although this study failed to confirm the utility of the D8/17 alloantigen in acute RF patients or TD patients, the finding of increased CD19-positive B cells in all patient groups is intriguing. The increased B cell percentage may be secondary to alterations in other lymphocyte subclasses or an increase in antibody machinery related to either antibody-mediated autoimmunity or a nonspecific reaction to a recent streptococcal infection.

EVIDENCE FOR MOLECULAR MIMICRY

Molecular mimicry refers to the phenomenon that occurs when a self protein and a microbial protein resemble each other. The self protein may become recognizable by the immune system following an injury and/or loss of a normally impermeable barrier. This similarity may lead to antibodies cross-reacting with both the pathogen and normal tissue. Molecular mimicry has been hypothesized to be a mechanism by which an autoimmune response is induced. The CNS manifestations characteristic of SC are thought to be related to the production of antibodies to the M protein of streptococcus that cross react with epitopes on neuronal tissue (4,66). Furthermore, a remarkable homology among various epitopes of the streptococcal M protein and tissue molecules (such as tropomyosin) has been noted in RF, suggesting a humoral-mediated mechanism of autoimmunity in the pathogenesis of this disease. Potential mechanisms by which autoantibodies cause clinical manifestations in CNS diseases such as SC and PANDAS include direct stimulation or blockade of receptors in the basal ganglia, or immune complexes promoting inflammation of these brain regions. Studies have found that the level of antineuronal antibody binding to basal ganglia tissue in SC patients correlates well with symptom severity (66,67), and there is support for antibody-mediated neuronal cell signaling in the pathogenesis of SC (68). Monoclonal antibodies in SC patients that were targeted to N-acetyl-beta-D-glucosamine—the dominant epitope of GAS—were found to bind specifically mammalian lysoganglioside, a CNS ganglioside that involved in neuronal signal transduction. Sera from SC patients further contained antibodies that targeted human neuronal cells and specifically induced calcium/calmodulin-dependent protein kinase II activity, whereas sera from patients convalescing or from patients with other streptococcal-related diseases lacked activation of this enzyme. Activation of calmodulin-dependent protein kinase II has been shown to cause increased dopamine release in brain tissue, a potential mechanism by which clinical symptoms might ensue (69).

There are organs in the human body that enjoy immune privilege; most notably, the brain, eye, testes, and fetal uterus (70). Due to a low level of complement, low major histocompatibility complex expression, tight junctions, and the relative lack of lymphatics, the cells of the immune system have great difficulty obtaining access to these tissues. The CNS is protected from the systemic circulatory and lymphatic systems by the blood-brain barrier (BBB). The exact mechanism by which the immune system could gain access to the CNS of PANDAS patients is not known, although it is known in other autoimmune diseases involving the CNS (multiple sclerosis, for example) that activation of the inflammatory cascade and resulting production of toxins leads to BBB breakdown and a massive influx of inflammatory cells (70). Despite the lack of defined lymphatics in the brain, 14% to 47% of radiolabeled albumin injected into the CNS can be recovered in cervical lymph (71), suggesting a connection between the CNS and the lymphatic system by which inflammatory cells could gain access to the CNS. Researchers have demonstrated the infusion of interferon (IFN-γ) and tumor necrosis factor (TNF-α) into the circulation induce the activation of inflammatory cells on the CNS side of the BBB (72). Within hours, enhanced major histocompatibility complex expression and synthesis of eicosinoids within the CNS can be detected and the endothelium is consequently activated, facilitating passage of lymphocytes through the BBB. Likewise, the cytokines interleukin-Iβ, interleukin-6, and TNF-α can cross the BBB via the circumventricular organs (the area postrema, median eminence of the pituitary,

and the organum vasculosum of the lamina terminalis of the forebrain), activating the endothelium and leading to further vascular permeability (70) Cross-reactive B cells, possibly to a CNS epitope, could lead to intrathecal productivity of antibody (73). The finding of increased antineuronal antibodies to the striatum in patients with TS (10,74) parallels findings of increased antineuronal antibodies in patients with SC (66,67). Evidence of antineuronal antibodies in patients with tic disorders implies a humorally-mediated mechanism of CNS pathology, but the mediating steps from a peripheral finding to CNS autoimmunity are unknown. At the minimum, it is clear that the immune system has access to the CNS via mechanisms that are complex and still not completely understood, and that, despite the BBB, the CNS has the ability to sense and respond to immunologically important substances in the periphery. Clearly, further research is needed to better define the means by which an autoimmune response can traverse the BBB and lead to the motor and behavioral disturbances seen in PANDAS.

EVIDENCE OF IMMUNE DYSFUNCTION

After streptococcal infections, titers may remain elevated for six months to a year. Murphy et al. (11) found evidence of persistent elevations in one or more strep titers in patients with a dramatically fluctuating neuropsychiatric symptom compared to those that had a course inconsistent with PANDAS. This finding may be due to the relative proximity of the streptococcal infection and repeated streptococcal exposures leading to more severe and turbulent symptoms. A corollary of this finding is the report of increased B cell percentages in patients with tic disorders that appear to be secondary to recent infection/immune activation (63).

Persistent immune activation to GAS is also a possibility and may be a consequence of multiple factors including developmental and/or environmental influences. Young age at time of streptococcal infection may alter future immune responses to GAS. An innate response to GAS antigens leading to higher than typical antibody levels may also be possible. This possibility has been reported in patients with RF (75) with evidence of streptococcal titer elevations many years after prophylactic antibiotics. Exclusive association to GAS is provisional because other types of infections are believed to trigger neuropsychiatric symptoms consistent with OCD/TS (76,77). Measurement of peripheral cytokine profiles, lymphocyte subsets, and antibodies to viruses and self-proteins have been the primary focus of efforts made to study alterations in immune indices in adults with OCD (78–81), following in the steps of studies that support the role of cell-mediated mechanisms in the pathogenesis of RF (36,82). Some studies found evidence of an altered or imbalanced immune function in adult OCD patients (80,83) whereas others failed to find humoral evidence of autoimmunity (79,80) or cytokine alterations (79,84,85). These studies highlight the need for further exploration of the role immune processes play in the development and maintenance of OCD and/or tic symptoms as previous study sample sizes have often been small, and the degree to which hypothalamo-pituitary-axis alterations (due to stress vs. autoimmunity) have affected results has yet to be resolved.

DIAGNOSIS AND TREATMENT ISSUES

As a definitive association between GAS and OCD/tics has yet to be established, protocols for diagnosis and treatment are provisional. During the history gathering process, careful attention should be given to reports of repeated, frequent infections, evidence of GAS in a young child (e.g., unexplained abdominal pain accompanied by fever), scarlet fever, brief episodes of tics, OCD, or compulsive urination that remitted, and especially sudden onset of OCD or tics accompanying an infectious illness. In patients with an abnormal neurologic examination evidenced by muscle weakness, abnormal reflexes (slow return of patellar reflex) or chorea, further workup is indicated. In patients with new onset OCD or tics, or recent symptom exacerbation, a throat culture is a relatively benign procedure that will help rule out the possibility of symptoms being triggered by a subclinical GAS infection. To maximize the utility of streptococcal titer measurement, streptococcal titers obtained at symptom onset

should be repeated to examine for a rise in titers 4 to 6 weeks later. In patients with onset exceeding 4 weeks prior, streptococcal titers add support but do not provide definitive proof of a streptococcal trigger.

A clinical trial involving the use of prophylactic penicillin in treating apparent episodes of PANDAS revealed no conclusive evidence that the antibiotic reduced clinical exacerbations (86). However, the lack of efficacy may have been due to the failure of antibiotic therapy to eliminate streptococcal colonization in the patients enrolled in the study. Since then, investigators have demonstrated a significant improvement in OCD symptoms following antibiotic treatment of acute exacerbations in PANDAS patients (27,87). Long-term follow-up further demonstrated continued improvement in symptoms, with antibiotic prophylaxis preventing recurrent streptococcal infections (87).

Given the pathophysiology proposed for PANDAS, immunomodulatory therapies that serve to interrupt the action of autoantibodies on the CNS would seem to be a reasonable course of treatment. Indeed, administration of intravenous immunoglobulin or plasma exchange was demonstrated in a clinical trial to lead to long-term (over one year) resolution of symptoms, with plasma exchange being better tolerated and providing greater relief in symptoms (47). The use of plasma exchange or intravenous immunoglobulin acutely for an exacerbation of neuropsychiatric symptoms in PANDAS patients requires further research, however, before being considered the standard of care. Further discussion of this topic is conducted elsewhere in this volume.

CONTROVERSY CONCERNING PANDAS

Spirited, academic debate exists concerning the clinical entity of PANDAS (13). The first PANDAS criterion of the presence of OCD/tics arguably is narrow and ignores the possible clinical spectrum of the disorder, which may include additional neuropsychiatric manifestations such as anorexia nervosa (88), ADHD (89), acute disseminated encephalomyelitis (90), myoclonus (91), dystonia (92), and paroxysmal dyskinesias (93). Additionally, the proposed age range of onset of PANDAS has been criticized as arbitrary and a waxing and waning clinical course described as unhelpful in distinguishing PANDAS from children with ordinary TS or OCD, although reasons for this waxing and waning course have not been established. Swedo et al. (94) reasons that PANDAS is a clinical entity that is easily distinguished if the clinical criteria are followed as originally described (sudden dramatic onset of tics and OCD in prepubertal children with 2 episodes of associated GAS). Clearly, although PANDAS remains a controversial entity it does provide an intriguing phenotypical and theoretical basis to study genetic, environmental, and immune-based triggers in childhood neuropsychiatric disorders.

ACKNOWLEDGMENTS

The author would like to acknowledge the support of her research by the Tourette Syndrome Association, Inc. grant award: *Characterization of Lymphocytic Diversity in Children with Tic Exacerbation*; the NARSAD Young Investigator Award: *Cellular Activation Markers in OCD and Tic Exacerbation*; the National Institute of Mental Health (NIMH) K23 Grant MH01739: *Neuroimmunology of Childhood Psychiatric Disorders* and NIMH RO1 MH/NS63914: *Prospective Study of PANDAS*. Personal and technical assistance were provided by Michael Bengtson MD, Wayne Goodman MD, Ohel Soto-Raices MD, Muhammad Sajid MD, Mark Yang PhD, Jane Mutch PhD, Pam Allen RN, and Annette Zaytoun.

REFERENCES

1. Steinman L. Elaborate interactions between the immune and nervous systems. *Nat Immunol.* 2004;5:575–581.
2. Hosier DM, Craenen JM, Teske DW, et al. Resurgence of acute rheumatic fever. *Am J Dis Child.* 1987;141: 730–733.
3. Ayoub EM. Resurgence of rheumatic fever in the United States. The changing picture of a preventable illness. *Postgrad Med.* 1992;92:133–142.
4. Bronze MS, Dale JB. Epitopes of streptococcal M proteins that evoke antibodies that cross-react with human brain. *J Immunol.* 1993;151:2820–2828.
5. Taranta A, Stollerman GH. The relationship of Sydenham's chorea to infection with group A streptococci. *Am J Med.* 1956;20:170–175.
6. Swedo SE, Rapoport JL, Cheslow DL, et al. High prevalence of obsessive-compulsive symptoms in patients with Sydenham's chorea. *Am J Psychiatry.* 1989;146: 246–249.
7. Swedo SE, Leonard HL, Schapiro MB, et al. Sydenham's chorea: physical and psychological symptoms of St Vitus dance. *Pediatrics* 1993;91:706–713.
8. Swedo SE. Sydenham's chorea. A model for childhood autoimmune neuropsychiatric disorders. *JAMA* 1994; 272:1788–1791.
9. Asbahr FR, Negrao AB, Gentil V, et al. Obsessive-compulsive and related symptoms in children and adolescents with rheumatic fever with and without chorea: a prospective 6-month study. *Am J Psychiatry.* 1998; 155:1122–1124.
10. Kiessling LS, Marcotte AC, Culpepper L. Antineuronal antibodies in movement disorders. *Pediatrics* 1993; 92:39–43.
11. Murphy TK, Sajid M, Soto O, et al. Detecting pediatric autoimmune neuropsychiatric disorders associated with streptococcus in children with obsessive-compulsive disorder and tics. *Biol Psychiatry.* 2004;55:61–68.
12. Mercadante MT, Busatto GF, Lombroso PJ, et al. The psychiatric symptoms of rheumatic fever. *Am J Psychiatry.* 2000;157:2036–2038.
13. Kurlan R, Kaplan EL. The pediatric autoimmune neuropsychiatric disorders associated with streptococcal infection (PANDAS) etiology for tics and obsessive-compulsive symptoms: hypothesis or entity? Practical considerations for the clinician. *Pediatrics* 2004; 113:883–886.
14. Selling L. The role of infection in the etiology of tics. *Arch Neurol Psychiatry.* 1929;22:1163–1171.
15. Murphy TK, Goodman WK, Ayoub EM, et al. On defining Sydenham's chorea: where do we draw the line? *Biol Psychiatry.* 2000;47:851–857.
16. Ahmed S, Ayoub EM, Scornik JC, et al. Poststreptococcal reactive arthritis: clinical characteristics and association with HLA-DR alleles. *Arthritis Rheum.* 1998; 41:1096–1102.
17. Jansen TL, Janssen M, van Riel PL. Grand rounds in rheumatology: acute rheumatic fever or post-streptococcal reactive arthritis: a clinical problem revisited. *Br J Rheumatol.* 1998;37:335–340.
18. Swedo SE, Leonard HL, Garvey M, et al. Pediatric autoimmune neuropsychiatric disorders associated with streptococcal infections: clinical description of the first 50 cases. *Am J Psychiatry.* 1998;155:264–271.
19. Murphy T, Goodman W. Genetics of childhood disorders: XXXIV. Autoimmune disorders, part 7: D8/17 reactivity as an immunological marker of susceptibility to neuropsychiatric disorders. *J Am Acad Child Adolesc Psychiatry.* 2002;41:98–100.
20. Giulino L, Gammon P, Sullivan K, et al. Is parental report of upper respiratory infection at the onset of obsessive-compulsive disorder suggestive of pediatric autoimmune neuropsychiatric disorder associated with streptococcal infection? *J Child Adolesc Psychopharmacol.* 2002;12:157–164.
21. Cardona F, Orefici G. Group A streptococcal infections and tic disorders in an Italian pediatric population. *J Pediatr.* 2001;138:71–75.
22. Singer HS, Giuliano JD, Zimmerman AM, et al. Infection: a stimulus for tic disorders. *Pediatr Neurol.* 2000; 22:380–383.
23. Perlmutter SJ, Garvey MA, Castellanos X, et al. A case of pediatric autoimmune neuropsychiatric disorders

associated with streptococcal infections. *Am J Psychiatry.* 1998;155:1592–1598.

24. Tucker DM, Leckman JF, Scahill L, et al. A putative poststreptococcal case of OCD with chronic tic disorder, not otherwise specified. *J Am Acad Child Adolesc Psychiatry.* 1996;35:1684–1691.

25. Kiessling LS, Marcotte AC, Culpepper L. Antineuronal antibodies: tics and obsessive-compulsive symptoms. *J Dev Behav Pediatr.* 1994;15:421–425.

26. Kerbeshian J, Burd L, Pettit R. A possible post-streptococcal movement disorder with chorea and tics. *Dev Med Child Neurol.* 1990;32:642–644.

27. Murphy ML, Pichichero ME. Prospective identification and treatment of children with pediatric autoimmune neuropsychiatric disorder associated with group A streptococcal infection (PANDAS). *Arch Pediatr Adolesc Med.* 2002;156:356–361.

28. Proft T, Webb PD, Handley V, et al. Two novel superantigens found in both group A and group C Streptococcus. *Infect Immun.* 2003;71:1361–1369.

29. Efstratiou A. Group A streptococci in the 1990s. *J Antimicrob Chemother.* 2000;45 Suppl:3–12.

30. Krause RM. Evolving microbes and re-emerging streptococcal disease. *Clin Lab Med.* 2002;22:835–848.

31. Schwartz B, Facklam RR, Breiman RF. Changing epidemiology of group A streptococcal infection in the USA. *Lancet* 1990;336:1167–1171.

32. Congeni BL. The resurgence of acute rheumatic fever in the United States. *Pediatr Ann.* 1992;21:816–820.

33. Abbott WG, Skinner MA, Voss L, et al. Repertoire of transcribed peripheral blood T-cell receptor beta chain variable-region genes in acute rheumatic fever. *Infect Immun.* 1996;64:2842–2845.

34. Kotb M. Bacterial pyrogenic exotoxins as superantigens. *Clin Microbiol Rev.* 1995;8:411–426.

35. Torres BA, Johnson HM. Modulation of disease by superantigens. *Curr Opin Immunol.* 1998;10:465–470.

36. Tomai M, Kotb M, Majumdar G, et al. Superantigenicity of streptococcal M protein. *J Exp Med.* 1990;172:359–362.

37. Tomai MA, Aelion JA, Dockter ME, et al. T cell receptor V gene usage by human T cells stimulated with the superantigen streptococcal M protein. *J Exp Med.* 1991;174:285–288.

38. Tomai MA, Beachey EH, Majumdar G, et al. Metabolically active antigen presenting cells are required for human T cell proliferation in response to the superantigen streptococcal M protein. *FEMS Microbiol Immunol.* 1992;4:155–164.

39. Beres SB, Sylva GL, Barbian KD, et al. Genome sequence of a serotype M3 strain of group A Streptococcus: phage-encoded toxins, the high-virulence phenotype, and clone emergence. *Proc Natl Acad Sci U S A.* 2002;99:10078–10083.

40. Pearson JA, Tyler MI, Retson KV, et al. Studies on the subunit structure of textilotoxin, a potent presynaptic neurotoxin from the venom of the Australian common brown snake (Pseudonaja textilis). 3. The complete amino-acid sequences of all the subunits. *Biochim Biophys Acta.* 1993;1161:223–229.

41. Chatellier S, Ihendyane N, Kansal RG, et al. Genetic relatedness and superantigen expression in group A streptococcus serotype M1 isolates from patients with severe and nonsevere invasive diseases. *Infect Immun.* 2000;68:3523–3534.

42. Haukness HA, Tanz RR, Thomson RB, Jr., et al. The heterogeneity of endemic community pediatric group a streptococcal pharyngeal isolates and their relationship to invasive isolates. *J Infect Dis.* 2002;185:915–920.

43. Medina E, Goldmann O, Rohde M, et al. Genetic control of susceptibility to group A streptococcal infection in mice. *J Infect Dis.* 2001;184:846–852.

44. Goldmann O, Chhatwal GS, Medina E. Immune mechanisms underlying host susceptibility to infection with group A streptococci. *J Infect Dis.* 2003;187:854–861.

45. Norrby-Teglund A, Chatellier S, Low DE, et al. Host variation in cytokine responses to superantigens determine the severity of invasive group A streptococcal infection. *Eur J Immunol.* 2000;30:3247–3255.

46. Rose NR, Bona C. Defining criteria for autoimmune diseases (Witebsky's postulates revisited). *Immunol Today.* 1993;14:426–430.

47. Perlmutter SJ, Leitman SF, Garvey MA, et al. Therapeutic plasma exchange and intravenous immunoglobulin for obsessive-compulsive disorder and tic disorders in childhood. *Lancet* 1999;354:1153–1158.

48. Church AJ, Dale RC, Lees AJ, et al. Tourette's syndrome: a cross sectional study to examine the PANDAS hypothesis. *J Neurol Neurosurg Psychiatry.* 2003;74:602–607.

49. Slattery MJ, Dubbert BK, Allen AJ, et al. Prevalence of obsessive-compulsive disorder in patients with systemic lupus erythematosus. *J Clin Psychiatry.* 2004;65:301–306.

50. Rohr W. Obsessive behavior and thoughts in patients with myasthenia gravis. *Schweiz Arch Neurol Psychiatr.* 1992;143:105–115.

51. Miguel EC, Stein MC, Rauch SL, et al. Obsessive-compulsive disorder in patients with multiple sclerosis. *J Neuropsychiatry Clin Neurosci.* 1995;7:507–510.

52. Dinn WM, Harris CL, McGonigal KM, et al. Obsessive-compulsive disorder and immunocompetence. *Int J Psychiatry Med.* 2001;31:311–320.

53. Lougee L, Perlmutter SJ, Nicolson R, et al. Psychiatric disorders in first-degree relatives of children with pediatric autoimmune neuropsychiatric disorders associated with streptococcal infections (PANDAS). *J Am Acad Child Adolesc Psychiatry.* 2000;39:1120–1126.

54. Lamers KJ, van Engelen BG, Gabreels FJ, et al. Cerebrospinal neuron-specific enolase, S-100 and myelin basic protein in neurological disorders. *Acta Neurol Scand.* 1995;92:247–251.

55. Persson L, Hardemark HG, Gustafsson J, et al. S-100 protein and neuron-specific enolase in cerebrospinal fluid and serum: markers of cell damage in human central nervous system. *Stroke* 1987;18:911–918.

56. van Passel R, Schlooz WA, Lamers KJ, et al. S100B protein, glia and Gilles de la Tourette syndrome. *Europ J Paediatr Neurol.* 2001;5:15–19.

57. Luo F, Leckman JF, Katsovich L, et al. Prospective longitudinal study of children with tic disorders and/or obsessive-compulsive disorder: relationship of symptom exacerbations to newly acquired streptococcal infections. *Pediatrics* 2004;113:e578–585.

58. Patarroyo ME, Winchester RJ, Vejerano A, et al. Association of a B-cell alloantigen with susceptibility to rheumatic fever. *Nature* 1979;278:173–174.

59. Zabriskie JB. Rheumatic fever: a model for the pathological consequences of microbial-host mimicry. *Clin Exp Rheumatol.* 1986;4:65–73.

60. Kemeny E, Husby G, Williams RC, et al. Tissue distribution of antigen(s) defined by monoclonal antibody

D8/17 reacting with B lymphocytes of patients with rheumatic heart disease. *Clin Immunol Immunopathol.* 1994;72:35–43.

61. Hoekstra PJ, Bijzet J, Limburg PC, et al. Elevated D8/17 expression on B lymphocytes, a marker of rheumatic fever, measured with flow cytometry in tic disorder patients. *Am J Psychiatry.* 2001;158:605–610.

62. Murphy TK, Benson N, Zaytoun A, et al. Progress toward analysis of D8/17 binding to B cells in children with obsessive compulsive disorder and/or chronic tic disorder. *J Neuroimmunol.* 2001;120:146–151.

63. Weisz JL, McMahon WM, Moore JC, et al. D8/17 and CD19 expression on lymphocytes of patients with acute rheumatic fever and Tourette's disorder. *Clin Diagn Lab Immunol.* 2004;11:330–336.

64. Singer HS, Loiselle C. PANDAS. A commentary. *J Psychosom Res* 2003;55:31–39.

65. Hamilton CS, Garvey MA, Swedo SE. Sensitivity of the D8/17 assay. *Am J Psychiatry.* 2003;160:1193–1194.

66. Husby G, van de Rijn I, Zabriskie JB, et al. Antibodies reacting with cytoplasm of subthalamic and caudate nuclei neurons in chorea and acute rheumatic fever. *J Exp Med.* 1976;144:1094–1110.

67. Kotby AA, El Badawy N, El Sokkary S, et al. Antineuronal antibodies in rheumatic chorea. *Clin Diagn Lab Immunol.* 1998;5:836–839.

68. Kirvan CA, Swedo SE, Heuser JS, et al. Mimicry and autoantibody-mediated neuronal cell signaling in Sydenham chorea. *Nat Med.* 2003;9:914–920.

69. Kantor L, Hewlett GH, Gnegy ME. Enhanced amphetamine- and K+-mediated dopamine release in rat striatum after repeated amphetamine: differential requirements for Ca2+- and calmodulin-dependent phosphorylation and synaptic vesicles. *J Neurosci.* 1999;19:3801–3808.

70. Ballabh P, Braun A, Nedergaard M. The blood-brain barrier: an overview: structure, regulation, and clinical implications. *Neurobiol Dis.* 2004;16:1–13.

71. Cserr HF, Harling-Berg CJ, Knopf PM. Drainage of brain extracellular fluid into blood and deep cervical lymph and its immunological significance. *Brain Pathol.* 1992;2:269–276.

72. Hickey WF, Vass K, Lassmann H. Bone marrow-derived elements in the central nervous system: an immunohistochemical and ultrastructural survey of rat chimeras. *J Neuropathol Exp Neurol.* 1992;51: 246–256.

73. Knopf PM, Harling-Berg CJ, Cserr HF, et al. Antigen-dependent intrathecal antibody synthesis in the normal rat brain: tissue entry and local retention of antigen-specific B cells. *J Immunol.* 1998;161:692–701.

74. Singer HS, Giuliano JD, Hansen BH, et al. Antibodies against human putamen in children with Tourette syndrome. *Neurology* 1998;50:1618–1624.

75. Shulman ST, Ayoub EM. Qualitative and quantitative aspects of the human antibody response to streptococcal group A carbohydrate. *J Clin Invest.* 1974;54:990–996.

76. Allen AJ, Leonard HL, Swedo SE. Case study: a new infection-triggered, autoimmune subtype of pediatric OCD and Tourette's syndrome. *J Am Acad Child Adolesc Psychiatry.* 1995;34:307–311.

77. Fallon BA, Nields JA. Lyme disease: a neuropsychiatric illness. *Am J Psychiatry.* 1994;151:1571–1583.

78. Black JL, Lamke GT, Walikonis JE. Serologic survey of adult patients with obsessive-compulsive disorder for neuron-specific and other autoantibodies. *Psychiatry Res.* 1998;81:371–380.

79. Carpenter LL, Heninger GR, McDougle CJ, et al. Cerebrospinal fluid interleukin-6 in obsessive-compulsive disorder and trichotillomania. *Psychiatry Res.* 2002; 112:257–262.

80. Marazziti D, Presta S, Pfanner C, et al. Immunological alterations in adult obsessive-compulsive disorder. *Biol Psychiatry.* 1999;46:810–814.

81. Ravindran AV, Griffiths J, Merali Z, et al. Circulating lymphocyte subsets in obsessive compulsive disorder, major depression and normal controls. *J Affect Disord.* 1999;52:1–10.

82. Hutto JH, Ayoub EM. Cytotoxicity of lymphocytes from patients with rheumatic carditis in vitro. In: Read SE, Zabriskie JB, eds. *Streptococcal Diseases and the Immune Response.* New York: Academic Press, 1987: 733–738.

83. Mittleman BB, Castellanos FX, Jacobsen LK, et al. Cerebrospinal fluid cytokines in pediatric neuropsychiatric disease. *J Immunol.* 1997;159:2994–2999.

84. Maes M, Meltzer HY, Bosmans E. Psychoimmune investigation in obsessive-compulsive disorder: assays of plasma transferrin, IL-2 and IL-6 receptor, and IL-1 beta and IL-6 concentrations. *Neuropsychobiology* 1994;30:57–60.

85. Monteleone P, Catapano F, Fabrazzo M, et al. Decreased blood levels of tumor necrosis factor-alpha in patients with obsessive-compulsive disorder. *Neuropsychobiology* 1998;37:182–185.

86. Garvey MA, Perlmutter SJ, Allen AJ, et al. A pilot study of penicillin prophylaxis for neuropsychiatric exacerbations triggered by streptococcal infections. *Biol Psychiatry.* 1999;45:1564–1571.

87. Leonard HL, Swedo SE. Paediatric autoimmune neuropsychiatric disorders associated with streptococcal infection (PANDAS). *Int J Neuropsychopharmacol.* 2001;4:191–198.

88. Sokol MS. Infection-triggered anorexia nervosa in children: clinical description of four cases. *J Child Adolesc Psychopharmacol.* 2000;10:133–145.

89. Swedo SE, Leonard HL, Mittleman BB, et al. Identification of children with pediatric autoimmune neuropsychiatric disorders associated with streptococcal infections by a marker associated with rheumatic fever. *Am J Psychiatry.* 1997;154:110–112.

90. Dale RC, Church AJ, Cardoso F, et al. Poststreptococcal acute disseminated encephalomyelitis with basal ganglia involvement and auto-reactive antibasal ganglia antibodies. *Ann Neurol.* 2001;50:588–595.

91. DiFazio MP, Morales J, Davis R. Acute myoclonus secondary to group A beta-hemolytic streptococcus infection: A PANDAS variant. *J Child Neurol.* 1998;13: 516–518.

92. Dale RC, Church AJ, Benton S, et al. Post-streptococcal autoimmune dystonia with isolated bilateral striatal necrosis. *Dev Med Child Neurol.* 2002;44:485–489.

93. Dale RC, Church AJ, Surtees RA, et al. Post-Streptococcal autoimmune neuropsychiatric disease presenting as paroxysmal dystonic choreoathetosis. *Mov Disord.* 2002;17:817–820.

94. Swedo SE, Leonard HL, Rapoport JL. The pediatric autoimmune neuropsychiatric disorders associated with streptococcal infection (PANDAS) subgroup: separating fact from fiction. *Pediatrics* 2004;113:907–911.

15

PANDAS: Overview of the Hypothesis

Gavin Giovannoni

Department of Neuroinflammation, Institute of Neurology, University College London, London, United Kingdom

There is an emerging concept that basal ganglia dysfunction, presenting as a movement disorder and/or psychiatric syndrome, is caused by an aberrant immune response triggered by streptococcal infection. Basal ganglia dysfunction has various manifestations, all of which fall into a relatively well defined symptom complex or syndrome. Therefore it is not sufficient to rely on the clinical manifestations to make an etiologic diagnosis with regard to a basal ganglia disorder. Antibasal ganglia antibodies (ABGA), which are strongly associated with serologic evidence of recent streptococcal infection, are a potential diagnostic marker for this group of disorders, which includes Sydenham chorea (SC) as the prototype. More recently subjects with pediatric autoimmune neuropsychiatric disorders associated with streptococcal infection (PANDAS), Tourette syndrome (TS), obsessive compulsive disorder (OCD) and other movement disorders have also been described in association with ABGA. The apparent overlap between the clinical phenotype of SC, PANDAS, TS, and OCD suggests that they may therefore represent one disease entity. The current working hypothesis is that antibodies induced in response to streptococcal infection cross-react with antigenic determinants in the basal ganglia resulting in basal ganglia dysfunction. Although the experimental evidence is incomplete there is sufficient evidence to support immune mediated basal ganglia dysfunction as an emerging clinical entity. This is important as it has implications for the diagnosis and treatment of subjects with these disorders.

THE WIDER PANDAS HYPOTHESIS

Basal ganglia dysfunction due to an aberrant immune response, triggered by streptococcal infection, underlies the pathogenesis of an emerging group of neuropsychiatric disorders of which PANDAS is an example (Fig 15-1).

How Wide Is the Clinical Phenotype?

The author of this chapter and other researchers have identified a wide range of movement disorders associated with ABGA and recent streptococcal infection. These include SC, PANDAS, TS, OCD, adult-onset tic disorders, dystonia, an encephalitis lethargica-like syndrome, and acute disseminated encephalomyelitis. ABGA appear to be specific to this group of disorders and identify similar antigens of 40, 45, 60, and 98 kDa bands. Immunofluorescence staining has identified ABGA as recognizing specific neuronal processes in the striatum. ABGA are associated with serological and microbiological evidence of recent or current streptococcal infection. These findings have raised the important question of whether or not this group of disorders is autoimmune and triggered by streptococcal infection.

What Is the Rationale for Widening the Clinical Phenotype of PANDAS?

To support the hypothesis that PANDAS is an autoimmune disease triggered by a streptococcal

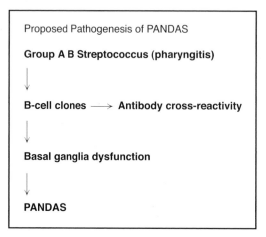

Proposed Pathogenesis of PANDAS

Group A B Streptococcus (pharyngitis)

↓

B-cell clones ⟶ **Antibody cross-reactivity**

↓

Basal ganglia dysfunction

↓

PANDAS

Fig. 15-1. Proposed pathogenesis of pediatric autoimmune neuropsychiatric disorders associated with streptococcal infection.

infection it is important to counter the argument that contemporary diagnostic criteria for PANDAS are too nonspecific for it to represent a distinct clinical entity. Basal ganglia dysfunction due to specific and well-defined causes, for example Huntington or Wilson disease, are characteristically associated with "classic phenotypes," but these diseases can present with the full phenotypic spectrum associated with basal ganglia dysfunction. It is therefore unlikely that basal ganglia dysfunction due to autoimmunity will be an exception. One would therefore expect a wider phenotype (possibly the full phenotypic spectrum of basal ganglia dysfunction) to be associated with basal ganglia autoimmunity and streptococcal infection. The author of this chapter therefore proposes that researchers shift their perspective when defining these disorders, at least the acute syndromes, to use broad clinical criteria and focus less on the clinical phenotype and more on biological markers, specifically ABGA. A shift in emphasis of this nature is not easy from within the fields of neurology and psychiatry that have a long tradition in "phenetics."

What Evidence Supports PANDAS as an Autoimmune Disease?

Before considering the evidence that PANDAS is an autoimmune disease caused by an infection

TABLE 15-1. *Modified Witesbsky criteria*

1. The presence of autoreactivity, i.e., an antibody or T-cell that is self-reactive.
2. Recognition of the specific autoantigen.
3. Induction of the disease in animal model.
4. Passive transfer of the disease to the animal. This criterion applies to auto-antibody mediated human disease only. It is not possible to transfer a human immune-mediated autoaggressive disease to animal via the passive transfer of autoreactive T-cells because they have to, by definition, see their "autoantigen" in context of the correct major histocompatibility complex molecule.

it is worth defining autoimmunity and reviewing current criteria for establishing disease causation.

The underlying concepts concerning autoimmunity have recently been challenged with the recognition that autoimmunity is a natural phenomenon and probably plays an important role in tissue homeostasis (1). Therefore immunologists prefer to use terms such as *immune-mediated autoaggressive disease* to describe autoimmune reactions that result in pathology. To establish whether a disease is an autoimmune disease, Witesbsky criteria have to be applied to the disease (Table 15-1) (2).

To establish a causal link between an infectious agent, such as streptococcus, and a specific disease one would traditionally apply Koch postulates (Table 15-2).

Koch postulates cannot be applied to postinfectious immune-mediated disorders because A) the organism may not persist long enough to be isolated when the patient presents with a neuropsychiatric syndrome, B) they are usually rare manifestations of relatively common infections, and C) several organisms may

TABLE 15-2. *Koch postulates*

1. The specific organism should be shown to be present in all cases of animals suffering from a specific disease but should not be found in healthy animals.
2. The specific microorganism should be isolated from the diseased animal and grown in pure culture on artificial laboratory media.
3. This freshly isolated microorganism, when inoculated into a healthy laboratory animal, should cause the same disease seen in the original animal.
4. The microorganism should be reisolated in pure culture from the experimental infection.

TABLE 15-3. *Bradford-Hill contemporary criteria to establish causation*

1. Consistency and unbiased findings
2. Strength of association
3. Temporal sequence
4. Biological gradient (dose-response relationship—more important for toxicology)
5. Specificity
6. Coherence with biological background and previous knowledge
7. Biological plausibility
8. Reasoning by analogy
9. Experimental evidence

From Bradford-Hill A. The Environment and Disease: Association or Causation? *Proc Royal Soc Med.* 1966;58:295.

trigger the same syndrome. Therefore one has to apply more contemporary criteria of causation, which have their roots in the field of occupational medicine but are now widely applied in other fields (3). These criteria serve as a general guide and are not meant to be inflexible. Importantly, they do not require all criteria to be fulfilled to establish "scientific causation." The Bradford Hill criteria required to establish causation are summarized in Table 15-3.

To make the case that PANDAS is an autoimmune disease triggered by streptococcal infection one has to consider the similarities between PANDAS and SC. The phenotypic overlap, from both a movement disorder and psychiatric perspective, between SC, PANDAS (Swedo syndrome), TS, and OCD is well described and beyond the scope of this review. The large overlap between the clinical phenotypes suggests that they may represent one disease entity. For example, patients with PANDAS usually have psychiatric features and frequently have choreiform movements. Patients with SC often have tics and OCD and patients with OCD often have tics and other subtle movement disorders. Therefore if researchers shift their perspective, as proposed, from the clinical phenotype to a biologic marker they note that a significant proportion of patients with TS, PANDAS, and/or OCD have a higher incidence of recent streptococcal infection and ABGA than controls and ABGA (Table 15-4). A temporal relationship between

the streptococcal infection and the onset of symptoms or an exacerbation in symptoms in patients with both PANDAS and OCD is often apparent (4,5).

SYDENHAM CHOREA: THE PROTOTYPE IMMUNE-MEDIATED AUTOAGGRESSIVE DISEASE OF THE BASAL GANGLIA

It is well accepted that SC is a neuropsychiatric immune-mediated disorder of the basal ganglia triggered by streptococcal infection. SC is strongly associated with rheumatic fever (RF) and is in fact included as one of the Jones major criteria in the diagnosis of RF (6). ABGA have been demonstrated in SC, using immunofluorescence microscopy, by several groups (Table 15-4). Although, several candidate autoantigens have been described in patients with SC, none have yet been shown to cause a similar disease in an appropriate animal model. However, disease with features similar to RF and SC can be induced in animals by inoculating the animal with "rheumatogenic" strains of streptococci. Whether or not a SC-like illness can be induced by the passive transfer of ABGA has not been definitively established. Other features that support SC as being an immune-mediated disorder is its delayed onset relative to the streptococcal infection, a female sex preponderance, familial and possible human leukocyte antigen associations, and the pathology. The pathology of SC is mostly localized to the basal ganglia, which included cellular mononuclear cell or lymphocyte infiltration, perivascular cuffs, and neuronal loss with relative sparing of other brain areas (6,7). It is important to note that there is no evidence of direct invasion of the nervous system with streptococci. In summary, SC is a relatively well defined clinical syndrome that is temporally related to streptococcal infection. It fulfils two out of four and possibly three out of four of the modified Witesbsky criteria for being an autoimmune disease. In addition, streptococcal infection is now a well established cause of SC. It can be argued that the causal link between SC and streptococcal infection was an easy one because of the relatively strong association between RF (an established post-streptococcal

TABLE 15-4. *Cross-sectional case-control studies investigating the presence of anti-streptococcal antibodies and antibasal ganglia antibodies in patients with neuropsychiatric disorders within the spectrum of immune-mediated autoaggressive disease of the basal ganglia associated with streptococcal infection*

Authors	Phenotype	Patients*/controls[#] (N)	Antistreptococcal antibodies	Antibasal ganglia antibodies
Husby G et al., 1976.[11]	SC	30/55	Not reported	$P < 0.005^a$
Kiessling LS et al., 1993.[12]	Movement disorders (tics/chorea)	45/38[#]	ASO and/or anti-DNAse B, ns	RR, 2.3 $P = 0.001^a$
Swedo SE et al., 1993.[13]	SC	11/18	ASO, mean of patients: 680 Todd units (normal values ≤480)	RR, 5.26, $P = 0.04^a$
Murphy et al., 1997.[14]	OCD TS	31*/21	ASO, ns; anti-DNAse B, ns ASO, ns; anti-DNAse B, ns	ns^a
Kotby AA et al., 1998.[15]	SC	40/40	ASO, >480 Todd units in 30% of patients (mean 600)	$P < 0.01^a$ only in patients with active chorea
Singer HS et al., 1998.[16]	TS	41/39	ASO, ns; anti-DNAse B, ns	$P = 0.006^b$; higher frequency among patients[c]
Singer HS et al., 1999.[17]	TS	41/39	Not performed	$P = 0.012^b$; similar frequency[c]
Muller N et al., 2000.[18]	TS	36*/52[#]	ASO, $P ≤ 0.01$ in children, ns in adults; anti-DNAseB, $P ≤ 0.0005$ in children, ns in adults	Not performed
Peterson BS et al., 2000.[19]	CTD	53/20	ASO, ns; anti-DNAse B, ns	Not performed
	OCD	27/20	ASO, ns; anti-DNAse B, ns	Not performed
	ADHD	41/20	ASO, $P = 0.03$; anti-DNAse B, $P = 0.03$	Not performed
Dale RC et al., 2001.[20]	Poststreptococcal ADEM	10/80[#]	ASO, $P = 0.002$; anti-DNAseB, $P < 0.001$ (both compared with the neurologic control)	$P < 0.001^b$ (compared with both groups) Western blotting: sensitivity 100%; specificity 92%
Muller N et al., 2001.[21]	TS	25*/25	ASO, $P = 0.025$; anti-DNAse B, $P < 0.001$	Not performed
Wendlandt JT et al., 2001.[22]	TS	20/21	Not performed	$P = 0.0007$ (using MANOVA and discriminant analysis)[c]
Morshed SA et al., 2001.[23]	TS	81*/67[#]	ASO, $P = 0.007$; anti-DNAseB, ns	$P = 0.006^a$
	SC	27*/67[#]	ASO, $P = 0.04$; anti-DNAseB, $P = 0.023$	$P = 0.0001^a$
Church AJ et al., 2002.[24]	SC	36/27[#]	Not performed	$P < 0.001^a$ (compared to both control groups) WI: sensitivity 100%; specificity 93%
Church AJ et al., 2003.[8]	TS	100*/190[#]	ASO, $P < 0.0001$ in children, $P < 0.05$ in adults	$P < 0.05^c$ in children and adults
Loiselle CR et al., 2003.[25]	TS	41/38	ASO, ns; anti-DNAse B, ns	Not performed
	ADHD	20/59	ASO, $P = 0.04$; anti-DNAse B, ns	Not performed
	OCB	8/71	ASO, ns; anti-DNAse B, ns	Not performed
Singer HS et al., 2003.[26]	SC	9/9	Not performed	$P < 0.0001$ (using MANOVA and discriminant analysis)[c]

TABLE 15-4. *Continued*

Authors	Phenotype	Patients*/ controls# (N)	Antistreptococcal antibodies	Antibasal ganglia antibodies
Dale RC et al., 2004.[27]	EL	20*/173#	ASO, *P* <0.005 compared with all control groups	*P* <0.0001[c]
Dale RC et al., 2003.	OCD	50/140#	Not performed	48% of patients and 4% of controls were positive[c]
Hoekstra PJ et al., 2003.[28]	Tics	82/83#	Not performed	67% of patients 40% to 42% of controls were positive
Rizzo R et al., 2003.[29]	TS	69/73#	59% of patients versus 19% of controls hadraised antistreptolysin-0 test	31% of patients versus 12% of controls had positive ABGA[d]
Church AJ et al., 2004.[9]	Chorea, tics, dystonia, and other movement disorders	40/190#	ASO, *P* <0.005 compared with all control groups, except the child streptococcal group elevated titers among selection criteria	ELISA: *P* <0.0001, sensitivity 82%, specificity 79%; WI: sensitivity 92%, specificity 95%

*Patient group includes both children and adults.
#Control groups include both pathological and healthy controls.
[a]Detected by indirect immunofluorescence; [b]detected by ELISA; [c]detected by Western immunoblotting; [d]method not reported

ABGA, antibasal ganglia antibodies; ADHD, attention deficit hyperactivity disorder; CTD, *Classification of Tic Disorders*; ELISA, enzyme-linked immunosorbent assay test; OCB, obsessive compulsive behavior; OCD, obsessive compulsive disorder; SC, Sydenham chorea; TS, Tourette syndrome.

Modified from Martino D, Giovannoni G. Antibasal ganglia antibodies and their relevance to movement disorders. *Curr Opin Neurol.* 2004;17:425–432. With permission.

disorder) and SC. RF, which is a systemic disorder, acts as a red flag and allows one to make the temporal association between the streptococcal infection and the neuropsychiatric disorder. What is very important, however, is that a diagnosis of SC does not necessarily rely on the subject also having RF. This implies, by inference, that the pathogenesis of RF and SC are different. This is a crucial point and needs to be kept in mind when considering the "PANDAS hypothesis."

Patients who are ABGA positive are more likely to have evidence of current or recent streptococcal infection (8,9). Preliminary studies suggest that ABGA may be cross-reactive with antigenic determinants on streptococci (10). ABGAs have been shown to recognize neuronal proteins of 40, 45, 60, and 98 kDa. Using proteomic methodology we have identified the 45 kDa antigen and the 98 kDa antigen as a monomer and dimer of the same protein and other two proteins as belonging to same functional class of proteins. All these neuronal proteins are cytosolic proteins. Unexpectedly,

these proteins are also located on the neuronal surface, where their function is unclear. Importantly, all three of the candidate autoantigens have protein homologues in streptococci.

If PANDAS and SC are the same disease, as recent data suggest, then extrapolating our knowledge from SC suggests that PANDAS is an autoimmune disease. At present it can be argued that 2 out of 4 of the modified Witesbsky criteria have been fulfilled for PANDAS. Now that potential autoantigens have been identified, experiments to create and animal model and to transfer the disease are required.

Does Streptococcal Infection Cause PANDAS? Are Contemporary Criteria for Causation Fulfilled?

In short, no, but causation is rarely a black-and-white issue and usually occurs as a gradual process, which is why the author of this chapter deliberately uses the term "*emerging disorder.*" At present the findings are not consistent. The strength of the association is debatable.

Adequately powered longitudinal studies need to be performed to demonstrate the temporal association between streptococcal infection, ABGA and the clinical onset. Unfortunately, with PANDAS, unlike RF, researchers do not have a flag to alert them to the possible diagnosis. Specificity depends on how the disease is defined. If a wider definition of PANDAS is accepted, then ABGA appear to be specific. The PANDAS hypothesis is consistent with current biologic and previous knowledge and as a hypothesis is plausible. By analogy one may consider PANDAS and SC to be the same disease. At present the experimental evidence in support of the PANDAS hypothesis is contentious. However, with the identification of specific autoantigens we are now in a position to investigate this disease or group of disorders in a systematic way.

CONCLUSIONS

The PANDAS hypothesis is plausible, particularly if the similarities between ABGA positive PANDAS, TS, OCD, and SC are accepted. The current working hypothesis is that antibodies induced in response to streptococcal infection cross-react with antigenic determinants in the basal ganglia, resulting in basal ganglia dysfunction. The experimental evidence is incomplete, and researchers have yet to define the autoantigens in full, create appropriate animal models, and reproducibly transfer disease with the passive transfer of autoantibodies. Despite this deficiency in experimental evidence there is a compelling case to accept immune-mediated basal ganglia dysfunction as an emerging clinical entity. The PANDAS hypothesis cannot be ignored or dismissed because of the implications it has for the diagnosis and treatment of patients with basal ganglia dysfunction. On the contrary, researchers need to embrace the hypothesis, apply their minds and resources to the problem, and investigate it methodically.

ACKNOWLEDGMENTS

The author would like to thank Tourette Syndrome Associations of the United States and United Kingdom, EU Marie Curie Fund, Action Research, Sophie Cameron Trust, and the University of London for their generous financial support. A special thanks to Andrew Church, Russell Dale, Paul Candler, Mark Edwards, Davide Martino, and Steven Lugsden for their hard work in the quest to answer some of these questions.

REFERENCES

1. Schwartz M, Cohen IR. Autoimmunity can benefit self-maintenance. *Immunol Today* 2000;21:265–268.
2. Rose NR, Bona C. Defining criteria for autoimmune disease (Witebsky's postulates revisted). *Immunol Today* 1993;114:426–430.
3. Bradford-Hill A. The environment and disease: association or causation? *Proc Royal Soc Med.* 1966;58:295.
4. Swedo SE, Leonard HL, Garvey M, et al. Pediatric autoimmune neuropsychiatric disorders associated with streptococcal infections: clinical description of the first 50 cases. *Am J Psychiatry* 1998;155:264–271.
5. Murphy ML, Pichichero ME. Prospective identification and treatment of children with pediatric autoimmune neuropsychiatric disorder associated with group A streptococcal infection (PANDAS). *Arch Pediatr Adolesc Med.* 2002;156:356–361.
6. Shiffman RN. Guideline maintenance and revision: fifty years of the Jones criteria for diagnosis of rheumatic fever. 1995;149:727–732.
7. Marie P, Tretiakoff C. Examen histologique de centres nerveux dans un cas de choree aigue de Sydenham. *Rev Neurol.* 1920;36:603–606.
8. Greenfield JG, Wolfsohn JM. The pathology of Sydenham's chorea. *Lancet* 1922;2:603–606.
9. Colony HS, Malamud N. Sydenham's chorea. A clinicopathologic study. *Neurology* 1956;6:672–676.
10. Church AJ, Dale RC, Lees AJ, et al. Tourette's syndrome: a cross sectional study to examine the PANDAS hypothesis. *J Neurol Neurosurg Psychiatry* 2003;74: 602–607.
11. Dale RC, Church AJ, Giovannoni G, et al. Obsessive-compulsive disorder: cross-sectional study for recent streptococcal infection and anti-basal ganglia antibodies [abstract]. *Eur Child Adolesc Psychiatry.* 2003;12 (suppl 2):I/24.
12. Church AJ, Dale RC, Giovannoni G. Anti-basal ganglia antibodies: a possible diagnostic utility in idiopathic movement disorders? *Arch Dis Child.* 2004;89: 611–614.
13. Bronze MS, Dale JB. Epitopes of streptococcal M proteins that evoke antibodies that cross-react with human brain. *J Immunol.* 1993;151:2820–2828.
14. Martino D, Giovannoni G. Antibasal ganglia antibodies and their relevance to movement disorders. *Curr Opin Neurol.* 2004;17:425–432.
15. Husby G, Van de Rijn I, Zabriskie JB, et al. Antibodies reacting with cytoplasm of subthalamic and caudate nuclei neurons in chorea and acute rheumatic fever. *J Exp Med.* 1976;144:1094–1110.
16. Kiessling LS, Marcotte AC, Culpepper L. Antineuronal antibodies in movement disorders. Pediatrics 1993; 92:39–43.

17. Swedo SE, Leonard HL, Schapiro MB, et al. Sydenham's chorea: physical and psychological symptoms of St Vitus dance. *Pediatrics* 1993;91:706–713.

18. Murphy TK, Goodman WK, Fudge MW, et al. B lymphocyte antigen D8/17: a peripheral marker for childhood-onset obsessive–compulsive disorder and Tourette's syndrome? *Am J Psychiatry*. 1997;154:402–407.

19. Kotby AA, El Badawy N, El Sokkary S, et al. Antineuronal antibodies in rheumatic chorea. *Clin Diag Lab Immunol*. 1998;5:836–839.

20. Singer HS, Giuliano JD, Hansen BH, et al. Antibodies against human putamen in children with Tourette syndrome. *Neurology* 1998;50:1618–1624.

21. Singer HS, Giuliano JD, Hansen BH, et al. Antibodies against a neuron-like (HTB-10 neuroblastoma) cell line in children with Tourette syndrome. *Biol Psychiatry*. 1999;46:775–780.

22. Muller N, Riedel M, Straube A, et al. Increased antistreptococcal antibodies in patients with Tourette's syndrome. *Psychiatry Res*. 2000;94:43–49.

23. Peterson BS, Leckman JF, Tucker D, et al. Preliminary findings of antistreptococcal antibody titers and basal ganglia volumes in tic, obsessive-compulsive, and attention deficit/hyperactivity disorders. *Arch Gen Psychiatry* 2000;57:364–372.

24. Dale RC, Church AJ, Cardoso F, et al. Poststreptococcal acute disseminated encephalomyelitis with basal ganglia involvement and auto-reactive antibasal ganglia antibodies. *Ann Neurol*. 2001;50:588–595.

25. Muller N, Kroll B, Schwarz MJ, et al. Increased titers of antibodies against streptococcal M12 and M19 proteins in patients with Tourette's syndrome. *Psychiatry Res*. 2001;101:187–193.

26. Wendlandt JT, Grus FH, Hansen BH, et al. Striatal antibodies in children with Tourette's syndrome: multivariate discriminant analysis. of IgG repertoires. *J Neuroimmunol*. 2001;119:106–113.

27. Morshed SA, Parveen S, Leckman JF, et al. Antibodies against neural, nuclear, cytoskeletal, and streptococcal epitopes in children and adults with Tourette's syndrome, Sydenham's chorea, and autoimmune disorders. *Biol Psychiatry*. 2001;50:566–577.

28. Church AJ, Cardoso F, Dale RC, et al. Anti-basal ganglia antibodies in acute and persistent Sydenham's chorea. *Neurology* 2002;59:227–231.

29. Loiselle CR, Wendlandt JT, Rohde CA, et al. Antistreptococcal, neuronal, and nuclear antibodies in Tourette syndrome. *Pediatr Neurol*. 2003;28:119–125.

30. Singer HS, Loiselle CR, Lee O, et al. Anti-basal ganglia antibody abnormalities in Sydenham chorea. *J Neuroimmunol*. 2003;136:154–161.

31. Dale RC, Church AJ, Surtees RAH, et al. Encephalitis lethargica syndrome: 20 new cases and evidence of basal ganglia autoimmunity. *Brain* 2004;127:21–33.

32. Hoekstra PJ, Horst G, Limburg PC, et al. Increased seroreactivity in tic disorder patients to a 60 kDa protein band from a neuronal cell line. *J Neuroimmunol*. 2003;141:118–124.

33. Rizzo R, Fogliani F, Gulisano M, et al. Tourette's syndrome: a study concerning recent streptococcal infection and anti-basal ganglia antibodies [abstract]. *Eur Child Adolesc Psychiatry* 2003;12 (suppl 2):I/30.

16

Autoimmunity and Pediatric Movement Disorders

Harvey S. Singer[1,2,3] and Phillip N. Williams[2]

[1]*Division of Pediatric Neurology, Johns Hopkins Hospital, Baltimore, Maryland;*
[2]*Departments of Neurology and* [3]*Pediatrics, Johns Hopkins University School of Medicine, Baltimore.*

Autoimmune disorders are those in which the host's natural defense mechanism turns against the person causing dysfunction of either a single organ or multiple organ systems. Several pediatric movement disorders, including Sydenham chorea (SC), pediatric autoimmune neuropsychiatric disorder associated with streptococcal infection (PANDAS), and Tourette syndrome (TS) have been hypothesized to fit in this category. In these disorders, it is proposed that antibodies produced against group A beta-hemolytic streptococcus (GABHS) cross-react with neuronal tissue (i.e., become antineuronal antibodies [ANAbs]) and, in turn, result in movement abnormalities (chorea or tics) and/or behavioral symptoms (obsessive compulsive behaviors, personality changes, and others). Although the proposal that immune responses directed against host neurons is controversial, the goals of this chapter are to provide an overview of immunology, a discussion of criteria required for confirmation of autoimmunity, and a review of existing data pertaining to SC, TS, and PANDAS.

IMMUNOLOGY

Principles of Immunology: Microbe to Antibodies

The proposed immune process in autoimmune pediatric movement disorders starts with a streptococcal infection and includes humoral immunity and molecular mimicry. For full appreciation of this process, this discussion begins by providing some basic knowledge of pathogens and the immune system in the context of a streptococcal infection.

Streptococcus pyogenes is a gram-positive bacterium with a cell wall surrounding a lipid bilayer plasma membrane. The Lancefield serologic grouping system for streptococci is based on immunological differences in cell wall polysaccharides (e.g., groups A, B, C, F, and G). The organism is further serologically separated into M-protein serotypes based on surface proteins that can be extracted from the bacteria. A variety of surface proteins have important roles in disease pathogenesis. For example, the streptococcal surface α-enolase, a 45-kDa protein that binds to plasmin(ogen), contributes to tissue invasion (1). Streptococci have the capacity to adhere to host epithelial cells lining the pharynx as well as to penetrate the tissue. Microbial damage is caused by either the production of a local infection or the secretion of exotoxin.

Once the streptococcus has created a local infection, the innate immune system responds. This response both precedes and is required for activation of the adaptive immune response. In brief, the innate immune response consists of the early arrival of macrophages and natural killer cells, as well as stimulation of the complement system. The macrophage has several important roles besides phagocytosis, including the secretion of chemokines (which activate vascular endothelial cells and attract more phagocytes), cytokines (which stimulate acute phase protein synthesis), and complement (which leads to osmotic lysis and opsonization). If the pathogen is not immediately eliminated, bacterial antigens are carried via the lymphatic system to lymph nodes. Portage of these antigens, which induce adaptive immunity (immunogens), is via linkage to the major histocompatibility complex (MHC) located on antigen-presenting cells (e.g., macrophages, dendritic cells, leukocytes). With the arrival of the antigen in the lymph node, lymphocytes are stimulated to become immune effector cells. Antigen type (polypeptides, carbohydrates, lipids), dose, route, timing, and immunogenicity can all affect the immune response. For example, immunogenicity is generally most pronounced for protein antigens and increases with greater molecular weight and complexity. After the primary contact with the streptococcus, there is a lag of several days before detection of increased antibody production or cellular immunity.

The pathway leading to induction of humoral (antibody) immunity by a specific antigen can vary, but typically involves the activation of T helper (Th) cells with subsequent induction of B lymphocytes (B cells), production of antibody, and the generation of memory B and T cells. In an early step, Th cells are activated to become either T helper 1 (Th1) or 2 (Th2) cells, depending on the local cytokine environment. This is a relatively important differentiation because cytokines produced by Th1 cells (interleukin 2 [IL-2], interferon alpha [INF-α], tumor necrosis factor beta [TNF-β]) activate the cell mediated immune system (cytotoxic T cells and macrophages), whereas cytokines produced by Th2 cells (IL-4 to 6, and IL-10) stimulate the humoral immune system.

Antibodies are immunoglobulins (Igs), which are synthesized in the rough endoplasmic reticulum within the cytoplasm of the B cell or plasma cell. They share a basic structure consisting of two identical heavy (H) polypeptide chains and two identical light (L) chains that are covalently bonded by interchain disulfide linkages. Antibody isotypes (IgA, IgG, IgM, IgE, IgD) have different H chain types that influence their function. The molecule is roughly shaped as a "Y," with the antigen recognition domains located at the extreme tips. Each IgG can cross-link two antigens, since it has two identical binding sites composed of a variable region from the H and L amino-terminal domains folded together. The binding can accommodate up to seven amino acid or sugar residues and binds to the antigen by various hydrogen and ionic bonds, hydrophobic interactions, and Van der Waals interactions. The strength of the binding is represented by the binding affinity. The portion of the antigen that binds to the antibody is the epitope. The stem of the "Y" (Fc region) is not involved in the recognition of antigens.

The predominant antibody produced during the primary immune response is IgM and it is the first antibody secreted during an immune response, whereas IgG is the prominent serum antibody with the longest half-life. The antibody has three main functions: to bind the antigen, activate other immune components, and stimulate phagocytes (2). The primary recognizable antigen on GABHS is the M protein. Once the antibody encounters this antigen, it stimulates the B cell to differentiate into a plasma cell which makes and secretes copious amounts of the parent antibody. B cells also differentiate into long-living memory cells that remain ready to mount a quick immune response upon re-exposure to the same antigen (3). Once the antibody coats the antigen, it is marked for destruction by phagocytes.

In addition to B cells, the immune system has a repertoire of T lymphocytes (T cells) that defend the body through cell-mediated mechanisms. Both T and B cells are derived from stem cells in the bone marrow, but T cells are developed in the thymus, in contrast to the lymph nodes. There are two types of T cells: cytotoxic T cells kill virus-infected cells whereas helper T cells communicate and stimulate B cells and other immune components.

Autoimmunity

Autoimmunity is caused by an adaptive immune response against "self" antigen. Autoimmunity is usually prevented during lymphocyte development in a process known as self tolerance. Some

TABLE 16-1. *Criteria for establishing a pathogenic role for autoantibodies*

1. Identification of autoantibodies
2. Presence of antibodies at the pathologic site
3. Induction of symptoms with autoantigens
4. Passive transfer of the disorder to animal models
5. Positive response to immunomodulatory therapy

autoreactive B-cells can escape this established tolerance mechanism; however, and produce autoantibodies that can contribute to tissue damage in immune-mediated disorders (3). Molecular mimicry is another proposed mechanism in which bacterial, viral, or other foreign antigenic epitopes with significant amino acid sequence homology to host epitopes cause antibody cross reactivity.

Even though the presence of autoantibodies may appear to indicate an autoimmune disorder, the reader must recognize that autoantibodies against brain epitopes are found even in healthy subjects (4–6). For example, autoantibodies can have important regulatory functions such as tissue repair and neuroprotection in the central nervous system (CNS) (3). Recent studies have even suggested that some inflammatory processes in the CNS may be a form of autoimmune neuroprotection that keeps a balance between the immune system and CNS (7).

Requirements for Autoimmunity

There are five basic criteria for experimentally establishing a pathogenic role for autoantibodies in a neurological disorder (Table 16-1) (3). Ideally all five criteria should be fulfilled to establish a causal link, although depending on the disorder the criteria may not all be of equal importance (3). Investigators use several laboratory techniques to identify autoantibodies quantitatively and qualitatively. Three well-accepted techniques include: enzyme-linked immunosorbent assay (ELISA), indirect immunofluorescence, and Western immunoblotting; however, each of these techniques may generate discrepant results (8).

Bypassing the Blood-Brain Barrier

Autoantibodies must gain access to the brain to cause dysfunction in autoimmune CNS movement disorders, but the presence of the blood-brain barrier (BBB) often complicates pathogenesis models. The BBB is a complex cellular system of endothelial cells, astroglia, pericytes, perivascular macrophages, and a basal lamina (9). The barrier permits selective exclusion or transport of substances on the basis of size and biochemical characteristics (10). This normally tight barrier is known to become increasingly permeable during immunologic distress. Nevertheless, determining whether a permeable BBB is necessary for inflammatory cell invasion, or whether these cells can gain outright access has been fuel for debate (11,12). Activated B and T cells have been found to cross the barrier easily (3). Cytokines such as TNF, IL-1, and IL-6 have been shown to enhance the permeability of cerebral endothelial cells (13). The endothelial cells themselves are also known to generate various factors that increase the permeability of the BBB (14).

Immune components, primarily in the form of microglia, are also found within the brain. Microglia are the resident immune cells and function in various roles. They were previously assumed to exist predominantly in a passive resting state; however, new evidence suggests that they are continually active in surveying their microenvironment (15). The presence of pathological signals activates microglia to proliferate, migrate, perform phagocytosis, present antigens, and secrete proinflammatory mediators (16). Despite their versatility, the activities of microglia are also associated with neuronal death (17). Future investigation into the numerous functions of microglia should provide a clearer picture of the nature of autoimmune processes in the brain.

PROPOSED POSTSTREPTOCOCCAL AUTOIMMUNE MOVEMENT DISORDERS

GABHS infections are proposed as the etiology for several postinfectious movement disorders, including SC, pediatric autoimmune neuropsychiatric disorder associated with streptococcal infection, and TS. The proposed pathophysiologic mechanism leading to the neurological condition is shown in Fig. 16-1. A description of each of

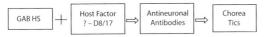

Fig. 16-1. Proposed mechanism for autoimmune movement disorders.

these disorders and evidence supporting an autoimmune mechanism is presented. It is clear that evidence supporting an immune disorder ranges from good to poor. Although others have speculated that a wide spectrum of movement disorders may be secondary to a similar subset of conserved antigens (18,19), the authors of this chapter believe that it is essential to focus on each disorder individually.

SYDENHAM CHOREA

SC is the prototype for an infectious agent (GABHS) triggering an autoimmune disorder that, in turn, causes a movement disorder. SC usually occurs between the ages 5 and 15 years, and a female predominance has been observed in all large studies. Chorea can range in severity, is usually generalized, but hemichorea occurs in about 20% of individuals. Associated neurologic symptoms may include dysarthria (about one-third), gait disturbances that correlate with severity of chorea, hypometric saccades, hypotonia, weakness, and hemiballismus (20,21). Most patients have concomitant psychological dysfunction presenting as personality changes, obsessive-compulsive symptoms, emotional irritability, distractibility, and age-regressed behaviors (22,23). Affected individuals may present with behavioral or emotional difficulties that predate the motor abnormalities by weeks to months. Motor or vocal tics and oculogyric crises have also been reported in patients with SC (20,24). Rheumatic valvular cardiac disease is seen in about one-third of patients, whereas arthritis is uncommon.

The diagnosis of SC is based on clinical observation and the lack of evidence for other disorders (25). No confirmatory test is available, although serological evidence of streptococcal infection is found in about 80% of patients. The outcome in SC is quite favorable, with most cases resolving in 1 to 6 months, although chorea (26) and neuropsychiatric problems may persist (22,23,27). About 20% to 42% of patients have recurrent episodes of chorea (28), which usually occurs within 1 to 2 years after the original event, but has been seen up to 10 years later (28,29). Reactivation may occur in association with a streptococcal infection, pregnancy (chorea gravidarum), or secondary to factors that are unrelated to streptococcal infection or rheumatic fever activity (28,30,31).

Despite its description more than 300 years ago by Sydenham, its defined association with rheumatic fever in 1838 (32), and linkage to a preceding GABHS infection (33), there are numerous unanswered questions about the underlying pathology and pathophysiology of SC. The number of postmortem studies has been limited by the overall good prognosis of the disorder. Nevertheless, a variety of widespread cerebral abnormalities have been reported, including acute and chronic neuronal degenerative (34) changes as well as vascular and inflammatory lesions (35–37). Indeed, pathologic changes identified in cerebral cortex, basal ganglia, and thalamus have included a reduction in neurons, cytoplasmic and nucleus changes in the cell, gliosis, hyperemia, endothelial swelling, perivascular round cell infiltration, and petechial hemorrhages. A magnetic resonance imaging volumetric study evaluating the size of the basal ganglia in children with SC showed a 10% increase in size of the caudate and a 7% increase in size of both putamen and globus pallidus (38). Focal areas of T2 hypersignal in the caudate, pallidum, putamen, and white matter have been noted in recurrent cases.

Since only a small percentage of individuals affected with GABHS infection develop rheumatic fever and a family history of rheumatic fever is present in about one-third of cases (29), it has been proposed that both pathogen and host-related factors influence the acquisition of this disorder. Increased expression of the monoclonal antibody D8/17 directed against a polymorphic protein on the surface of B lymphocytes has been found in individuals with rheumatic fever and is hypothesized to be a trait marker for susceptibility (39,40). The monoclonal antibody reacts with epitopes present on a significantly higher proportion of B lymphocytes in patients with acute rheumatic fever or rheumatic heart disease (100%) than in controls (12%). A significantly higher frequency of D8/17 positive cells has also been identified in children with SC (89%) compared with healthy children (17%). How this marker relates to the disease process is unknown, especially since it has been reported in patients with other neuropsychiatric disorders of childhood onset who have not been diagnosed with rheumatic fever or SC (41,42). Researchers have also failed to reproduce some correlations by using automated techniques, rather than manual counting of stained cells with a fluorescent microscope.

An autoimmune hypothesis has been proposed as the underlying mechanism in SC, that is, after a streptococcal infection in susceptible individuals, antibodies directed against bacterial antigens cross-react (molecular mimicry) with epitopes on neurons of the basal ganglia, causing chorea and behavioral disturbances. The streptococcal M protein serotypes most often associated with SC are 5, 6, 19, and 24 (43). Several lines of evidence support the involvement of immune mechanisms in this disorder: improvement of symptoms after immunomodulatory therapies (44–46); documentation of autoreactive antibodies against human basal ganglia (47–49) or rat striatum (5); correlation of the severity and duration of the chorea with ANAbs and the loss of immunoreactivity after preabsorption of sera against streptococci (47,50); a modest up-regulation of cytokine production in cerebrospinal fluid and serum (51); and the demonstration that monoclonal antibodies, obtained from B clones derived from a patient with acute SC, cross-react with mammalian lysoganglioside GM1 and N-acetyl-α-D-glucosamine, a dominant epitope of the group A streptococcal carbohydrate (52). Additional support for the hypothesis of molecular mimicry comes from the finding that antibodies to streptococcal M protein can cross-react with human brain tissue (43).

Several of the criteria necessary to establish a definitive causal link between autoantibodies and SC have yet to be fulfilled (passive transfer of disease to animals and disease induction with autoantigen) and there are several areas with conflicting data (53). Studies of human lymphocyte antigen report conflicting results in detecting associations between classes I or class II MHC antigens and acute rheumatic fever; specific human lymphocyte antigen alleles were overrepresented in rheumatic carditis and arthritis subgroups, but were not increased in frequency in a subgroup with SC only (54). Intravenous immunoglobulin (IVIG) treatment has failed to alter the natural history of acute rheumatic fever, with no detectable difference in the clinical, laboratory, or echocardiographic parameters of the disease process during the subsequent 12 months (55). Furthermore, it remains unexplained by proposed mechanisms why the onset of chorea is delayed for 3 to 5 months after GABHS infection, unlike the other features of rheumatic fever. In summary, however, even though there are existing issues, SC remains the accepted standard for poststreptococcal neuropsychiatric disease.

Tourette Syndrome

The clinical features and course of TS are fully described in this text and will not be reviewed in this chapter. A hypothesized role for streptococcal infections as the etiology for tics is not new. Several early case reports described children with tic disorders and associated acute sinusitis (56–58). Kiessling (59), in an outpatient clinic setting, identified current or recent GABHS infections in eight out of 14 children with initial or recurrent tics. Researchers have sought to determine whether individuals with a tic disorder have increased levels of streptococcal antibodies. In several studies, higher antistreptolysin O titers were present in adult TS subjects as compared with controls (5,60,61). In each study, however, there was no association between levels of antistreptococcal titers and clinical symptoms. In other studies, no association was detected between streptococcal markers and tics in pediatric (5,6,62) or mixed pediatric/adult populations (63). One study suggested that antistreptolysin O (ASO) and antiDNAse-B titers correlated with the presence of attention deficit hyperactivity disorder (63).

Studies of ANAbs in children with tics and TS have been reported. ANAbs against human basal ganglia and human neuroblastoma cells have been quantified by ELISA and those against human basal ganglia and rat striatum by immunofluorescent methods. One ELISA study showed that, compared with control subjects ($N = 39$), children with TS ($N = 41$) had a significant increase in the mean and median optical density levels of serum antibodies against the putamen, but not the caudate or globus pallidus (6). Total antineural antibodies, measured by immunofluorescence on frozen sections of rat striatum, were higher in 81 subjects with TS (age 8 to 51 years) compared with controls. The difference in antibody titers, however, was not significant when children and adolescents with TS ($N = 54$) were compared with normal controls (5). Western immunoblotting analyses, performed in order to identify disease-specific changes in regional brain epitopes, have identified abnormalities in sera from patients with TS, but results are extremely variable. One study showed positive binding in 20 to 30% with a common band located at 60 kDa (64), a second indicated that 23% of children with TS had reactivity against striatal antigens at either 40, 45, or 60 kDa (65), and a third study showed that numerous bands with different molecular weights contributed to changes in TS antibody repertoires (66). In TS, although several studies have reported elevated serum autoantibodies, the source of these antibodies is unclear, especially since the majority of study subjects had no evidence of a preceding infection (5,6,62,64,65,67).

Because the passive transfer of the disorder to animal models is one of the required criteria to establish an autoimmune etiology, animal models have been used to study whether sera from TS subjects can induce stereotypies in rodents. To date, four studies have evaluated the effect of infusing sera or IgG containing elevated levels of ANAb from individuals with TS into rodent striatum. Hallett et al. (68) compared

the effect of dilute serum (1:6) infused into the ventral striatum, from 5 TS patients and controls. Sera from TS subjects, selected on the basis of antibody titers against a solubilized neuroblastoma cell membrane fraction, significantly increased stereotypic behaviors in Fischer 344 rats (e.g., licks and forepaw shakes) as well as episodic utterances. Abnormal behaviors were identified during the 3-day period of microinfusion and on days eight to 10 after microinfusion. Taylor et al. (67) infused sera from TS patients, ranked for autoantibody levels by use of an immunofluorescent technique against rat striatum, into the ventrolateral striatum of male Sprague-Dawley rats. In this study, behavioral abnormalities coincided with the 5 days of serum infusion. Results showed a significant increase of oral stereotypies in 12 rats receiving higher-titer sera as compared to 12 rats infused with lower-titer patient sera and 12 controls. In a third study, Loiselle et al. (53) microinfused serum from 5 subjects with TS, each with elevated ANAb titers against fresh human postmortem putamen, and 5 children with PANDAS, bilaterally into Fischer 344 ventral striatum or ventrolateral striatum. Despite infusion of patient sera at the same coordinates that were used in the Hallett and Taylor protocols, no rat developed any audible abnormality and there was no significant increase in stereotypic behaviors.

Because of the importance of establishing a model useful for evaluating autoimmune hypotheses, a tripartite collaborative effort among the previously reporting institutions (Brown, Yale, and Johns Hopkins) was undertaken and designed to clarify discrepancies in prior results. ANAbs were measured in subjects with TS, attention deficit hyperactivity disorder and/or obsessive compulsive disorder. Sera containing the highest and the lowest levels of ANAbs were identified, re-encoded and sent back to each center for infusion into the ventrolateral striatum of male Sprague-Dawley rats by using a specific protocol. Animals were observed for behavioral abnormalities for 3 days before the start of infusion, during infusion on days two to four, and for 2 days after infusion. Combined stereotypy scores increased after antibody infusion; however, there was no significant effect based on serum titer ($P = 0.85$). Scores differed among centers, but analyses based on individual institutional data again failed to show an effect based on elevated or low ANAb values (Brown, $P = 0.95$; Yale and Johns Hopkins, $P = 0.81$). Post hoc studies with sham surgery and phosphate-buffered saline (PBS) infusion support suggestions of nonspecific behavioral effects unrelated to antibody titer. This report emphasizes that any conclusions about antibody-mediated movement disorders that are based upon results from the rodent infusion model must be considered with caution.

The role of the cytokines in early-onset OCD and tic disorders has been investigated by measurement of serial serum concentrations of those associated with T-cell activation (INF-γ, IL-2, 4,5,6,10) or local inflammation (IL-12, INF-α, TNF-α) and brain-derived neurotrophic factor, bDNF (69). IL-12 and TNF-α were elevated at baseline and increased during periods of exacerbation. Of interest, however, was the finding that IL-12 levels were increased in TS subjects who did not have a history of a preceding streptococcal infection. Readers should also be aware that studies have shown little correlation between levels of cytokines in sera and cerebrospinal fluid (70).

PANDAS (Pediatric Autoimmune Neuropsychiatric Disorder Associated with Streptococcal Infection)

In 1998 Swedo et al. (71) proposed that SC was not the only immune-mediated CNS manifestation of GABHS and described their diagnostic criteria for PANDAS. They suggested that a systematic clinical evaluation of children with obsessive compulsive disorder (OCD) and tic disorders, including TS, would define a homogeneous subgroup. Hence, based on 50 cases recruited from a nationwide search, they established the existence of a subset of children with tic disorders and/or OCD who had the abrupt onset/exacerbation of symptoms that were temporally associated with a streptococcal infection. Diagnostic criteria include: the presence of OCD and/or tic disorder; prepubertal

TABLE 16-2. *PANDAS criteria*

1. Presence of obsessive compulsive disorder and/or tic disorder
2. Prepubertal age at onset
3. Sudden, "explosive" onset of symptoms and a course of sudden exacerbations and remissions
4. Temporal relationship between symptom onset and exacerbations and group A beta-hemolytic streptococcus infections
5. The presence of neurologic abnormalities including tics, hyperactivity, and choreiform movements during exacerbations

PANDAS, pediatric autoimmune neuropsychiatric disorders associated with streptococcal infection.

age at onset; sudden, "explosive" onset of symptoms and/or a course of sudden exacerbations and remissions; a temporal relationship between symptoms and GABHS infection; and the presence of neurological abnormalities, including hyperactivity and choreiform movements. In subsequent reports, proponents have clarified several requirements (72). For example, diagnosis necessitates at least two exacerbations of neuropsychiatric symptoms with distinct intervening periods of remission during which throat cultures and antistreptococcal antibody titers are negative. Explosive tic exacerbations are defined as the simultaneous appearance of several different motor and phonic tics with an intensity that causes parents to seek immediate medical attention. These acute recurrences must begin simultaneously with a positive throat culture or within 7 to 14 days after the infection. Lastly, choreiform movements are described as fine piano-playing finger movements (Table 16-2).

The existence of PANDAS remains controversial, with advocates and opponents taking firm positions on either side of the clinical issue (72–76). Support for PANDAS is derived from the following: the description of additional cohorts (77); familial studies showing that first degree relatives of children with PANDAS have higher rates of tic disorders and OCD than do those in the general population (78); expanded expression of a trait marker for susceptibility in rheumatic fever (the monoclonal antibody D8/17) in individuals with PANDAS (42); and magnetic resonance imaging volumetric analyses showing that the average size of the caudate, putamen, and globus pallidus, but not thalamus or total cerebrum, was significantly greater in PANDAS than it was in healthy children (79). Despite these findings, concerns continue to be raised about the existence of PANDAS. For example, no prospective epidemiologic study has confirmed that an antecedent GABHS infection is specifically associated with either the onset or exacerbation of tic disorders or OCD. Diagnostic criteria established for PANDAS are potentially confounded by the phenotypic variability commonly associated with tic disorders, such as a normal fluctuation in the frequency and severity of symptoms, exacerbation of tics by stress, fatigue, and illness, occurrence of "sudden, abrupt" onset and/or recurrence of tics in non-PANDAS subjects (80), and lack of a precise definition for associated neurological conditions (75). Additionally, longitudinal laboratory data, rather than studies that use only a throat culture or only a single antistreptolysin O or antideoxyribonuclease B titer, are necessary to confirm the presence of a previous GABHS infection.

In rheumatic fever, the reduction of recurrences by antibiotic prophylaxis against GABHS was an important factor in confirming a pathogenic association with streptococci. Hence, the effectiveness of oral penicillin prophylaxis has been evaluated in patients with PANDAS and tic disorders. In a double-blind, placebo-controlled crossover trial with oral penicillin (250 mg penicillin V) undertaken to prevent recurrences of PANDAS, no significant change in severity of either obsessive compulsive or tic symptoms occurred between the active and placebo arms (81). Unfortunately, since an acceptable level of streptococcal prophylaxis was not achieved, no firm conclusions were possible. Two prospective longitudinal studies have shown no clear relationship between new GABHS infections and the development or exacerbation of tic/OCD symptoms (82,83). One recent study has shown that penicillin and azithromycin decreased streptococcal infections and neuropyschiatric symptoms (84), but several investigators have raised concerns about serious shortcomings in design and suggested that

the results be interpreted with great caution. Clearly, an adequately powered, double-blind randomized trial that includes true placebo therapy, proper blinding, careful operational criteria for clinical exacerbations, intensive microbiologic and serologic assessment and appropriate confirmation of GABHS infection will be required to determine whether chronic antibiotic therapy can influence the PANDAS constellation of symptoms.

Similar to SC, an immune-mediated mechanism involving molecular mimicry has been proposed for PANDAS. Indirect support for an immune hypothesis is derived from a single study showing that a small number of patients with PANDAS responded to immunotherapy with IVIG and plasmapheresis (PEX) (85). Twenty-nine children with PANDAS recruited from a nationwide search were randomized in a partially double-blind fashion (no sham apheresis) to an IVIG, IVIG placebo (saline), and PEX group. One month after treatment, the obsessive-compulsive symptoms were reduced by 58% and 45% in the PEX and IVIG groups, respectively, compared with only 3% in the IVIG control. In contrast, tic scores were significantly improved only after PEX treatment, with reductions of 49% (PEX), 19% (IVIG), and 12% (IVIG placebo). The NIH has recommended that immunotherapy be reserved for patients participating in controlled double-blind protocols.

ANAbs have been assessed in patients with PANDAS with variable results. Investigators using ELISA and Western immunoblotting methodologies to evaluate sera from 40 children with movement disorders associated with streptococcal infections (including 16 with PANDAS), suggested that this cohort could be readily differentiated from a variety of disease controls (64). ELISA results were significantly elevated in this cohort compared with those in control populations. Further, immunoblotting, by use of a colorimetric assay with frozen postmortem basal ganglia tissue as the epitope, detected limited reactivity in controls, but significantly more bands (at 60, 45, and 40 kDa) in poststreptococcal patients. In contrast, other researchers using ELISA assays with several human postmortem epitopes, including

A

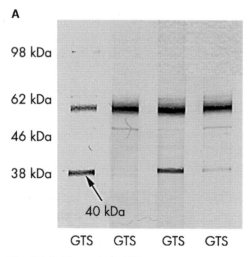

B

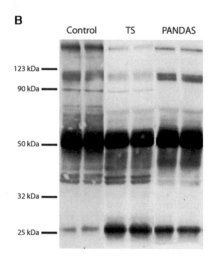

Fig. 16-2. Examples of Western blots. Blot A (Church et al.) (64) was performed on frozen, delipidated postmortem brain tissue using a colorimetric detection method. Blot B (Singer et al.) (87) was performed on fresh, non-delipidated postmortem brain tissue using an electrochemiluminescent detection method. These two methods produce distinctly different results.

supernatant, pellet, and synaptosomal fractions from fresh caudate, putamen, and globus pallidus, were unable to distinguish 15 PANDAS subjects from controls (86). Immunoblotting assays in this cohort, with the use of supernatant and pellet fractions from the caudate and putamen and an electrochemiluminescent method, showed that no molecular weight bands had measurable activity exclusive to either PANDAS or controls for any of the antigenic tissues (86).

In a larger study from the laboratory of the authors of this chapter, ANAb profiles in subjects with TS ($N = 48$) and PANDAS ($N = 46$) were compared with those of age-matched controls ($N = 43$) (87). Autoantibodies were measured by use of ELISA and Western immunoblotting methodologies against a variety of epitopes, including human postmortem caudate, putamen, and prefrontal cortex (Brodmann area 10). Results confirmed that ELISA optical density readings were similar among the groups. Immunoblotting showed complex staining patterns in both patient and control groups with no differences in any tissue. Thus, the number of bands with reactivity peaks at molecular weights 98, 60, 45, and 40 kDa, and total area under ScanPack-derived peaks were not different. Additionally, we sought to determine

the presence of serum antibodies against several commercially obtained specific antigens including pyruvate kinase M1, α- and γ-enolase, and aldolase C. These antigens are reported to be the purified epitopes identified in poststreptococcal patients at MW 60, 45 (a doublet), and 40 kDa, respectively (18). Nevertheless, despite prior claims of their potential specificity (64,65,88), our investigation identified no difference in the frequency of serum antibodies (Fig. 16-2, Fig. 16-3). In order to determine whether detected antibodies cross-react with streptococcal proteins, several assays were repeated after preabsorption with homogenized GABHS. The failure to alter immunoreactivity by the prior exposure of sera to streptococcal antigens further suggests a lack of association between antibodies against these putative antigens and a preceding GABHS infection. Lastly, the microinfusion of sera from children with PANDAS into rodent striatum did not change the number of observed motor stereotype behaviors (53) (Table 16-3).

CONCLUSION

Investigations have shown that methodologic variables, including tissue selection and preparation,

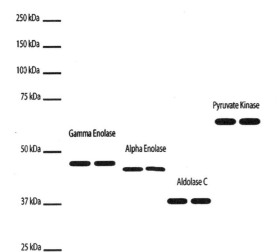

Fig. 16-3. Western blot immunoreactivity composite against gamma and alpha enolase, aldolase C, and pyruvate kinase. Specific proteins were electrophoresed, exposed to patient sera, and developed with ECL methods. Preabsorption of serum with streptococcal antigens did not change observed reactivity.

TABLE 16-3. *Subjects (%) with reactivity to putative antigens and postmortem caudate (at 60, 45, and 40 kDa)**

Molecular weight	TS	PANDAS	Control
60 kDa			
PK M1 ($N = 40$)	43%	55%	37%
Caudate	89%	100%	75%
45 kDa			
α-Enolase ($N = 40$)	0%	3%	0%
γ-Enolase ($n = 40$)	3%	3%	2%
Caudate	54%	48%	44%
40 kDa			
Aldolase C ($N = 40$)	95%	98%	91%
Caudate	43%	35%	30%

*No significant difference was identified among groups. PANDAS, pediatric autoimmune neuropsychiatric disorders associated with streptococcal infection; TS, Tourette syndrome.

antibody source, and Western blot methods can be significant factors in the measurement of ANAbs (8). Thus, until a universally accepted antineuronal detection method is implemented, readers can expect continued variation in reported results from such studies. Further, weaknesses of many cited studies include the analysis of antibody patterns at a single point in time, rather than in serial samples, the failure to correlate ANAb alterations with clinical symptomatology, and the unknown status of a streptococcal infection. Thus, we await the results of longitudinal analyses in well characterized patients (currently in progress). Other important points include recognition that: A) an antibody titer incorporates both antibody affinity and avidity and that a low concentration of high affinity antibodies can be significant; B) measured autoantibody repertoires can be secondary immune responses to components of damaged tissue rather than to an inciting pathological factor (89); and C) immunologic factors other than antibodies can be important.

Lastly, Plato's metaphor of the cave, found in *The Republic*, may provide a fitting analogy to the current situation (90). Plato describes unenlightened life as lying in a cave, watching images displayed on a screen. The source of these images is a fire behind the viewer, illuminating the true objects. Most individuals accept the images as the genuine objects, drawing conclusions from altered reflections of reality. It is only a rare individual that actually questions the image and turns around to see the truth. Similar to those in the cave, researchers may be watching flickering images and basing conclusions on them. Indeed, this is an unsettling prospect.

In summary, the authors of this chapter believe that, to date, there remains no consistent evidence that an autoimmune process is the underlying pathophysiological mechanism in either TS or PANDAS. The authors recognize, however, that confirmation of the concept of a postinfectious autoimmune tic/OCD disorder would have broad neurobiologic, epidemiologic, and treatment implications; consequently, these authors continue to pursue studies in this area with enthusiasm.

REFERENCES

1. Pancholi V, Fischetti VA. Alpha-enolase, a novel strong plasmin(ogen) binding protein on the surface of pathogenic streptococci. *J Biol Chem.* 1998;273: 14503–14515.
2. Sehgal A, Berger MS. basic concepts of immunology and neuroimmunology. *Neurosurgery Focus.* 2000;9:1–6.

3. Archelos JJ, Hartung HP. Pathogenetic role of auto-antibodies in neurological diseases. *Trends Neurosci.* 2000;23:317–327.

4. Lacroix-Desmazes S, Kaveri SV, Mouthon L, et al. Self-reactive antibodies (natural autoantibodies) in healthy individuals. *J Immunol Methods.* 1998;216:117–137.

5. Morshed SA, Parveen S, Leckman JF, et al. Antibodies against neural, nuclear, cytoskeletal, and streptococcal epitopes in children and adults with Tourette's syndrome, Sydenham's chorea, and autoimmune disorders. *Biol Psychiatry.* 2001;50:566–577.

6. Singer HS, Giuliano JD, Hansen BH, et al. Antibodies against human putamen in children with Tourette syndrome. *Neurology* 1998;50:1618–1624.

7. Tabakman R, Lecht S, Sephanova S, et al. Interactions between the cells of the immune and nervous system: neurotrophins as neuroprotection mediators in CNS injury. *Prog Brain Res.* 2004;146:387–401.

8. Rippel CA, Hong JJ, Yoon DY, et al. Methodological factors affect the measurement of anti-basal ganglia antibodies. *Ann Clin Lab Sci.* 2005;35:121–130.

9. Swedo SE. Sydenham's chorea. A model for childhood autoimmune neuropsychiatric disorders. *JAMA* 1994; 272:1788–1791.

10. Gilman S, Newman SW. *Mantz and Gatz's Essentials of Clinical Neuroanatomy and Neurophysiology.* Philadelphia, Pa: PA Davis; 2003.

11. Bendszus M, Bartsch A, Stoll G. Is the disruption of the blood-brain barrier a prerequisite for cellular infiltration in autoimmune encephalitis? *Brain* 2005;128:E25.

12. Floris S, blezer EL, Schreibelt G, Dopp E, et al. blood-brain barrier permeability and monocyte infiltration in experimental allergic encephalomyelitis: a quantitative MRI study. *Brain* 2004;127:616–627.

13. de Vries HE, Blom-Roosemalen MC, van Oosten M, et al. The influence of cytokines on the integrity of the blood-brain barrier in vitro. *J Neuroimmunol.* 1996;64:37–43.

14. de Vries HE, Kuiper J, de boer AG, et al. The blood-brain barrier in neuroinflammatory diseases. *Pharmacol Rev.* 1997;49:143–155.

15. Nimmerjahn A, Kirchhoff F, Helmchen F. Resting microglial cells are highly dynamic surveillants of brain parenchyma in vivo. *Science* 2005;308:1314–1318.

16. Vilhardt F. Microglia: phagocyte and glia cell. *Int J Biochem Cell Biol.* 2005;37:17–21.

17. Gao HM, Hong JS, Zhang W, et al. Distinct role for microglia in rotenone-induced degeneration of dopaminergic neurons. *J Neurosci.* 2002;22:782–790.

18. Dale RC, Candler PM, Church AJ, et al. Neuronal surface glycolytic enzymes are autoantigen targets in post-streptococcal autoimmune CNS disease. *J Neuroimmunol.* 2005, Dec. 11 [Epub ahead of print].

19. Giovannoni G. Anti-neuronal antibodies and movement disorders. *J Neuroimmunol.* 2005;163:5–7.

20. Cardoso F, Eduardo C, Silva AP, et al. Chorea in fifty consecutive patients with rheumatic fever. *Mov Disord.* 1997;12:701–703.

21. Vidakovic A, Dragasevic N, Kostic VS. Hemiballism: report of 25 cases. *J Neurol Neurosurg Psychiatry.* 1994;57:945–949.

22. Freeman JM, Aron AM, Collard JE, et al. The emotional correlates of Sydenham's chorea. *Pediatrics* 1965;35:42–49.

23. Swedo SE, Leonard HL, Schapiro MB, et al. Sydenham's chorea: physical and psychological symptoms of St Vitus dance. *Pediatrics* 1993;91:706–713.

24. Mercadante MT, Campos MC, Marques-Dias MJ, et al. Vocal tics in Sydenham's chorea. *J Am Acad Child Adolesc Psychiatry.* 1997;36:305–306.

25. Stollerman GH. Rheumatic fever. *Lancet* 1997;349: 935–942.

26. Cardoso F, Vargas AP, Oliveira LD, et al. Persistent Sydenham's chorea. *Mov Disord.* 1999;14:805–807.

27. Swedo SE, Rapoport JL, Cheslow DL, et al. High prevalence of obsessive-compulsive symptoms in patients with Sydenham's chorea. *Am J Psychiatry.* 1989;146:246–249.

28. Korn-Lubetzki I, Brand A, Steiner I. Recurrence of Sydenham chorea: implications for pathogenesis. *Arch Neurol.* 2004;61:1261–1264.

29. Nausieda PA, Grossman BJ, Koller WC, et al. Sydenham chorea: an update. *Neurology* 1980;30:331–334.

30. Taranta A. Relation of isolated recurrences of Sydenham's chorea to preceding streptococcal infections. *N Engl J Med.* 1959;260:1204–1210.

31. Berrios X, Quesney F, Morales A, et al. Are all recurrences of "pure" Sydenham chorea true recurrences of acute rheumatic fever? *J Pediatr.* 1985;107:867–872.

32. Bright R. Cases of spasmodic disease accompanying affections of the pericardium. *Medico-Chirurgical Transactions* 1838;22:1–19.

33. Schwartzman JD, McDonald DH. Sydenham's chorea: report of 140 cases and review of the recent literature. *Arch Pediatr.* 1948;65:6–24.

34. Comrie JD. *Selected Works of Thomas Syndenham*, New York: Willam Wood and Co., 1922.

35. Marie P, Tretiakoff C. Histology of acute chorea of Sydenham. *Rev Neurol.* 1920;36:428.

36. Greenfield JG, Wolfsohn JM. The pathology of Sydenham's chorea. *Lancet* 1922;2:603–606

37. Colony HS, Malamud N. Sydenham's chorea. A clinicopathologic study. *Neurology* 1956;6:672–676.

38. Giedd JN, Rapoport JL, Kruesi MJ, et al. Sydenham's chorea: magnetic resonance imaging of the basal ganglia. *Neurology* 1995;45:2199–2202.

39. Zabriskie JB, Lavenchy D, Williams RC Jr, et al. Rheumatic fever-associated B cell alloantigens as identified by monoclonal antibodies. *Arthritis Rheum.* 1985; 28(9):1047–1051.

40. Kemeny E, Husby G, Williams RC Jr., et al. Tissue distribution of antigen(s) defined by monoclonal antibody D8/17 reacting with B lymphocytes of patients with rheumatic heart disease. *Clin Immunol Immunopathol.* 1994;72:35–43.

41. Murphy TK, Goodman WK, Fudge MW, et al. B lymphocyte antigen D8/17: a peripheral marker for childhood-onset obsessive-compulsive disorder and Tourette's syndrome? *Am J Psychiatry.* 1997;154:402–407.

42. Swedo SE, Leonard HL, Mittleman BB, et al. Identification of children with pediatric autoimmune neuropsychiatric disorders associated with streptococcal infections by a marker associated with rheumatic fever. *Am J Psychiatry.* 1997;154:110–112.

43. Bronze MS, Dale JB. Epitopes of streptococcal M proteins that evoke antibodies that cross-react with human brain. *J Immunol.* 1993;151:2820–2828.

44. Cardoso F, Maia D, Cunningham MC, et al. Treatment of Sydenham chorea with corticosteroids. *Mov Disord.* 2003;18:1374–1377.

45. Garvey MA, Swedo SE. Sydenham's chorea. Clinical and therapeutic update. *Adv Exp Med Biol.* 1997;418: 115–120.

46. Barash J, Margalith D, Matitiau A. Corticosteroid treatment in patients with Sydenham's chorea. *Pediatr Neurol.* 2005;32:205–207.

47. Husby G, van de Rijn I, Zabriskie JB, et al. Antibodies reacting with cytoplasm of subthalamic and caudate nuclei neurons in chorea and acute rheumatic fever. *J Exp Med.* 1976;144:1094–1110.

48. Church AJ, Cardoso F, Dale RC, et al. Anti-basal ganglia antibodies in acute and persistent Sydenham's chorea. *Neurology* 2002;59:227–231.

49. Singer HS, Loiselle CR, Lee O, et al. Anti-basal ganglia antibody abnormalities in Sydenham chorea. *J Neuroimmunol.* 2003;136:154–161.

50. Dale RC, Church AJ, Cardoso F, et al. Poststreptococcal acute disseminated encephalomyelitis with basal ganglia involvement and auto-reactive antibasal ganglia antibodies. *Ann Neurol.* 2001;50:588–595.

51. Church AJ, Dale RC, Cardoso F, et al. CSF and serum immune parameters in Sydenham's chorea: evidence of an autoimmune syndrome? *J Neuroimmunol.* 2003; 136:149–153.

52. Kirvan CA, Swedo SE, Heuser JS, et al. Mimicry and autoantibody-mediated neuronal cell signaling in Sydenham chorea. *Nat Med.* 2003;9:914–920.

53. Loiselle CR, Lee O, Moran TH, et al. Striatal microinfusion of Tourette syndrome and PANDAS sera: Failure to induce behavioral changes. *Mov Disord.* 2004; 19:390–396.

54. Donadi EA, Smith AG, Louzada-Junior P, et al. HLA class I and class II profiles of patients presenting with Sydenham's chorea. *J Neurol.* 2000;247:122–128.

55. Voss LM, Wilson NJ, Neutze JM, et al. Intravenous immunoglobulin in acute rheumatic fever: a randomized controlled trial. *Circulation* 2001;103:401–406.

56. Selling L. The role of infection in the etiology of tics. *Arch Neurol Psychiatry.* 1929;22:1163–1171.

57. Brown EE. Tics (habit spasms) secondary to sinusitis. *Arch Pediatr.* 1957;74:39–46.

58. Kondo K, Kabasawa T, Greenberg BD, et al. Improvement in Gilles de la Tourette syndrome after corticosteroid therapy Symptom exacerbation of vocal tics and other symptoms associated with streptococcal pharyngitis in a patient with obsessive-compulsive disorder and tics Lyme disease presenting as Tourette's syndrome Tourette's syndrome and mycoplasma pneumoniae infection. *Ann Neurol.* 1978;4:387.

59. Kiessling LS. Tic disorders associated with evidence of invasive group A beta hemolytic streptococcal disease, abstracted. *Dev Med Child Neurol.* 1989; 31(suppl 59):48.

60. Muller N, Riedel M, Straube A, et al. Increased anti-streptococcal antibodies in patients with Tourette's syndrome. *Psychiatry Res.* 2000;94:43–49.

61. Muller N, Kroll B, Schwarz MJ, et al. Increased titers of antibodies against streptococcal M12 and M19 proteins in patients with Tourette's syndrome. *Psychiatry Res.* 2001;101:187–193.

62. Loiselle CR, Wendlandt JT, Rohde CA, et al. Antistreptococcal, neuronal, and nuclear antibodies in Tourette syndrome. *Pediatr Neurol.* 2003;28:119–125.

63. Peterson BS, Leckman JF, Tucker D, et al. Preliminary findings of antistreptococcal antibody titers and basal ganglia volumes in tic, obsessive-compulsive, and attention deficit/hyperactivity disorders. *Arch Gen Psychiatry.* 2000;57:364–372.

64. Church AJ, Dale RC, Lees AJ, et al. Tourette's syndrome: a cross sectional study to examine the PANDAS hypothesis. *J Neurol Neurosurg Psychiatry.* 2003;74:602–607.

65. Martino D, Church A, Dale R, et al. Anti-basal ganglia antibodies and Tourette syndrome: a phenotype analysis. *Mov Disord.* 2005;20 (suppl 10):S165.

66. Wendlandt JT, Grus FH, Hansen BH, et al. Striatal antibodies in children with Tourette's syndrome: multivariate discriminant analysis of IgG repertoires. *J Neuroimmunol.* 2001;119:106–113.

67. Taylor JR, Morshed SA, Parveen S, et al. An animal model of Tourette's syndrome. *Am J Psychiatry.* 2002; 159:657–660.

68. Hallett JJ, Harling-berg CJ, Knopf PM, et al. Antistriatal antibodies in Tourette syndrome cause neuronal dysfunction. *J Neuroimmunol.* 2000;111:195–202.

69. Leckman JF, Katsovich L, Kawikova I, et al. Increased serum levels of interleukin-12 and tumor necrosis factor-alpha in Tourette's syndrome. *Biol Psychiatry.* 2005;57:667–673.

70. Zimmerman AW, Jynouchi H, Comi AM, et al. Cerebrospinal fluid and serum markers of inflammation in autism. *Pediatr Neurol.* 2005;33:195–201.

71. Swedo SE, Leonard HL, Garvey M, et al. Pediatric autoimmune neuropsychiatric disorders associated with streptococcal infections: clinical description of the first 50 cases. *Am J Psychiatry.* 1998;155:264–271.

72. Swedo SE, Leonard HL, Rapoport JL. The pediatric autoimmune neuropsychiatric disorders associated with streptococcal infection (PANDAS) subgroup: separating fact from fiction. *Pediatrics* 2004;113:907–911.

73. Kurlan R, Kaplan EL. The pediatric autoimmune neuropsychiatric disorders associated with streptococcal infection (PANDAS) etiology for tics and obsessive-compulsive symptoms: hypothesis or entity? Practical considerations for the clinician. *Pediatrics* 2004; 113:883–886.

74. Singer HS, Loiselle C. PANDAS: a commentary. *J Psychosom Res.* 2003;55:31–39.

75. Singer HS. [PANDAS—Pediatric autoimmune neuropsychiatric disorders associated with streptococcal infection: is it a specific clinical disorder?]. *Rev Bras Psiquiatr.* 2004;26:220,221.

76. Snider LA, Swedo SE. Post-streptococcal autoimmune disorders of the central nervous system. *Curr Opin Neurol.* 2003;16:359–365.

77. Murphy ML, Pichichero ME. Prospective identification and treatment of children with pediatric autoimmune neuropsychiatric disorder associated with group A streptococcal infection (PANDAS). *Arch Pediatr Adolesc Med.* 2002;156:356–361.

78. Lougee L, Perlmutter SJ, Nicolson R, et al. Psychiatric disorders in first-degree relatives of children with pediatric autoimmune neuropsychiatric disorders associated with streptococcal infections (PANDAS). *J Am Acad Child Adolesc Psychiatry.* 2000;39:1120–1126.

79. Giedd JN, Rapoport JL, Garvey MA, et al. MRI assessment of children with obsessive-compulsive disorder or tics associated with streptococcal infection. *Am J Psychiatry.* 2000;157:281–283.

80. Singer HS, Giuliano JD, Zimmerman AM, et al. Infection: a stimulus for tic disorders. *Pediatr Neurol.* 2000;22:380–383.

81. Garvey MA, Perlmutter SJ, Allen AJ, et al. A pilot study of penicillin prophylaxis for neuropsychiatric exacerbations

triggered by streptococcal infections. *Biol Psychiatry*. 1999;45:1564–1571.

82. Perrin EM, Murphy ML, Casey JR, et al. Does group A beta-hemolytic streptococcal infection increase risk for behavioral and neuropsychiatric symptoms in children? *Arch Pediatr Adolesc Med*. 2004;158:848–856.

83. Luo F, Leckman JF, Katsovich L, et al. Prospective longitudinal study of children with tic disorders and/or obsessive-compulsive disorder: relationship of symptom exacerbations to newly acquired streptococcal infections. *Pediatrics* 2004;113:E578–585.

84. Snider LA, Lougee L, Slattery M, et al. Antibiotic prophylaxis with azithromycin or penicillin for childhood-onset neuropsychiatric disorders. *Biol Psychiatry*. 2005;57:788–792.

85. Perlmutter SJ, Leitman SF, Garvey MA, et al. Therapeutic plasma exchange and intravenous immunoglobulin for obsessive-compulsive disorder and tic disorders in childhood. *Lancet* 1999;354:1153–1158.

86. Singer HS, Loiselle CR, Lee O, et al. Anti-basal ganglia antibodies in PANDAS. *Mov Disord*. 2004;19:406–415.

87. Singer HS, Hong JJ, Yoon DY, et al. Serum autoantibodies do not differentiate PANDAS and Tourette syndrome from controls. *Neurology* 2005;65:1701–1707.

88. Church AJ, Dale RC, Giovannoni G. Anti-basal ganglia antibodies: a possible diagnostic utility in idiopathic movement disorders? *Arch Dis Child*. 2004;89:611–614.

89. Bornstein NM, Aronovich B, Korczyn AD, et al. Antibodies to brain antigens following stroke. *Neurology* 2001;56:529,530.

90. Plato, *The Republic*, 1991. Dent/Everyman, translated by A.D. Lindsay.

17

PANDAS: To Treat or Not to Treat?

Robert A. King

Tourette's/OCD Clinic, Yale Child Study Center, New Haven, Connecticut

The validity of the pediatric autoimmune neuro-psychiatric disorders associated with strepto-coccal infection (PANDAS) concept remains controversial as does its relative prevalence, potential pathogenic mechanisms, and appropriate diagnostic criteria (1–3). In addition to these uncertainties, the inherently longitudinal nature of the core PANDAS criteria presents the clinician with significant practical challenges concerning treatment.

The working research criteria proposed by Swedo et al. (1,4) characterize PANDAS as: A) cases of obsessive compulsive disorder (OCD) and/or tic disorder, B) with prepubertal onset; C) a history of sudden, severe symptom onset and an episodic course characterized by remissions and abrupt exacerbations; D) evidence that the onset or exacerbation of symptoms is "temporally related" to group A beta-hemolytic streptococcus (GABHS) infection; and E) adventitious movements or clumsiness. Using these criteria to confirm or disconfirm a potential PANDAS diagnosis is difficult in many individual cases, especially early in the course of illness.

AMBIGUITY AND POTENTIAL NONSPECIFICITY OF THE "TEMPORAL ASSOCIATION" PANDAS CRITERIA

The first difficulty encountered is that the criterion of "temporal association" between symptom onset and GABHS infection is ambiguous. Based on the observation that Sydenham chorea can occur 3 to 6 months after a streptococcal infection, Swedo et al. (4) specified a time window of 12 weeks between infection and symptom onset for their PANDAS criteria, with a more stringent limit of no more than 7 to 14 days between infection and exacerbation, which Swedo et al. (1) note "usually occur simultaneously."

A second and more intractable difficulty in identifying PANDAS cases is that the PANDAS diagnosis can only be established *over time*, on the basis of an episodic course characterized by remissions and abrupt exacerbations that are also temporally related to GABHS infection. In other words, the PANDAS diagnosis can only be determined on the basis of longitudinal history. In the clinical experience of the author of this chapter, in most established cases of tic disorder or OCD it is very difficult to establish retrospectively a definite temporal relationship between exacerbations and GABHS infection.

Furthermore, given the current absence of any reliable biological marker for PANDAS, it is impossible to tell in the short run in any individual *new* case of Tourette syndrome (TS) or OCD whether the connection between a streptococcal infection and an acute onset (or exacerbation) of symptoms is causal or merely coincidental. GABHS pharyngitis and carrier states are very common in the general school-age population (5). Given prevalence estimates of 1% to 3% for childhood OCD (6) and up to 10% to 25% for transient motor tics in early school-age children (7), many children will experience the co-occurrence of GABHS infection and tic/OCD symptom onset purely by coincidence. Furthermore, like other stressors, GABHS (and other febrile illnesses) may exacerbate pre-existing tics or obsessive-compulsive symptoms in a non-specific manner.

A recent prospective study from our group at Yale (8) illustrates this dilemma. A group of 47 children with TS or OCD and 19 healthy controls, all age 7 to 17 years were followed longitudinally with regular monitoring of tic/OCD symptom severity, streptococcus culture, and antibody titer status. Using empirically derived criteria for symptom exacerbation, the overall rate of tic/OCD exacerbations was 0.56 per patient per year. The average rate of new GABHS infection was 0.42 per subject per year. However, the temporal association between tic/obsessive-compulsive symptom exacerbation and new GABHS infection was no greater than expected by chance. Although these findings do not preclude the existence of a small subgroup of PANDAS, they suggest that the symptom fluctuations in the majority of this unselected sample were not related to GABHS.

AMBIGUITY OF THE "NATURAL HISTORY" CRITERION

Swedo et al. (1,4) suggest natural history as another putative PANDAS criterion. They describe PANDAS as characterized by explosive "overnight" onset ("reaching maximal, clinically significant impairment in 24 to 48 hours") of severe symptoms or abrupt exacerbation, e.g., "simultaneous onset of (multiple) tics of such intensity and frequency that emergency treatment is often sought" (1). However, Singer et al. (9) noted that in a group of 80 consecutive unselected children with TS, the parents of 53% of the subjects described their child as having "sudden explosive onset or worsening of tic symptoms." Because even abrupt onset of tics/OCD with a positive throat culture may be coincidental, Swedo et al. (1) caution that "a single positive throat culture or elevated antibody titer is not sufficient to determine that a child's neuropsychiatric symptoms are associated with streptococcal infections.... Instead the determination that a child fits the PANDAS profile is made through prospective evaluation and documentation of streptococcal infections in conjunction with at least 2 episodes of

neuropsychiatric symptoms, as well as demonstrating negative throat culture or stable titers during times of ... symptom remission ..."

CURRENT ABSENCE OF BIOLOGICAL MARKERS FOR PANDAS

The absence of specific biological markers for PANDAS complicates diagnosis, especially at the onset of symptoms. Many lay people and even physicians mistakenly believe that elevated antistreptolysin O antibody or anti-streptococcal DNAase B antibody titers are "markers" for PANDAS. Elevation of these antibodies, however, indicates nothing more than that a child has had a streptococcal infection and mounted a normal immunologic response to it. There is *no* evidence that these antibodies play any pathogenic role in PANDAS or other autoimmune poststreptococcal disease or that they constitute a specific marker for PANDAS, rather than merely a garden-variety GABHS infection.

THE ROLE OF ANTIBIOTICS

What is the clinician to do when confronted with a child with a positive GABHS throat culture and sudden onset of tics or OCD? To minimize the risk of rheumatic fever, infectious disease guidelines (10) clearly mandate a 10-day course of antibiotic treatment, irrespective of tic or OCD symptoms. A more difficult decision is called for in children who have had a recent onset of tics or OCD and are found to have a positive GABHS throat culture but no history recent of pharyngitis or antibody elevation. As many as 10% of children may be such asymptomatic carriers, often for many weeks. Although there is debate as to whether asymptomatic streptococcus carriers in the general pediatric population require antibiotic treatment, treatment is probably advisable if there has been a recent onset or change in tic/OCD symptoms.

Long-term prophylactic antibiotic treatment should be reserved for only those children with a longitudinal course clearly compatible with PANDAS. The hazard of fostering antibiotic resistance is a serious one, as many communities have seen the explosive emergence of erythro-mycin-resistant strains of GABHS in recent years (11). Low levels of adherence to antibiotic treatment, even in children prescribed 10-day courses for acute streptococcus pharyngitis (12), underline the practical problems of adherence to longer-term prophylactic regimens. An initial National Institute of Mental Health (NIMH) placebo-controlled cross-over study of penicillin prophylaxis failed to find significant differences between active treatment and placebo (13). In addition to other methodologic limitations of this study, the rate of GABHS in the penicillin prophylaxis group was 38% versus 54% in the placebo group, suggesting that missed doses of the short-acting antibiotic permitted streptococcal infection even in what was supposed to be the active treatment group. Although longer-acting intramuscular benzathine penicillin eliminates the problem of missed doses, 3% to 6% of patients receiving long-term benzathine penicillin G for rheumatic fever prophylaxis develop penicillin allergy (14). In addition, 30% to 50% of patients receiving benzathine penicillin G have moderately to severely painful local reactions (15). A second-generation NIMH trial is currently underway comparing placebo with prophylaxis with azithromycin, a long-acting macrolide that need be given only once a day.

IMMUNOMODULATORY INTERVENTIONS

The apparently promising results of the small NIMH trial of plasmapheresis (PEX) and intravenous immunoglobulin (IVIG) in children meeting PANDAS criteria (16) has led many parents to seek out these treatments for their children. (A long-term follow-up study of the subjects from the NIMH trial is now underway [Swedo, personal communication]). However, PEX was *not* helpful for a group of somewhat older (and perhaps more chronic) children with tic/OCD who did *not* meet the PANDAS criteria (17). Similarly, a study of 30 unselected tic disorder patients (mean age 28.71, range 14–53), randomized to placebo or IVIG, found no differences between the

two groups in terms of improvement in tic severity scores (18).

These interventions are not without their hazards. PEX usually requires central venous line placement, with all its attendant hazards. In the NIMH trial, PEX was well-tolerated, with the principal side effects being pallor, dizziness, nausea, or vomiting, all limited to the duration of procedure. In large series of adult patients treated with PEX for various disorders, adverse event rates run 3% to 25% (with severe reactions occurring in 0.5% to 3.1% of procedures) and include complications of venous access (sepsis, hemorrhage), alteration of clotting factors, hypotension, and fluid imbalance (19–21). Given their small intravascular volume, children may be even more prone to hypotension and fluid imbalance when treated with PEX.

Perhaps contrary to initial expectations, Perlmutter et al. (16) found that children tolerated IVIG more poorly than they did PEX, with six of nine children receiving IVIG having mild-moderate adverse effects (nausea and vomiting; headache; and low-grade fever) that persisted for 12 to 24 hrs.

Because of the uncertainties surrounding immunomodulatory treatments in children with apparent PANDAS, these interventions should be used only in the context of properly reviewed research protocols. The NIMH Intramural Program study of these treatments is no longer active, and the author of this chapter is unaware of any active clinical trials of these treatments.

UNRESOLVED ISSUES OF PATHOGENESIS AND POTENTIAL THERAPEUTIC ACTION

It is often presumed that the pathogenesis of PANDAS probably involves auto-immune antibodies triggered by GABHS that cross-react with basal ganglia tissues on the basis of "molecular mimicry" (21,22). However, a host of other processes may theoretically be at work, including an altered balance of inflammatory and anti-inflammatory cytokines and chemokines; superantigens; skewing of lymphocyte subpopulations; and other forms of immune dysregulation, such as are found at work in other

GABHS-related disorders, (e.g., guttate psoriasis [23]). Similarly, it is often assumed that PEX and IVIG work by washing out presumed pathogenic auto-antibodies or modulating their production. Here too, however, numerous other ameliorative processes may be at work. For example, in addition to removing pathogenic auto-antibodies, PEX may A) remove other pathogenic circulating factors such as immune complexes, inflammatory mediators, and cytokines; B) enhance immunoregulation and splenic functioning; C) and influence the profile of T-cell subsets (24). In addition to modulating antibody production, IVIG may interfere with co-stimulatory molecules; inhibit complement activation and membrane attack complex formation; modulate the balance of inflammatory and anti-inflammatory cytokines and chemokines; and modulate macrophage Fc receptors (25). Hence, even if replicated, the efficacy of IVIG or PEX for PANDAS would still leave open the pathogenic and therapeutic mechanisms involved, as well as the indications and counter-indications for these treatments.

Other, less well-studied, potential immunomodulatory interventions for PANDAS exist. Some, such as omega-3 fatty acid (fish oil) supplementation, currently the subject of an ongoing trial by Gabbay et al., (26) for children with TS, are probably benign. Others, such as monoclonal antibodies have proven effective in other pediatric autoimmune illnesses (27,28), e.g., juvenile rheumatoid arthritis and inflammatory bowel disease, but have potentially severe side effects (29), including anergy, lymphoma, and reactivation of tuberculosis.

CONCLUSION

While awaiting greater clarity concerning the role of streptococcal infection in tic and OCD, the clinician must deal in the here-and-now with the exigencies of patients and families seeking treatment. Despite the uncertainties reviewed here, the prudent clinician will: A) obtain throat cultures of children with abrupt onset or dramatic exacerbation of tic/OC symptoms and B) treat positive GABHS cultures with the standard antibiotic regimens. Beyond these two

clear mandates, the clinician will have to A) use clinical judgment in more chronic cases and consider antibiotic prophylaxis in those cases with a clear longitudinal course of recurrent abrupt exacerbations linked to GABHS as well as B) reserve immunomodulatory treatments for only those cases meeting the PANDAS criteria and unresponsive to standard treatments.

ACKNOWLEDGMENT

This work was supported by the Tourette's Syndrome Association and National Institutes of Health grants MH61940 and MH493515.

REFERENCES

1. Swedo SE, Leonard HL, Rapoport JL. The pediatric autoimmune neuropsychiatric disorders associated with streptococcal infection (PANDAS) subgroup: separating fact from fiction. *Pediatrics* 2004;113:907–911.
2. Kurlan R, Kaplan EL. The pediatric autoimmune neuropsychiatric disorders associated with streptococcal infection (PANDAS) etiology for tics and obsessive-compulsive symptoms: hypothesis or entity? Practical considerations for the clinician. *Pediatrics* 2004;113:883–886.
3. March JS. Pediatric autoimmune neuropsychiatric disorders associated with streptococcal infection (PANDAS): implications for clinical practice. *Arch Pediatr Adolesc Med.* 2004;158:927–929.
4. Swedo SE, Leonard HL, Garvey M, et al. Pediatric autoimmune neuropsychiatric disorders associated with streptococcal infections: clinical description of the first 50 cases. *Am J Psychiatry.* 1998;155:264–271.
5. Shulman ST. Streptococcal pharyngitis: clinical and epidemiologic factors. *Pediatr Infect Dis J.* 1989;8:816–819.
6. Zohar AH. The epidemiology of obsessive-compulsive disorder in children and adolescents. *Child Adolesc Psychiatr Clin N Am.* 1999;8:445–460.
7. Snider LA, Seligman LD, Ketchen BR, et al. Tics and problem behaviors in schoolchildren: prevalence, characterization, and associations. *Pediatrics* 2002;110:331–336.
8. Luo F, Leckman JF, Katsovich L, et al. Prospective longitudinal study of children with tic disorders and/or obsessive-compulsive disorder: relationship of symptom exacerbations to newly acquired streptococcal infections. *Pediatrics* 2004;113:E578–E585.
9. Singer HS, Loiselle C. PANDAS: a commentary. *J Psychosom Res* 2003;55:31–39.
10. American Academy of Pediatrics, Group A streptococcal infections. In: Pickering LK ed. *2003 Red Book Report of the Committee on Infectious Diseases*, 26th ed., Elk Grove, IL: American Academy of Pediatrics; 2003.
11. Green M, Martin JM, Barbadora KA, et al. Reemergence of macrolide resistance in pharyngeal isolates of Group A Streptococci in Southwestern Pennsylvania. *Antimicrob Agents Chemother.* 2004;48:473–476.

12. Dajani AS. Adherence to physicians' instructions as a factor in managing streptococcal pharyngitis. *Pediatrics* 1996;97:976–980.

13. Garvey MA, Perlmutter SJ, Allen AJ, et al. A pilot study of penicillin prophylaxis for neuropsychiatric exacerbations triggered by streptococcal infections. *Biol Psychiatry.* 1999;45:1564–1571.

14. Markowitz M, Lue HC. Allergic reactions in rheumatic fever patients on long-term benzathine penicillin G: the role of skin testing for penicillin allergy. *Pediatrics* 1996;97:981–983.

15. Bass JW. A review of the rationale and advantages of various mixtures of benzathine penicillin G. *Pediatrics* 1996;97:960–963.

16. Perlmutter SJ, Leitman SF, Garvey MA, et al. Therapeutic plasma exchange and intravenous immunoglobulin for obsessive-compulsive disorder and tic disorders in childhood. *Lancet* 1999;354:1153–1158.

17. Nicolson R, Swedo SE, Lenane M, et al. An open trial of plasma exchange in childhood-onset obsessive-compulsive disorder without poststreptococcal exacerbations. *J Am Acad Child Adolesc Psychiatry.* 2000;39:1313–1315.

18. Hoekstra PJ, Minderaa RB, Kallenberg CG. Lack of effect of intravenous immunoglobulins on tics: a double-blind placebo-controlled study. *J Clin Psychiatry.* 2004; 65:537–542.

19. Madore F. Plasmapheresis: technical aspects and indications. *Crit Care Clin.* 2002;18:375–392.

20. Mokrzycki MH, Kaplan AA. Therapeutic plasma exchange: complications and management. *Am J Kidney Dis.* 1994;23:817–827.

21. Norda R, Stegmayr BG. Swedish Apheresis Group. Therapeutic apheresis in Sweden: update of epidemiology and adverse events. *Transfus Apher Sci.* 2003;29:159–166.

21. Swedo SE. Genetics of childhood disorders: XXXIII. Autoimmunity, part 6: poststreptococcal autoimmunity. *J Am Acad Child Adolesc Psychiatry.* 2001;40: 1479–1482.

22. Kirvan CA, Swedo SE, Heuser JS, et al. Mimicry and autoantibody-mediated neuronal cell signaling in Sydenham chorea. *Nat Med.* 2003;9:914–920.

23. Leung DYM, Travers JB, Giorno R, et al. Evidence for a streptococcal superantigen-driven process in acute guttate psoriasis. *J Clin Invest.* 1995;96:2106–2112.

24. Braun-Moscovici Y, Furst DE. Plasmapheresis for rheumatic diseases in the twenty-first century: take it or leave it. *Curr Opin Rheumatol.* 2003;15:197–204.

25. Dalakas MC. Intravenous immunoglobulin in autoimmune neuromuscular diseases. *JAMA.* 2004;291: 2367–2375.

26. Gabbay V, Coffey B, Castellanos F, et al. The Efficacy of Fish Oil in Children with Tourette's Disorder. Poster presented at: American Academy of Child and Adolescent Psychiatry Annual Meeting; 2004; Miami Beach, FL.

27. Olsen NJ, Stein CM. New drugs for rheumatoid arthritis. *N Engl J Med.* 2004;350:2167–2179.

28. Schwartz RS. Shattuck lecture: diversity of the immune repertoire and immunoregulation. *N Engl J Med.* 2003; 348:1017–1026.

29. Keane J, Gershon S, Wise RP, et al. Tuberculosis associated with infliximab, a tumor necrosis factor (alpha)-neutralizing agent. *N Engl J Med.* 2001;345: 1098–1104.

30. Kurlan R. The PANDAS hypothesis: losing its bite? *Mov Disord.* 2004;19:371–374.

31. Snider LA. Swedo SE. Post-streptococcal autoimmune disorders of the central nervous system. *Curr Opin Neurol.* 2003;16:359–365.

18

Disruptive Behavior Problems in a Community Sample of Children with Tic Disorders

Lawrence Scahill,[1] Susan Williams,[1] Mary Schwab-Stone,[1] Judy Applegate,[2] James F. Leckman[1]

[1]*Yale Child Study Center, Yale University School of Medicine, New Haven, Connecticut;*
[2]*Yale University, School of Nursing, New Haven.*

Tic disorders are neurologic conditions of childhood onset characterized by abnormal movements (motor tics) and/or vocalizations (vocal tics). Tic disorders are defined by the type and duration of the tic symptoms. For example, transient tic disorder is defined by the presence of tic symptoms that do not persist for a full year. When either motor or vocal tics are present for more than 1 year, the child is diagnosed with chronic motor tic disorder or chronic vocal tic disorder. Tourette syndrome (TS) is defined by the presence of motor and vocal tics that persist for more than 1 year. Follow-up studies in clinical samples show that tics often peak between 10 and 12 years of age followed by a gradual decline by age 18 years (1). Thus, from a public health perspective, knowing accurately the prevalence of tic disorders and level of associated disability in school-age children (ages 6 to 12 years) would be most informative for planning health services and secondary prevention strategies.

Tics are relatively common, affecting 12% to 24% of school-age children (2,3). For most of these children, however, the tics are isolated (consisting only of a single tic) and transitory. The prevalence of multiple and enduring tics ranges from 4% to 6% (3–6). Traditionally, the prevalence of TS has been viewed as rare disorder in the range of 1 per 2,000 (7–8). More recent studies have used community sampling methods and better methods of assessment. Current estimates derived from the largest available community-based suggest that the prevalence of TS in school-age children is between 1 and 11 per 1000 (4–6,9–10). The purpose of the current study is to estimate the prevalence of tic disorders and to examine the clinical characteristics in a community sample of young school age children.

METHODS

This assessment of tic disorders was part of a two-stage mental health needs assessment completed in 1991 in the State of Connecticut (12–14). In the first stage survey, parents were asked to complete the Child Behavior Checklist (CBCL) and teachers were asked to complete the companion Teacher's Report Form (TRF). In addition, parents and teachers were also asked to comment on whether the child "needed help" for emotional or behavioral problems. A positive screen was defined both quantitatively and qualitatively. Using norms from Achenbach & Edelbrock (15), the quantitative criterion was the 90th percentile on the CBCL or the TRF. The qualitative criterion was an indication by a parent or teacher that the child "needs help" for a behavioral or emotional problem. The first stage sample consisted of 910 children who were randomly selected from classroom rosters in 83 public and private schools from 25 rural and semi-rural communities in eastern

Connecticut. Written informed consent was obtained from a parent for all 910 children. All screen positive cases ($N = 460$) and a 20% random sample ($N = 115$) of the screen negatives were invited to participate in the second stage (total, $N = 575$).

The second stage sample consisted of 449 children (241 boys and 208 girls) who were between the ages of 6 and 12 years (mean 9.2 ± 1.78). Of these 449 children, 359 screened positive at the first stage and 90 were screen negative (response rate was 78% for both screen positives and screen negatives). The 449 subjects recruited for the second stage children were systematically assessed for psychiatric disorders and mental health service utilization.

Procedures

The *Diagnostic Interview Schedule for Children-Revised* (DISC-R) was administered to the parents of the 449 children. The reliability and validity of the DISC-R are well established (13,16). The interview, which was keyed to DSM-III-R, provides a systematic method of collecting data about the full range of child psychiatric disorders including tic disorders (17). Each disorder was surveyed with a set of initial queries. If the initial queries were negative, the interviewer moved on to the next section. If the opening questions were positive, the interviewer was guided by the DISC-R to elicit a fuller description of the symptoms for that disorder and to identify impairment in school, home or with friends. Parents were also asked whether they sought treatment for their child's symptoms.

Conners Teacher and Conners Parent Questionnaires

Since their introduction more than three decades ago (18), these rating scales have been used in numerous clinical and epidemiological studies. The 48-item Conners Parent Questionnaire (CPQ) yields several scores including five factor scores and the 10-item Hyperactivity Index, which is often used as a dimensional measure of attention deficit hyperactivity disorder

(ADHD). The Conners Teacher Questionnaire (CTQ) is a 28-item questionnaire that consists of three statistically-derived factors, as well as the same 10-item Hyperactivity Index in the CPQ (19–21).

Family Assessment Device

The General Functioning Scale of the Family Assessment Device is a 12-item self-report measure of family functioning (22,23). Scale items are scored from 1 to 4 (strongly agree to strongly disagree), a score of 27 on this scale is often used as a cutoff for family dysfunction (12,24).

Diagnostic Determination and Group Definition

For most axis I diagnoses (e.g., ADHD, major depression, overanxious disorder, separation anxiety disorder, conduct disorder, and oppositional defiant disorder), diagnostic determinations were made by computer algorithms. These computer algorithms consider the number of DSM-III-R symptoms and the impairment caused by those symptoms (13,16). Based on this algorithm, 200 of the 449 children in stage 2 were deemed free of a tic disorder or any psychiatric disorder, 89 children were classified as having ADHD (12).

The major advantage of the computer algorithm method is efficiency. However, for some childhood disorders, particularly those in which subclinical variants may be of interest, this method has potential drawbacks. Because the delineation of tic symptoms from idiosyncratic mannerisms of childhood can be a thorny problem, we used a combined approach of a computerized algorithm and case-by-case review of the actual interviews to make a best estimate diagnosis of tic disorders. The computer algorithm selected all children ($N = 58$) whose parent answered "yes" to any of the initial DISC-R probes about tics. The interviews included more detailed questions about the onset, duration, type, and frequency of tics as well as a written description of the reported abnormal movement or vocalization. A case-by-case review of all 58 interviews was then conducted. Using DSM-III-R criteria, two raters classified all 58 children into five diagnostic categories: no tic disorder, transient tic disorder, chronic motor tic disorder, chronic vocal tic disorder, or TS. Differences were resolved by consensus. Following the consensus conference, 32 subjects were identified as having a possible or definite tic disorder in a hierarchical fashion (e.g., a case of possible TS could be classified as definite chronic motor tic disorder if the presence of vocal tics was not clearly documented).

Contrast Groups

Definite cases with tic disorders ($N = 21$) were compared to a sample of 41 children with ADHD (50% of the children with ADHD who did not have tics) and 43 normal controls (randomly selected from the pool 200 children with no psychiatric diagnosis).

RESULTS

The independent review of 58 cases by the two clinicians achieved an average Kappa coefficient of agreement between raters of .60, corresponding with good agreement. Following the consensus discussion: 26 children did not have a tic disorder; 11 youngsters were identified as having a possible tic disorder only and were excluded from further analyses. Twenty-one were diagnosed with a probable or definite tic disorder ($N = 21$). Of the 21 children: three children met definite criteria for TS; 11 with probable or definite chronic motor or chronic vocal tic disorder; and seven with probable or definite transient tic disorder. Table 18-1 provides a conservative estimate of prevalence for TS and other tic disorders in that it assumes no missed cases among the screen negatives.

Eight of the 21 (38%) children with a tic disorder also met criteria for ADHD. Table 18-2 compares demographic characteristics as well as service utilization and family functioning across the diagnostic groups compared to unaffected controls. These data suggest, not surprisingly, that ADHD is more common in boys compared to controls (chi = 7.35; $P = 0.007$; odds

TABLE 18-1. *Frequency of tic disorders in community sample of 910 children**

Diagnosis	N (%)	Prevalence per 1000
Definite TS	3 (0.33)	3
Possible or probable TS	6 (0.66)	6
Chronic motor tic disorder	7 (0.77)	8
Chronic vocal tic disorder	4 (0.44)	4
Transient tic disorder	7 (0.77)	8
Total for all tic disorders	21 (2.31)	23

*Eleven children classified as possible tic disorder are not included. Possible or probable TS is *not* included in prevalence estimate for TS. Five of these subjects were placed in other categories (e.g., chronic motor or transient tic disorder) when they met probable or definite criteria for that diagnosis; one subject was classified as possible tic disorder due to incomplete information about the duration of tics. TS, Tourette syndrome.

ratio = 3.4 (95% confidence interval = 1.3 to 9.5). The percentage of boys with tic disorders was not significantly different from the percentage in controls (chi = 0.67; $P = 0.4$; odds ratio = 1.5 (95% confidence interval = 0.5 to 5.1). Similarly, compared with the control group, there was no difference in the percentage of boys within the subgroup with tic disorder and ADHD (chi = 0.35; $P = 0.4$; odds ratio = 1.6 (95% confidence interval = 0.3 to 9.7) or those with a tic disorder and no ADHD (chi = 0.44; $P = 0.5$; odds ratio = 1.5 (95% confidence interval = 0.4 to 6.5). This failure to observe significant differences in the percentage of boys with tic disorders compared to controls may be due to the small sample sizes.

As measured by the Peabody Picture Vocabulary Test (25), all four groups appeared to be functioning in the average range of intelligence. However, there were significant group differences on the analysis of variance ($F_{(3,95)} = 3.78$, $P < 0.05$). Post hoc analysis showed a difference between children with tic disorder without ADHD (mean Peabody Picture Vocabulary Test score = 92.3 ± 19.10) compared with the control group (mean Peabody Picture Vocabulary Test score = 110.9 ± 21.16).

The presence of ADHD was associated with mental health service use. Children with a tic disorder and ADHD were nine times more likely to use mental health services than

TABLE 18-2. *Demographic characteristics and service use across diagnostic groups and controls*

Domain	All	Tics	Tics plus	ADHD	Unaffected
	Tic N=21 *N* (%)	No ADHD N=13 *N* (%)	ADHD N=8 *N* (%)	No Tics N=46 *N* (%)	Controls N=45 *N* (%)
Males	13 (61.9)	8 (61.5)	5 (62.5)	36 (78.3)	23 (51.1)
PPVT	97.9 (20.61)	92.3 (21.10)	108.2 (16.53)	98.9 (21.11)	110.9 (19.16)
Standard scores					
Single mother	2 (9.5)	1 (7.7)	1 (12.5)	9 (19.6)	3 (6.7)
Welfare	1 (4.8)	0 (0)	1 (12.5)	3 (6.5)	0 (0)
Mental health					
Service use*	7 (33.3)	2 (15.4)	5 (62.5)	20 (43.5)	7 (15.5)
Family dysfunction	5 (25)	3 (23)	2 (25)	12 (26.1)	5 (11.1)

*Tics plus ADHD versus controls: chi = 8.6, *P* = .01; ADHD versus controls: chi = 8.5, *P* = .004.

ADHD, attention deficit hyperactivity disorder; Family Dysfunction, Family Assessment Device (FAD) global score >26 (usual cutoff for family dysfunction); PPVT, Peabody Picture Vocabulary Test; Single Mother, household headed by single mother; Welfare, family reported receiving public assistance.

controls (chi = 8.6, *P* = 0.01 by Fisher exact test; odds ratio = 9.05 (95% confidence interval = 1.4 to 65). Children with ADHD but no tic disorder were four times more likely to use mental health services than controls (chi = 8.5, *P* = 0.004; odds ratio = 4.2 (95% confidence interval = 1.4 to 12.8). There was no difference in the rate of mental health service use in any other pair-wise comparison. There were no significant differences across the groups in the other demographic characteristics: family headed by single mother (χ^2 = 3.35, ns), family on welfare (χ^2 = 4-75, ns), or family dysfunction (χ^2 = 3.00, ns).

CPQ scales are presented in Table 18-3. The pattern for externalizing subscales (conduct problems, hyperactivity/impulsive problems, and the hyperactivity index) is remarkably consistent. Children with tic disorders and no ADHD show parent ratings that are similar to unaffected controls. Children with tics plus ADHD have a pattern that is similar to those with ADHD without tics. The learning problem scale shows a slightly different pattern. Children with a tic disorder show higher scores than controls even in the absence of ADHD ($F_{(3, 107)}$ = 13.01, *P* <0.01; post hoc test tic disorder versus controls P <0.05).

Similarly, teacher responses suggest that in the absence of ADHD, children with tic disorders show few differences from unaffected controls. Using analysis of variance, group differences were observed on all CTQ scales (Table 18-4). Post hoc analyses showed that

the hyperactivity index for the tic-only group was indistinguishable from that of the controls: 4.8 ± 6.0 compared with 4.6 ± 4.64 (*P* >0.05), respectively. By contrast, the hyperactivity index for the tic disorder plus ADHD was significantly higher than the unaffected controls (8.4 ± 5.35 versus 4.60 ± 4.64) (*P* <0.05), and, although lower, was not statistically different from the ADHD group without tic disorders 12.62 ± 7.47) (*P* >0.05). On the conduct and impulsive scales children with tic disorders plus ADHD were more hyperactive, impulsive, and disruptive than those with a tic disorder only and than unaffected controls. The one exception to this pattern was the learning problems scale, which was higher in those with tic disorders with and without ADHD than the control group (*P* >0.05 on post hoc test).

DISCUSSION

In the present study, we observed a prevalence estimate of 2.3% for all tic disorders in a community sample of children between the age of 6 and 12 years of age. The prevalence of TS was estimated at three cases per 1000. These estimates are consistent with the study by Costello et al., (4) which reported a prevalence of 4.2% for all tic disorders and one per 1000 for TS. The upper bound of prevalence for TS, however, ranges from 11 per 1000 observed by Kadesjo and Gillberg (10) to 30 cases per 1000

TABLE 18-3. *Comparison of raw scores on Conner's parent questionnaire across diagnostic groups and controls*

	Subscale	All	Tics	Tics plus	ADHD	Unaffected
	Tics (N = 20)	No ADHD (N = 12)	ADHD (N = 8)	No tics (N = 46)	Controls (N = 45)	$F_{(3, 107)}$
Anxiety	1.50 (1.24)	1.67 (1.23)	1.25 (1.28)	1.04 (1.43)	0.71 (0.92)	2.18
Conduct disorder	4.10 (4.30)	2.67 (1.72)	6.25 (6.07)	6.46 (4.76)	3.24 (2.82)	6.57*
Hyperactivity index	8.85 (5.82)	6.67 (4.44)	12.13 (6.36)	11.28 (6.04)	4.18 (3.60)	17.24*
Impulsive/Hyperactive	4.15 (2.87)	2.75 (2.42)	6.25 (2.19)	6.07 (3.12)	2.80 (2.41)	13.68*
Learning problems	3.90 (2.73)	3.17 (1.99)	5.00 (3.42)	4.72 (2.99)	1.64 (1.69)	13.01*
Psychosomatic	1.55 (1.88)	1.50 (1.51)	1.63 (2.45)	1.07 (1.73)	0.69 (1.00)	1.55

*P <0.001
Post-hoc tests at alpha <0.05, using Tukey HSD procedure:
Conduct disorder: ADHD > tic-only group; ADHD > control
Hyperactivity index: Tic plus ADHD, ADHD group > control; ADHD group > tic-only group
Impulsive/Hyperactive: Tic plus ADHD, ADHD group > control; tic plus ADHD, ADHD group > tic-only group
Learning problems: Tic plus ADHD, ADHD group > control
ADHD, attention deficit hyperactivity disorder.

Table 18-4. *Comparison of raw scores on Conner's teacher questionnaire across diagnostic groups and controls*

	All	Tics	Tics plus	ADHD	Unaffected	
	Tics (N = 18)	No ADHD (N = 11)	ADHD (N = 7)	No Tics (N = 37)	Controls (N = 35)	$F_{3,86}$
Conduct disorder	2.83 (4.16)	2.18 (2.96)	3.86 (5.70)	7.00 (6.58)	3.11 (4.48)	4.07*
Hyperactivity index	6.22 (5.88)	4.82 (6.00)	8.43 (5.35)	12.62 (7.47)	4.60 (4.64)	11.42**
Impulsive/Hyperactive	4.06 (4.28)	2.55 (4.20)	6.43 (3.41)	8.35 (6.38)	2.91 (3.80)	8.27**
Learning problems	7.67 (6.93)	6.55 (7.59)	9.43 (5.83)	10.24 (5.83)	4.14 (4.14)	7.84**

*P <0.01; **P <0.001
Post-hoc tests at alpha <0.05, using Tukey HSD procedure:
Conduct disorder: ADHD > control
Hyperactivity index: ADHD > tic-only group, control
Impulsive/Hyperactive: ADHD > tic only, control
Learning problems: ADHD > control

reported by Mason et al. (26). Mason et al. (26) based their estimate on a small sample in a single school district and their finding has not been replicated in any subsequent study, suggesting that this estimate is untrustworthy. Several other surveys, however, provide good agreement in a much narrower range from six to eight per 1000 for TS (5,6,9,11). Thus, the prevalence of TS in the present study may be an underestimate.

Indeed, there are several reasons to support the notion that the estimate is conservative. First, the authors assumed no missed cases among nonparticipants or screen negatives, which is a potential source of error. Second, although trained interviewers directly observed the children, the interviewers did not receive extensive training on the recognition of tics.

Third, the sample was younger than the participants in the other studies and it is likely that the children in this sample had not passed through the peak age of risk for onset of tics or worse-ever tics (1). For example, the study classified six additional children as possible TS. This classification was often used when the subject did not meet the duration criterion. Given more time, perhaps some of these children would have become clear cases of TS.

When the tic disorder group was divided into those with ADHD and those without ADHD, those with a tic disorder plus ADHD were more likely to have used mental health services. Children with ADHD and no tics were also more likely to use mental health services than the nonpsychiatrically ill controls. In the absence of ADHD, however, children with tic disorders were not more likely to use mental health services than unaffected controls. Whether these children with tic disorder only were unrecognized as needing mental health services or whether such services were not indicated is not clear from this study. Indeed, as shown in Table 18-2, the presence of ADHD with or with a tic disorder did not guarantee that the child would be treatment. Thus, it seems likely that some children with tic disorders (such as those with ADHD) are unrecognized and untreated. Given the functional impairment associated with the combination of a tic disorder and ADHD, this lack of recognition is an important public health concern.

Across several scales on the CPQ and CTQ, the group with a tic disorder and no ADHD were similar to the control group and the tic disorder plus ADHD group was similar to the ADHD group. Taken together, the data from the CPQ and the CTQ suggest that, as observed in clinical samples, tic disorders plus ADHD commonly co-occur in community samples as well. Moreover, in the absence of ADHD, a tic disorder alone does not appear to be associated with disruptive behavior and functional impairment (27,28). Nonetheless, even in the absence of ADHD, parents and teachers identified children with tic disorders as having learning problems. This finding may be an artifact of this sample or it may suggest that the presence of tics carries with it some neurodevelopmental vulnerability.

Over the past two decades the estimated prevalence of TS in children has varied from 5 to 300 per 10,000 (29). From a health policy perspective, this level of imprecision is unsatisfactory as it provides insufficient guidance for allocation of resources and suggests fundamental disagreement about the boundaries of the condition. This range of estimates is almost certainly due to differences in sample ascertainment, assessment methods and diagnostic threshold. Using better sampling techniques, more systematic assessment methods and clearer diagnostic thresholds, several recent studies have narrowed the estimated prevalence of TS in children. The emerging consensus ranges from one to eleven per 1000, with several studies falling in an even tighter range

of three to eight per 1000. According to the most recent census data, there are 53 million children between the ages of 5 and 17 years in the United States (30), a prevalence of one per 1000 would result in an estimated 53,000 children with TS. By contrast, if the true estimate is 10 per 1000, that would increase the tally of TS cases to 530,000 (i.e., an additional 477,000 children). In the current sample, nearly 40% of the children with a tic disorder (TS, chronic tic disorder or transient tic disorder) also had ADHD. This group appears to be more impaired than those with a tic disorder only. Nonetheless, even in the absence of ADHD, tic disorders were associated with some degree of impairment. Large-scale, community-based case finding efforts may help to tease apart the sources of functional impairment in children with tics and tic disorders including TS. This information may be especially useful in planning mental health services and educational programs.

Limitations

The screen for tics (affirmative response by a parent on any one of the DISC probe questions) was broad and offered protection against missing true cases. However, it is possible that parents did miss some cases. In addition, although the yield from stage 1 was almost 1000 children, the subgroups available for comparison were relatively small.

ACKNOWLEDGMENTS

This work was supported in part by the following federal grants: Program Project MH-49351; Children's Clinical Research Center grant (M01-RR06022); the Mental Health Research Center grant (MH-30929). RUPP-MH70009-04 to Dr. Scahill. This study also received support from gifts give by the Smart Family Foundation and by Jean and Jay Kaiser.

The authors acknowledge the advice and collaboration of Drs. Robert A. King, M.D., Paul J. Lombroso, M.D., Diane Findley, Ph.D., Denis Sukhodolsky, PhD, and Donald J. Cohen, M.D., Thanks also to Erin Kustan and Allison Lancor for assistance in preparing this manuscript.

REFERENCES

1. Leckman JF, Zhang H, Vitale A, et al. Course of tic severity in Tourette syndrome: the first two decades. *Pediatrics* 1998;102:14–19.
2. Lapouse R, Monk MA. Behavior deviations in a representative sample of children: variation by sex, age, race, social class and family size. *Am J Orthopsychiatry.* 1962;34:436–446.
3. Snider LA, Seligman LD, Ketchen BR. Tics and problem behaviors in schoolchildren: prevalence, characterization, and associations. *Pediatrics* 2002;110:331–336.
4. Costello EJ, Angold A, Burns BJ, et al. The Great Smoky Mountains study of youth: goals, design, methods, and the prevalence of DSM-III-R disorders. *Arch Gen Psychiatry.* 53:1129–1136.
5. Khalifa N, von Knorring AL. Prevalence of tic disorders and Tourette syndrome in a Swedish school population. *Dev Med Child Neurol.* 2003;45:315–319.
6. Wang HS, Kuo MF. Tourette's syndrome in Taiwan: an epidemiological study of tic disorders in an elementary school at Tapei County. *Brain Develop.* 2003;25(suppl):S29–31.
7. Burd L, Kerbeshian J, Wikenheiser M, et al. Prevalence of Gilles de la Tourette's syndrome in North Dakota children. *J Am Acad Child Adolesc Psychiatry.* 1986; 25:552–553.
8. Apter A, Pauls DL, Bleich A, et al. An epidemiologic study of Gilles de la Tourette's syndrome in Israel. *Arch Gen Psychiatry.* 1993;50:734–738.
9. Hornsey H, Banerjee S, Zeitlin H, et al. The prevalence of Tourette syndrome in 13-14-year-olds in mainstream schools. *J Child Psychol Psychiatry.* 2001;42:1035–1039.
10. Kadesjo B, Gillberg C. Tourette's Disorder: epidemiology and comorbidity in primary school children. *J Am Acad Child Adolesc Psychiatry.* 2000;39:548–555.
11. Kurlan R, McDermott MP, Deeley C, et al. Prevalence of tics in schoolchildren and association with placement in special education. *Neurology* 2003;57:1383–1388.
12. Scahill L, Schwab-Stone M, Merikangas K, et al. Psychosocial and clinical correlates of ADHD in a community sample of young school-age children. *J Am Acad Child Adolesc Psychiatry.* 1999;38:976–983.
13. Schwab-Stone M, Fallon T, Briggs M, et al. Reliability of diagnostic reporting for children aged 6-11 years: a test-retest study of the Diagnostic Interview Schedule for Children-Revised. *Am J Psychiatry.* 1994;151:1048–1054.
14. Zahner GE, Jacobs JH, Freeman DH, Jr, et al. Rural-urban child psychopathology in a Northeastern U.S. state: 1986–1989. *J Am Acad Child Adolesc Psychiatry.* 1993;32:378–387.
15. Achenbach TM, Edelbrock CS. Behavioral problems and competencies reported by parents of normal and disturbed children aged four through sixteen. *Monogr Soc Res Child Dev.* 1981;46:1–82.
16. Piacentini J, Shaffer D, Fisher P, et al. The Diagnostic Interview Schedule for Children-Revised Version (DISC-R): III. Concurrent criterion validity. *J Am Acad Child Adolesc Psychiatry.* 32:658–665.
17. American Psychiatric Association. *Diagnostic and Statistical Manual, Third Edition-Revised (DSM-III-R).* Washington, DC: American Psychiatric Association; 1987.
18. Conners CK. A teacher rating scale for use in drug studies with children. *Am J Psychiatry.* 1969;126: 884–888.
19. Barkley RA. *Attention deficit hyperactivity disorder: A handbook for diagnosis and treatment.* New York: Guilford; 1998.
20. Conners CK. *Conners' Rating Scales Manual.* North Tonowanda, NY: Multi-Health Systems; 1989.
21. Goyette CH, Conners CK, Ulrich RF. Normative data on revised Conners Parent and Teacher Rating Scales. *J Abnorm Child Psychol.* 1978;6:221–236.
22. Epstein NB, Baldwin LM, Bishop DS. The McMaster Family Assessment Device. *J Marital Fam Ther.* 1983;9:171–180.
23. Miller IW, Epstein NB, Bishop DS, et al. The McMaster Family Assessment Device: reliability and validity. *J Marital Fam Ther.* 1985;11:345–356.
24. Byles J, Byrne C, Boyle MH, et al. Ontario Child Health Study: reliability and validity of the general functioning subscale of the McMaster Family Assessment Device. *Fam Process.* 1988;27:97–104.
25. Dunn LM, Dunn LM. *Peabody Picture Vocabulary Test,* 3rd ed. Circle Pines, MN. American Guidance Service; 1997.
26. Mason A, Banerjee S, Eapen V, et al. The Prevalence of Tourette syndrome in a mainstream school. *Dev Med Child Neurol.* 1998;40:292–296.
27. Spencer T, Biederman J, Coffey BJ, et al. Tourette disorder and ADHD. *Adv Neurol.* 2001;85:57–77.
28. Sukhodolsky D, Scahill L, Zhang H, et al. Disruptive behavior in children with Tourette's syndrome: association of ADHD comorbidity, tic severity, and functional impairment. *J Am Acad Child Adolesc Psychiatry.* 2003;42:98–105.
29. Scahill L, Sukhodolsky D, Williams S, et al. Public health significance of tic disorders in children and adolescents. *Adv Neurol.* 2005. In press.
30. United States Census Bureau. Population estimates NC-EST2003-01. Available at: http://www.census.gov/. Accessed July 25, 2004.

19

Treatment of Tics

Leon S. Dure IV and Jennifer DeWolfe

Tics and tic disorders are conditions that are familiar to most pediatricians, neurologists, and psychiatrists. Despite the frequency of clinical encounters with patients who have tics, clear and concise guidelines addressing the decisions relating to the type of treatment or when to begin treatment have not been formulated. The following discussion aims primarily to elucidate the problems relating to how clinicians may interpret the extant views regarding the treatment of tic disorders, and suggests some areas of further investigation.

DEFINITIONS

Tics may manifest clinically as either motor or vocal types, although some investigators prefer the term *phonic tic* as opposed to *vocal tic* because not all sounds involve the vocal cords. Tics are quite interesting when considered among other movement disorders for a variety of reasons. One aspect unique to tics is that they are suppressible yet irresistible. This refers to the fact that tics may be much more apparent in some situations rather than others. Tics may not be obvious in a clinical setting, but patients or their families will report a marked increase in tics in a variety of settings, or after a period of suppression. In children and adults who are capable of articulating the sensation, conscious suppression of a tic may be associated with an increasing need to perform the activity. This need is at times manifested as a premonitory sensation or urge. Some patients relate a need to perform the tic

"just right," or in some particular way that is necessary to achieve relief. This feature is reminiscent of patients with compulsive behaviors and indeed underscores the similarities between tics and obsessive compulsive disorder (OCD).

Another feature of tics that renders them distinct from other movement disorders is the extremely wide repertoire of behaviors that tics represent. A list of potential activities that would be consistent with tics includes almost any type of purposeful behavior, from simple eye blinking and head shaking to complex, orchestrated motor behaviors. This aspect is in contrast to other disorders such as chorea or dystonia, both of which have mild, moderate, and severe manifestations. However, these latter conditions are often essentially the same movement of worsening degree related to duration and distribution rather than the number of types of activity. Suffice it to say that tics have the appearance of normal behaviors "gone wrong," in that they are repeated abnormally, and this repetition of movements has characteristics that are distinct from other movement disorders for the reasons above.

TICS IN CHILDHOOD

As mentioned in the introduction, health professionals frequently encounter patients with tics. Studies of tic prevalence indicate that anywhere from 4% to 15% of school age children will exhibit tics (1). However, the number of children with tics that can be classified as manifesting a tic disorder is unknown. Transient tic disorder (TTD) is a well-described entity used to characterize a child with no history of a medical disorder or drug ingestion that could cause tics, who manifests tic activity for less than 6 months. In many ways, the prevalence of TTD is hard to gauge, as large cohorts of tic patients do not typically distinguish TTD from other chronic conditions (2).

Tourette syndrome (TS) is paradigmatic of chronic tic disorders (3). It is defined as the presence of both motor and vocal tics that occur on a regular basis for more than a 12-month period. These tics typically wax and wane in severity over time and characteristically migrate from one part of the body to another. It has been argued that the requirement for both motor and vocal tics is somewhat artificial because chronic motor tic disorder (an equivalent disorder to TS, without vocal tics) is often seen in families who manifest TS. Indeed, the Tourette Syndrome Study Group has included both chronic motor tic disorder as well as TS in clinical and observational studies (4).

The prevalence of TS has apparently increased, at least in the extant literature. Estimates of TS as high as 3% to 7% have been reported in carefully studied populations (5,6). Consonant with Study Group criteria, studies have typically defined TS by the presence of tics, but inclusion criteria may not necessarily include specific measures of impairment or disability. However, impairment in school, family, or peer relations is often the major determinant of whether or not to begin therapy for tics. To date, there is still no widely accepted criteria for impairment in TS thus resulting in a disconnection between the growing recognition of tic disorders on the one hand, and how the clinician decides on a treatment plan on the other.

It is clear that there are significant unknowns when considering treatment of tics in the context of an increasing number of patients who manifest tics. This is especially important when considering treatment options for tics. The following discussion will attempt to point out issues relating to interpretation of the literature regarding tic therapy, as well as to provide some information from the clinic of the authors of this chapter dealing with a primary population of children with tic disorders.

TICS AND IMPAIRMENT

One of the most difficult issues to investigate is that relating the contribution of tics themselves to morbidity in TS. Although there are data indicating a relationship between tic severity and associated psychopathology (7), causality is far from proven. In a study of 186 children with TS who completed the Child Behavior Checklist, Rosenberg et al. (8) illustrated that there were children who manifested severe tic behaviors but little evidence of other co-morbidity as well as a group with mild tics and a relatively high degree of co-morbidity. The authors considered that in TS, there may be populations of "resilient" and "vulnerable" children, and pointed out the need to better characterize these subgroups. More recently, in a longitudinal study of TS patients in a specialty clinic, Coffey et al. (9) reported that the rate of impairment as indicated by the Yale Global Tic Severity Scale (YGTSS) and Kiddie Schedule for Affective Disorders and Schizophrenia (KSADS) declined over time while tic characteristics did not change. Their results are consonant with others reporting an overall abatement of tics over time and underscore the concept that tics are not the only determinant of impairment in TS (10). Interestingly, in the context of parental perception of children with TS, tics have been shown to be less significant than other behavioral manifestations (11).

Nonetheless, a child with a tic disorder who presents to a clinician is often accompanied by a parent with an appropriate level of anxiety, and the child's own concerns regarding the self perception of a medical problem can also complicate matters. On the other hand, most clinicians who see children with TS are often confronted with the 6- or 7-year-old child with very frequent tics who is oblivious to them and not endorsing any problems in school or at home. Health care professionals are then faced with the situation in which they must address a condition that is defined by the cardinal symptom of tics, but the chief contribution to disability may lie elsewhere.

There are a variety of instruments used to characterize the extent and frequency of tics, and one of the most widely used instruments is the YGTSS (12). The YGTSS rates number, frequency, complexity, intensity, and interference of both motor and vocal tics. The maximal score for this portion of the scale is 50, with 25 being attributed to motor tics and 25 for vocal tics. There is also a 50-point subjective score for impairment, but as mentioned previously, this score is often not used in clinical studies.

Although clearly an excellent means of capturing a variety of characteristics about tics at a given point in time and also helpful for longitudinal assessment, there is a question about whether this instrument actually rates tic severity, as the name implies. Smaller children may manifest a variety of tics and be unaware of them, whereas adolescents may be particularly troubled by, for example, a simple blinking tic. Similarly, it has not been demonstrated that tic complexity is directly correlated to severity. On the other hand, the equal weight given to motor and vocal tics may actually underestimate the severity of tics, especially if a child is manifesting solely motor tics without any vocalization. These issues related to the YGTSS give some cause for concern with respect to its utilization in treatment trials for TS. There is currently no accepted score on the YGTSS for inclusion or exclusion in clinical treatment trials. Likewise, there is no threshold score that has been correlated with any other measure of global function, except in the studies cited previously.

PHARMACOTHERAPY FOR TICS

Since the seminal observation of Seignot that haloperidol reduces the tic symptoms in TS (13), it is clear that agents which block dopamine (D_2) receptors can have a beneficial effect (3,14–23). Other agents demonstrated to be of benefit include Δ-9 tetrahydrocannabinol (24,25), pergolide (26), clonidine (27), mecamylamine (28,29), and tetrabenazine (14), among others. Although these reports indicate a beneficial effect in tic disorders, the issue remains to determine for whom these agents are effective in a context outside of a clinical trial setting. As an example of this issue, in two of the most recent studies, examining the role of risperidone and ziprasidone, respectively, for the treatment of tics, there was no minimal YGTSS score for inclusion (18,30). In those studies the

reduction in tics was on the order of 20%, but what this translates to in terms of clinical effect is uncertain. Another issue with respect to inclusion in clinical trials is the fact that there does appear to be a greater impairment with patients who have a larger number of co-morbidities, specifically attention deficit disorder and OCD. In some studies, these are considered exclusion criteria, as children should not be taking other medications that might affect tic expression. Thus one could argue that patients most in need of therapy and those who are among the most difficult treatment challenges are least likely to be studied in a clinical trial setting.

Given the complexities of interpreting the results of clinical trials for the treatment of TS, it would seem important to try and assess the features of children who ultimately require therapy. Large clinics that specialize in the diagnosis and management of TS may function as excellent laboratories in which to carry out treatment trials. However, it could be argued that there is an inherent bias towards more complicated patients in these settings. A very different situation exists at the University of Alabama at Birmingham, where the Movement Disorders Clinic at the Children's Hospital of Alabama serves as the primary referral center for children with a variety of disorders affecting movement, and captures patients from the State of Alabama as well as surrounding regions. In this clinic, children are often being evaluated by a neurologist for the first time. It functions as the next step of evaluation for a child after having been seen by a primary caregiver such as a pediatrician or family practitioner. Because of these attributes, it has the potential to provide a relatively broad view of the types of children who present for evaluation of tics, and thus a unique opportunity to address rather basic questions regarding therapeutic interventions.

As part of a broader survey of the scope of movement disorders in the pediatric neurology practice at the University of Alabama at Birmingham, the authors of this chapter determined that almost two thirds of the referrals to the Movement Disorders Clinic manifested either TS or a chronic tic disorder. This determination was made by a single neurologist using study group criteria (4). The authors of this chapter elected to perform a retrospective analysis, in order to address the following issues. First of all, the frequency of treatment interventions that had been instituted prior to presentation to the clinic was ascertained, as well as any other related comorbidities assessed by the referring physician to the goal was to determine how often general practitioners elected to treat tic disorders and also to get an indication of how many children had been diagnosed with other conditions that are associated with TS. Secondly, the authors examined clinical records to assess the frequency in which therapy was instituted after evaluation in the clinic. The hope was to begin to determine a rough estimation of how often children with tic disorders presenting to the clinic had symptoms of a severity to merit pharmacologic intervention.

Records were reviewed from the years 1994 to 2002. From these records, the following data were obtained: A) age and gender; B) medications taken by patients for the treatment of tics, attention deficit hyperactivity disorder (ADHD), anxiety, OCD, or depression; C) the diagnosis formulated as a result of the visit to the clinic; and D) documentation of pharmacologic interventions with agents affecting tics and started at the first clinic visit. Diagnosis of a chronic tic disorder or TS was made on the basis of criteria put forward by study group criteria, and other co-morbid diagnoses were made on the basis of the clinical history obtained by the neurologist. The typical agents used included clonidine, pimozide, and atypical antipsychotic agents such as risperidone.

Table 19-1 illustrates the age and gender of patients with a diagnosis of chronic tic disorder (includes motor or vocal tics, but not both), or TS. The mean age of chronic tic disorder and TS patients was comparable, and there was a bias towards males, consistent with other

TABLE 19-1. *Characteristics of tic disorder patients at the university of Alabama at Birmingham, 1994 to 2002*

Condition	Number	Gender (Male/Female)	Age ± SD, (Range)
Chronic tic disorder*	120	3.14	10.1 ± 0.5 (2–42)
Tourette syndrome	536	4.96	11.3 ± 0.5 (3–70)

*Includes chronic motor tic disorder and chronic vocal tic disorder.

studies (3). A total of 656 patients were identified, 375 of whom were felt to have uncomplicated tics with no co-morbid conditions (Table 19-2). Of that group, one third of patients were on medications, two thirds had never been treated. A second group ($N = 281$) was identified that was felt to manifest a chronic tic disorder associated with co-morbidities such as ADHD, OCD, anxiety, or depression. Of this group, 28% were on no medications, 11% were being treated for tics, and 38% treated for the comorbidity. Combination therapy with more than one drug was identified in 23% of children with tics and a co-morbidity.

Therefore, out of 656 children with chronic tic disorder or TS, 332 had never been treated with any medication for their tics or co-morbidities. In this group, 253 were felt to have solely a chronic tic disorder, and 79 were diagnosed with a chronic tic disorder and co-morbidity. In the children who had solely a chronic tic disorder, 11 (4%) were treated for tics with agents such as clonidine or a neuroleptic. Of the 79 patients with chronic tics and co-morbidity, 31 (40%) were treated for tics. In the never treated population ($N = 332$), a total of 8% ($N = 42$) of children were treated with agents that would affect tics at the time of their first visit to the clinic.

TABLE 19-2. *Pharmacologic interventions in tic disorder patients*

Condition	Pretreatment, N (%)	Untreated	Treatment Started
Uncomplicated tics ($N = 375$)	122 (33%)	253 (67%)	11 (4% of untreated)
Tics plus comorbidity ($N = 281$)	Tics, 30 (11%) Co-morbidity, 107 (38%) Combination, 65 (23%)	79 (28%)	31 (39% of untreated)

There are, of course a number of limitations of this type of analysis. First of all, it is primarily a retrospective chart review, and limitations in documentation could certainly have an impact on the data obtained. Referring physician's records did not often indicate the specific reason for treatment with some medications. However, the relatively basic questions asked in this study could be addressed because the purpose was not so much to determine if an accurate diagnosis or intervention was present, but rather that any intervention at all was felt to be necessary. Perhaps a more significant criticism is the fact that determination of the diagnosis as well as co-morbidities was made by one neurologist, and would therefore reflect only a single treatment bias. In addition, treatment strategies often overlap, as certain drugs may have beneficial effects on tics as well as co-morbidities (e.g., clonidine). These authors would argue, however, this is actually a fairly good approximation of typical clinical practice in the community. Whereas, on the one hand, there is no attempt at correlating clinical rating scales to interventions, clinicians often must make decisions based on the clinical situation with which they are faced. Finally, a point must be made about the unique nature of this clinic, as this contributes to the most salient point of the analysis. The fact that almost all of these children had never seen a neurologist or psychiatrist prior to their evaluation in the clinic would seem to support the idea that there is indeed a broad spectrum of clinical severity to which the diagnosis of a chronic tic disorder can be applied. However, the data would suggest that few of these children actually require any specific pharmacologic intervention. Indeed, when an intervention is undertaken, more often it would appear to be in the situation in which co-morbidities are present.

The data presented here in no way could be applied to more complex questions regarding the relationship of tics to co-morbidities, and the best approaches to management. One could certainly argue that the standards for therapy applied by this clinic may not be typical for other clinicians managing chronic tic disorders.

This criticism, however, precisely underscores the issue previously raised with respect to clinical criteria addressing be management of TS and tic disorders. It is the lack of any clear clinical guidelines that really contributes to the complexity of such decisions.

CONCLUSIONS

Most reviews of pharmacologic interventions in TS focus on specific clinical trials using a variety of medications. The clinical experience of the authors of this chapter, however, would seem to indicate that there is a need for a more thorough determination of when and why a particular patient would require therapy for the treatment of tics. As has been stated previously, the impairment scale of the YGTSS is not uniformly applied in clinical treatment trials. However, there is data that indicate the relationship between tics and co-morbidities. Likewise, it is becoming clearer that it is the presence of co-morbidities which often contributes significantly to overall disability. Thus, the fact that exclusion criteria for most clinical trials will bar patients with ADHD, OCD, anxiety, or depression can incorrectly inform clinicians of the efficacy of agents used to treat tics in TS.

How then, should clinical investigators work to rectify the situation? New initiatives are underway to better characterize the epidemiology of TS. It is hoped that these efforts will bring us a better understanding of the determinants of impairment in TS, and by extension, guidelines for clinical situations in which treatment is indicated. In addition, clinical trials need to be designed in such a way as to include patients who meet treatment criteria that can be applied to community settings. Finally, researchers should perhaps be more flexible in the thinking about TS. It has been suggested that the concept of "full-blown" TS be used to describe patients who manifest tics as well as significant co-morbidities, and that researchers should perhaps reserve that diagnosis for patients with some evidence of a particular disability. Efforts should be put in motion to develop a consensus on these and other issues.

REFERENCES

1. Scahill L, Tanner C, Dure L. The epidemiology of tics and Tourette syndrome in children and adolescents. *Adv Neurol.* 2001;85:261–271.
2. Costello EJ, Angold A, Burns BJ, et al. The Great Smoky Mountains Study of Youth. Goals, design, methods, and the prevalence of DSM-III-R disorders. *Arch Gen Psychiatry.* 1996;53:1129–1136.
3. Jankovic J. Tourette's syndrome. *N Engl J Med.* 2001; 345:1184–1192.
4. The Tourette Syndrome Classification Study Group. Definitions and classification of tic disorders. *Arch Neurol.* 1993;500:1013–1016.
5. Kurlan R, McDermott MP, Deeley C, et al. Prevalence of tics in school children and association with placement in special education. *Neurology* 2001;57:1383–1388.
6. Mason A, Banerjee S, Eapen V, et al. The prevalence of Tourette syndrome in a mainstream school population. *Dev Med Child Neurol.* 1998;40:292–296.
7. Nolan EE, Sverd J, Gadow KD, et al. Associated psychopathology in children with both ADHD and chronic tic disorder. *J Am Acad Child Adolesc Psychiatry.* 1996;35:1622–1630.
8. Rosenberg LA, Brown J, Singer HS. Behavioral problems and severity of tics. *J Clin Psychol.* 1995;51:760–767.
9. Coffey BJ, Biederman J, Geller D, et al. Reexamining tic persistence and tic-associated impairment in Tourette's disorder: Findings from a naturalistic follow-up study. *J Nerv Ment Dis.* 2004;192:776–780.
10. Leckman JF, Zhang H, Vitale A, et al. Course of tic severity in Tourette syndrome: the first two decades. *Pediatrics* 1998;102:14–19.
11. Dooley JM, Gordon KE. Parent perceptions of symptom severity in Tourette's syndrome. *Arch Dis Child.* 1999;81:440–441.
12. Scahill L, King RA, Schultz RT, et al. Selection and use of diagnostic and clinical rating instruments. In: Leckman JF, Cohen DJ, eds. *Tourette's Syndrome—Tics, Obsessions, Compulsions.* New York: John Wiley & Sons, Inc.; 1999:310–324.
13. Rickards H, Hartley N, Robertson MM. Seignot's paper on the treatment of Tourette's syndrome with haloperidol. *Hist Psychiatry.* 1997;8:433–436.
14. Sandor P. Pharmacological management of tics in patients with TS. *J Psychosom Res.* 2003;55:41–48.
15. Mukaddes NM, Abali O. Quetiapine treatment of children and adolescents with Tourette's disorder. *J Child Adolesc Psychopharmacol.* 2003;13:295–299.
16. Gaffney GR, Perry PJ, Lund BC, et al. Risperidone versus clonidine in the treatment of children and adolescents with Tourette's syndrome. *J Am Acad Child Adolesc Psychiatry.* 2002;41:330–336.
17. Dion Y, Annable L, Sandor P, et al. Risperidone in the treatment of Tourette syndrome: a double-blind, placebo-controlled trial. *J Clin Psychopharmacol.* 2002; 22:31–39.
18. Sallee F. Ziprasidone treatment of children and adolescents with Tourette's syndrome: a pilot study. *J Am Acad Child Adolesc Psychiatry.* 2000;39:292–299.
19. Saccomani L, Rizzo P, Nobili L. Combined treatment with haloperidol and trazodone in patients with tic disorders. *J Child Adolesc Psychopharmacol.* 2000;10: 307–310.
20. Onofrj M, Paci C, D'Andreamatteo G, et al. Olanzapine in severe Gilles de la Tourette syndrome: a 52-week double-blind cross-over study vs. low-dose pimozide. *J Neurol.* 2000;247:443–446.
21. Short-term versus longer term pimozide therapy in Tourette's syndrome: a preliminary study. *Neurology* 1999;52:874–877.
22. Sallee FR, Nesbitt L, Jackson C, et al. Relative efficacy of haloperidol and pimozide in children and adolescents with Tourette's disorder. *Am J Psychiatry.* 1997;154: 1057–1062.
23. Shapiro AK, Shapiro E, Fulop G. Pimozide treatment of tic and Tourette disorders. *Pediatrics* 1987;79: 1032–1039.
24. Muller-Vahl KR, Schneider U, Prevedel H, et al. Delta 9-tetrahydrocannabinol (THC) is effective in the treatment of tics in Tourette syndrome: a 6-week randomized trial. *J Clin Psychiatry.* 2003;64:459–465.
25. Muller-Vahl KR, Schneider U, Koblenz A, et al. Treatment of Tourette's syndrome with delta9-tetrahydrocannabinol (THC): a randomized crossover trial. *Pharmacopsychiatry* 2002;35:57–61.
26. Gilbert DL, Dure L, Sethuraman G, et al. Tic reduction with pergolide in a randomized controlled trial in children. *Neurology* 2003;60:606–611.
27. Jimenez-Jimenez FJ, Garcia-Ruiz PJ. Pharmacological options for the treatment of Tourette's disorder. *Drugs* 2001;61:2207–2220.
28. Silver AA, Shytle RD, Sheehan KH, et al. Multicenter, double-blind, placebo-controlled study of mecamylamine monotherapy for Tourette's disorder. *J Am Acad Child Adolesc Psychiatry.* 2001;40:1103–1110.
29. Silver AA, Shytle RD, Sanberg PR. Mecamylamine in Tourette's syndrome: a two-year retrospective case study. *J Child Adolesc Psychopharmacol.* 2000;10:59–68.
30. Scahill L, Leckman JF, Schultz RT, et al. A placebo-controlled trial of risperidone in Tourette syndrome. *Neurology* 2003;60:1130–1135.

20

Attention Deficit Hyperactivity Disorder, Chronic Tic Disorder, and Methylphenidate

Kenneth D. Gadow and Jeffrey Sverd

Department of Psychiatry and Behavioral Science, State University of New York at Stony Brook, Stony Brook, New York

Psychostimulants are the most commonly prescribed drugs for the treatment of what is now termed attention deficit hyperactivity disorder (ADHD). They have been prescribed to millions of school-aged children in the United States and are considered to be among the safest psychoactive agents in current use in child psychiatry. When work on the safety and efficacy of stimulant medication for children with ADHD plus tics began at State University of New York at Stony Brook, there were three controlled case studies of the effects of dextroamphetamine on tics, which collectively showed tic exacerbation in seven of nine patients studied (1–3), and only one controlled case study of the efficacy of stimulants for the treatment of hyperactivity in a child with tic disorder (1). At that time it was a widely held belief that methylphenidate (MPH) exacerbated tics and was therefore contraindicated for the treatment of ADHD in child patients with tic disorder (4,5). Although Stony Brook researchers, and others, questioned these assertions (6–11), it was not until the results of controlled studies were published that sentiment began to change (12–24).

Nevertheless, some experts continued to caution practitioners about the serious risk of stimulant-induced tic exacerbations (25) and state their preference for non-stimulant medications as the initial treatment for ADHD symptoms in this clinical population (26).

The goals of the studies of the authors of this chapter were to examine A) the safety and efficacy of MPH for the treatment of ADHD and associated disruptive behaviors and its effect on motor and vocal tics, B) the effects of long-term drug exposure using regularly scheduled follow-up visits, C) the relation between tic severity and psychopathology and developmental changes in the frequency and severity of motor and vocal tics and co-morbid psychopathology, and D) the implications of tic disorder and various comorbidities for clinical outcome in children with ADHD with or without tics. This chapter presents a brief synopsis of the program research that was initiated in 1987 beginning with the findings of short- and long-term drug studies and concluding with co-morbid symptomatology. At the onset, however, these authors wish to acknowledge the efforts of other distinguished researchers (and their colleagues) working in the area of ADHD, tic disorder, and stimulant medication, including Xavier Castellanos (now at New York University), Roger Kurlan (University of Rochester), Samuel Law and Russell Schachar (University of Toronto), James Lechman and the late Donald Cohen (Yale University), Thomas Spencer (Harvard Medical School), and in particular, the important pioneering work of David Comings (City of Hope), Martha Denckla (Johns Hopkins), Gerald Ehrenberg (Cleveland Clinic), and the late Arthur Shapiro (Mt. Sinai School of Medicine), arguably the father of modern tic disorder research.

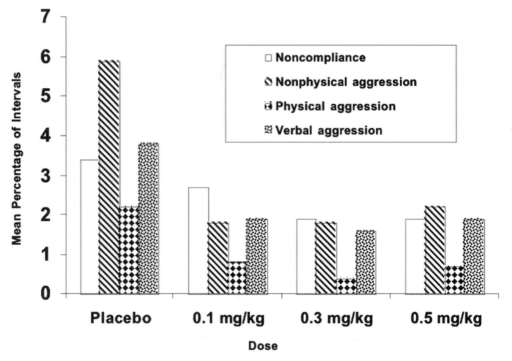

Fig. 20-1. Lunchroom observations of aggressive and noncompliant behaviors as a function of dose of methylphenidate. Copyright 2004 by K.D. Gadow. Reprinted with permission.

DRUG RESPONSE

Short-Term Drug Effects

In the first 8-week study by these authors (17–18), 34 children (31 boys and three girls) were entered into a double-blind, placebo-controlled, crossover trial of three doses of MPH (0.1, 0.3, and 0.5 mg/kg). Each dose sequence was randomly assigned, and each dose was administered twice daily for 2 weeks. All children showed dramatic clinical improvement consequent to MPH treatment; there were no "nonresponders." MPH was highly effective in the amelioration of inattentive, disruptive, and aggressive behaviors in children with ADHD plus tics as assessed by teacher- and parent-completed behavior rating scales, direct observations, and a computer-presented continuous performance task evaluation in the clinic. In public school settings, behavioral improvement was most dramatic during structured classroom academic activities, but there was clear evidence of decreased levels of aggressive behaviors in the lunchroom and on the playground (18). In the lunchroom, for example, MPH was associated with significantly lower levels of noncompliance and physical and nonphysical aggression (Fig. 20-1). Trend analyses of most dependent measures indicated dose effects to be linear; however, the magnitude of clinical improvement associated with the 0.5-mg/kg dose compared with the 0.3-mg/kg dose was minimal for many children. The 0.5-mg/kg dose was associated with more side effects, but fortunately these were generally of limited clinical significance.

Even more gratifying than the finding that MPH was effective for the management of ADHD behaviors in this clinical population was the compelling evidence supporting its benign impact on the severity of tics. During the course of this short-term drug evaluation, physician, teacher, and parent ratings were in uniform agreement that MPH did not lead to a worsening in the severity of the children's tic disorder (group data). In fact, teacher ratings actually suggested improvement in the frequency and severity of motor and vocal tics when children were receiving MPH compared with placebo. The only clinician measure that indicated tic exacerbation was the physician's 2-minute tic count of motor tics (0.5-mg/kg dose only), which was consistent with the initial report on a subsample of subjects (14). Given the fact that 23 different tic measures were used that included information from five different sources (parent, teacher, clinician, school observers, clinic observers), this could be a spurious finding, but it is also possible that stimulant medication interacts with specific somatic (e.g., level of arousal) and environmental variables to produce "tic exacerbations" in certain situations, a hypothesis that warrants further study. For example, the children were present in the room as the physician interviewed the parent about changes in tic status, and occasionally, some even performed mock tics in response to specific questions when the physician was interviewing the parent.

Observations of the children in public school settings indicated that the 0.1-mg/kg dose of MPH was associated with a statistically significant increase in the frequency of occurrence of motor tics in the classroom (but not lunch or recess), but the magnitude of this "tic exacerbation" effect (effect size = 0.34 SD) was relatively small (18), and evidently beyond the detection of care providers (17). There is, however, an ironic twist to the clinical significance of this finding. Given the fact that the frequency of tic occurrence in the classroom was only 3% higher during the 0.3-mg/kg dose condition compared with placebo, it may not be prudent to abandon a MPH trial when a patient experiences a modest increase in motor tic frequency on a low dose (0.1 mg/kg) of medication. It is also interesting that when subjects were videotaped in the clinic's simulated classroom, no significant dose effects on the frequency of motor tics were noted. Furthermore, although individual subject analyses indicated that seven children (out of 34) exhibited a higher frequency of motor tics when receiving their minimal effective dose than placebo, it is difficult to know if this represents "true" drug-induced tic exacerbation in specific individuals or simply

what would be expected on the basis of chance alone if tic frequency normally fluctuates over time. The fact that the frequency of motor tics emitted during clinic videotaping sessions conducted at diagnosis and on placebo differed by at least 0.5 SD (diagnostic) in 61% of the children does not bode well for the former interpretation. In other words, given the moderately high reliability of this type of assessment, this finding indicates a great deal of instability over time (several weeks) and provides strong support for the natural waxing and waning in the frequency of tic symptoms during the course of a short-term drug study.

Purported Cases of Methylphenidate-Induced Tic Exacerbations

In the course of these authors' research and collaborations with a child psychiatry outpatient service, a number of cases of seeming stimulant-induced tic exacerbation or tic induction *de novo* were noted. Needless to say, these occurrences can create an enormous amount of stress and conflict for the child patient, his/her family, the school, and the clinician. Four such cases were carefully re-examined to determine if stimulant medication really played a key role in these occurrences (16). To address this issue at the individual patient level, the authors used either dose reversals or placebo substitutions and reliable and valid measures of tic frequency and severity to help determine if tic worsening was related to pharmacotherapy. In all four instances, treatment with stimulant medication was not a likely explanation for changes in tic severity. Patient A was a child with severe ADHD whose tic disorder gradually became worse during MPH treatment. He was found to have less severe tic symptoms when the dose of medication was increased. Patient B evidenced apparent MPH-induced Tourette syndrome, but with careful observation in controlled settings, pretreatment videotapes, and repeated questioning about developmental history, a preexisting but undiagnosed tic disorder was established. Patients C and D illustrated how standard dose titration procedures commonly

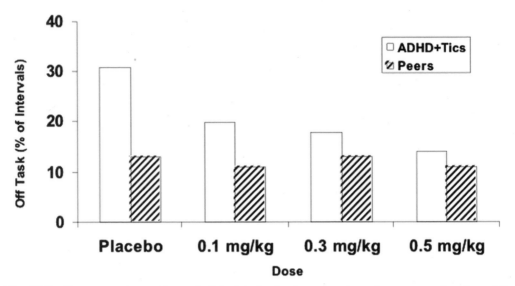

Fig. 20-2. Classroom observations of off task behavior in probands and peers as a function of the probands' dose of methylphenidate. Copyright 2004 by K.D. Gadow. Reprinted with permission.

used in everyday clinical settings can lead to erroneous conclusions about medication and fluctuations in tic frequency.

Behavioral Normalization and Spillover Effects

The short-term drug trial examined A) behavioral differences between children with ADHD plus tics and their peers in school, B) whether effective treatment with methylphenidate normalized ADHD, oppositional, and aggressive behavior, and C) if clinical improvement in the proband consequent to drug therapy was associated with concurrent socially appropriate changes in the behavior of peers (20). Children with ADHD plus tics and their peers were observed for approximately 20 hours in the school setting (classroom seatwork activities, lunchroom, and playground). The former were more inattentive and more disruptive in the classroom and more aggressive in all settings than their peers. Although treatment with methylphenidate made probands less easily distinguished from their peers (normalization), many children still scored in the deviant range for at least one ADHD behavior when receiving the 0.5-mg/kg dose. There was little evidence that peer behavior

improved as a function of the proband's dose of medication, i.e., treatment spillover effect (Fig. 20-2). It was concluded that although conventional doses of MPH produced dramatic improvement in ADHD-related behavior, behavioral normalization is often not attained.

Co-Occurring Anxiety and Depression Symptoms

Studies of differential responsiveness to MPH in children with ADHD with or without anxiety are mixed (27–30). These authors examined this issue in the sample of children with ADHD plus tics who participated in the short-term drug study (31). There was little evidence (group data) that children with anxiety or depression symptoms responded in a clinically different manner to MPH than children who did not exhibit these symptoms, particularly with regard to school observations of the core features of ADHD. Seeming differences between children with and without co-morbid anxiety or depression symptoms and drug response are likely explained by differences in pretreatment levels of negativistic behaviors (i.e., symptoms of oppositional defiant disorder or conduct disorder). It was concluded that MPH appears to

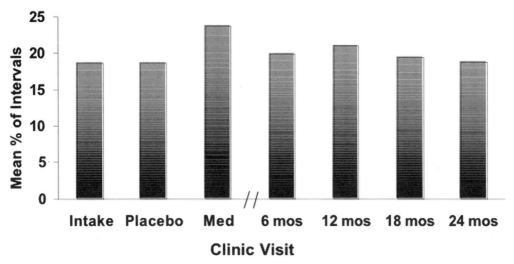

Fig. 20-3. Simulated classroom observations of motor tics for eight time intervals (MED = minimal effective dose). Copyright 2004 by K.D. Gadow. Reprinted with permission.

be an effective treatment for the management of ADHD behaviors in children with mild to moderate anxiety or depression symptoms; nevertheless, much research remains to be done in this area.

Long-Term Treatment Effects

Children with ADHD plus tics were evaluated at 6-month intervals for 2 years following their participation in the short-term MPH trial (23). During the course of the follow-up study, attrition was limited. There was no evidence (group data) that motor tics or vocal tics changed in frequency or severity during maintenance therapy compared with diagnostic or initial placebo evaluations. In fact, the overall rate of tic occurrence as documented with videotapes of children in a simulated clinic classroom indicated that after 2 years of ongoing MPH therapy, the average tic frequency of this sample was virtually identical to the day on which they were first seen in the clinic (Fig. 20-3). Behavioral improvements demonstrated during the acute drug trial were maintained during follow-up. There was no evidence (group data) of clinically significant adverse drug effects on cardiovascular function. Norm-adjusted scores for height and weight (i.e., growth tables) were used to conduct comparisons between actual and expected growth at the end of 2 years of treatment. There was no evidence of drug effects on these outcome variables. It was concluded that long-term treatment with MPH does not appear to be associated with exacerbation of tics, although individual subject sensitivity to MPH remains a possibility.

Medication Withdrawal

Subjects were 19 children with ADHD plus tics who had received MPH for a minimum of one year (22). Children were switched to placebo and MPH (crossover design) under double-blind conditions. Findings failed to support improvement in tic status when children were switched to placebo (Fig. 20-4). In other words, MPH did not cause tic exacerbation. Even more important, however, was the finding that the discontinuation of medication did not result in tic worsening (i.e., there was little evidence for tic exacerbation as a withdrawal phenomenon), which is consistent with the case reports of Riddle et al. (26). There was also no evidence of tic exacerbation in the evening as a rebound effect. Treatment with the maintenance dose was also associated with behavioral improvement in ADHD behaviors, indicating continued efficacy. It was concluded that abrupt withdrawal of

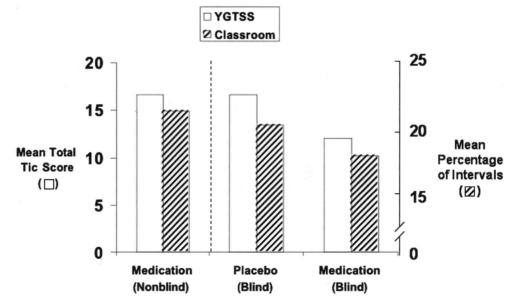

Fig. 20-4. Yale Global Tic Severity Scores (YGTSS) and simulated classroom observations of motor tics during methylphenidate/placebo crossover during long-term stimulant drug therapy for attention deficit hyperactivity disorder. Copyright 2004 by K.D. Gadow. Reprinted with permission.

MPH in children receiving long-term maintenance therapy does not appear to result in worsening of tic frequency or severity.

COMORBIDITY

Numerous studies have reported relatively high rates of psychopathology in children with chronic multiple tic disorder referred for evaluation to tic disorder specialty clinics or child psychiatry clinics. The most commonly associated comorbidity in these children is ADHD (7–8,10,32–33). In this regard, the authors of this chapter conducted several studies of co-occurring tic disorder in children with and without ADHD that involved both referred and clinic-based samples.

Tic Severity

To better understand potential implications of tic characteristics and comorbidities for long-term clinical outcome, a systematic examination of the relation between the severity of tic disorder and comorbidity (as assessed at referral)

was conducted that used multiple measures of child psychopathology (parent- and teacher-completed behavior rating scales, structured psychiatric interviews, and direct observations of ADHD/aggressive behavior in clinic and public school settings) to provide independent verification of the presence of psychopathology and confirmation of reported relations with measures of established ecological validity (34). Of primary interest was whether severity of tic disorder is an indicator of more complex psychopathology and the need to inquire about a broad band of symptoms when conducting clinical evaluations. The parents of all the children in this investigation were seeking clinical evaluation and treatment for ADHD symptoms, and most children had not previously received a diagnosis of tic disorder; therefore, the potential for ascertainment bias was minimized. Subjects were 47 prepubertal children with chronic, multiple tic disorder who were referred for clinical evaluation of and treatment for ADHD, oppositional, and aggressive behaviors. Parents completed the Child Behavior Checklist (CBCL) (35) and teachers completed the Teacher's Report

Form (TRF) (36) for each child. Seventy-five percent of the sample was in the clinical range for at least two categories of psychopathology. When the children were divided into two groups on the basis of tic severity, those with more severe tics had significantly higher scores on the narrowband depressed, uncommunicative, obsessive-compulsive, and aggressive scales, and the broadband Internalizing scale of the CBCL. The severity groups did not differ on TRF scores. Children who were more aggressive also received higher CBCL scores. It was concluded that the severity of chronic tics was a clinical indicator of complex psychopathology in children with ADHD who are referred for psychiatric evaluation.

Attention Deficit Hyperactivity Disorder With or Without Tics

To determine if children with ADHD plus tics were at greater risk for associated psychopathology than children with ADHD without tics, these authors conducted a study of 37 boys with ADHD plus tics (29 of whom had participated in the aforementioned short-term drug study) and 60 boys with ADHD-tics, all of whom were referred for clinical evaluation (37). Parents and teachers completed the CBCL and TRF, respectively. Findings were that boys with ADHD plus tics, compared with boys with ADHD and without tics, evidenced higher rates of aggressive behavior and internalizing symptoms. Depressive symptoms were associated with aggressive behavior in both samples. Children with mild tic disorder were more similar on CBCL scale scores to boys with ADHD and without tics than they were to children with more severe tic disorder. It was concluded that the relatively higher rate of comorbidity in the ADHD plus tics group suggests that tics are a marker for more severe symptomatology in clinic-referred samples of children with ADHD. Furthermore, these data suggest that it is not the presence, per se, but rather the severity of tic disorder that is associated with higher rates of emotional and behavioral disturbance. These findings also provide support for the notion that aggression and

depression are associated irrespective of the presence of tic disorder.

These authors also examined the relation of tics, ADHD, and co-occurring psychiatric symptoms in a large community-based sample of children and adolescents (38). The study sample was comprised of a total of 3,006 children in preschool ($N = 413$; 3 to 5 years; 57% male), elementary school ($N = 1,520$; 5 to 12 years; 52% male), and secondary school ($N = 1,073$; 12 to 18 years; 53% male), all of whom were attending regular education programs. Children were evaluated with a teacher-completed, DSM-IV-referenced rating scale. The sample was divided into four groups: ADHD with or without tics, tics without ADHD, and a comparison group (i.e., neither ADHD nor tics). The percentage of children with tic behaviors varied with age: preschoolers (22.3%), elementary school children (7.8%), and adolescents (3.4%). Screening prevalence rates of tics and ADHD behaviors are plotted in Fig. 20-5. Tic behaviors were more common in males than females, regardless of co-morbid ADHD symptoms. For many psychiatric symptoms, screening prevalence rates were highest for the ADHD groups (ADHD plus tics > ADHD > tics > comparison). However, obsessive-compulsive and simple and social phobia symptoms were more common in the tic behavior groups. Findings for the community-based sample showed many similarities with studies of clinically-referred samples suggesting that teacher-completed ratings of DSM-IV symptoms may be a useful methodology for investigating the phenomenology of tic disorders.

Tics, Attention Deficit Hyperactivity Disorder, and Pervasive Developmental Disorder

Although there is a voluminous literature supporting a relation between tic disorder and co-occurring psychiatric symptoms, this topic has received scant attention in children with pervasive developmental disorder (PDD) owing to the controversy surrounding the existence of psychiatric disorders in this clinical population. Nevertheless, for at least two decades, investigators have commented on a possible

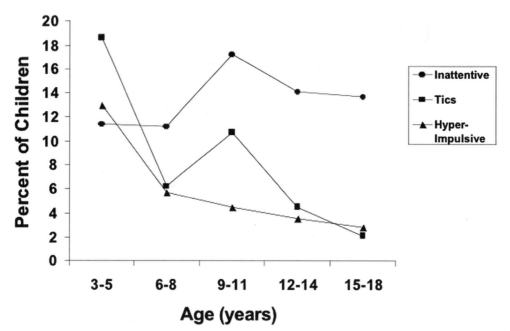

Fig. 20-5. Screening prevalence rates of tics, attention deficit hyperactivity disorder inattentive type, and attention deficit hyperactivity disorder hyperactive-impulsive type symptoms in 3006 school children. (From Gadow KD, Nolan EE, Sprafkin J, et al. Tics and psychiatric comorbidity in children and adolescents. *Dev Med Child Neurol.* 2002;44:331–338. With permission.)

relation between PDD and tic disorders (39–43). Researchers suggest that the co-occurrence of these two disorders may constitute a unique clinical entity and that the two disorders possibly share causal mechanisms, but it is also possible that there is a tic disorder phenocopy in PDD. To examine the clinical significance of co-occurring tics and ADHD as indicators of more complex symptomatology in children with and without PDD, these authors conducted a study in which parents and teachers completed a DSM-IV-referenced rating scale for 3- to 5-year-old ($N = 182/135$) and 6 to 12-year-old ($N = 301/191$) children with PDD and clinic controls, respectively (44). The PDD and non-PDD samples were divided into four groups: ADHD with or without tics, tics without ADHD, and a comparison group (i.e., neither ADHD or tics). In the PDD sample, the percentage of children with tic behaviors varied with age: preschoolers (25%,44%) versus elementary school children (60%,66%), parents and teachers, respectively. For many psychiatric

symptoms, screening prevalence rates were highest for the ADHD plus tics group, and lowest for the control group, but the pattern of group differences varied by age group and informant. In general, there were few differences between the ADHD-only and tics-only groups. It is noteworthy that the pattern of group differences was similar for both PDD and non-PDD children. The conclusion was that these findings support the notion that the co-occurrence of ADHD and tics is an indicator of more complex psychiatric symptomatology in children with PDD.

Natural History

Although there are a number of published reports (primarily chart reviews or retrospective follow-up studies) of developmental changes in the symptomatology of patients with chronic tic disorder (45), these data are saddled with numerous well-known methodologic problems (which is not to say that they are not

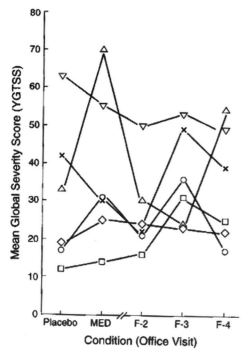

Fig. 20-6. Yale Global Tic Severity Scores (YGTSS) for six representative children (two each of low, moderate, and high severity at intake) during a short-term methylphenidate trial (placebo, MED = minimal effective dose) and three follow-up assessments (F-2 = 12 months, F-3 = 18 months, F-4 = 24 months). Copyright 2004 by K.D. Gadow. Reprinted with permission.

useful). Because the follow-up study gathers data at regularly scheduled intervals, actual reports of symptom frequency and severity at the time of evaluation are obtained. The goal is to better understand developmental changes in ADHD, tics, and co-occurring psychiatric symptoms and their interrelationships. Although much of this work is still in progress, at this writing preliminary plots of individual subject data for the frequency and severity of tics during 2-year follow-up shows considerable variability over time (Fig. 20-6), although correlations of physician ratings of tic severity between various time intervals were in the moderate range. Furthermore, the data show a relatively stable profile (group data) of tic severity as assessed with the Yale Global Tic Severity Scale from age 7 (32.5) through age

12 (31.0) years (range 29.4 to 32.5). Whether this developmental pattern will remain the same during adolescence is unknown, and the clarification of this question is one of the primary objectives of ongoing research.

CONCLUSIONS

The findings of the Stony Brook program of research into stimulant drug therapy for ADHD in children with chronic, multiple tic disorder suggest that MPH is safe and effective for most children. Although MPH may result in tic exacerbation in specific individuals, research into this phenomenon has failed to support the notion that this is a common occurrence or an indication not to use MPH in this clinical population. Findings also suggest that tics are an indicator of more complex psychiatric symptomatology in children, and as such have clinical implications for diagnosis and patient management. In spite of this growing knowledge, much remains to be learned about developmental changes in these disorders and the role of specific risk and protective factors (both biological and environmental) in their manifestation, exacerbation, and remission.

ACKNOWLEDGMENTS

The preparation of this manuscript was supported, in part, by grants from the Tourette Syndrome Association and the National Institute of Mental Health (MH 45358). The authors wish to thank Dr. Joyce Sprafkin, Dr. Edith Nolan, Linda Volkersz, and Dr. Joseph Schwartz for their collaboration in these studies.

Reprint requests for Figures 1–4 and 6 can be sent to Dr. Ken Gadow, Ph.D., Department of Psychiatry and Behavioral Science, Putnam Hall-South Campus, SUNY at Stony Brook, Stony Brook, NY 11794–8790.

REFERENCES

1. Meyerhoff JL, Snyder SH. Gilles de la Tourette's disease and minimal brain dysfunction: amphetamine isomers reveal catecholamine correlates in an affected patient. *Psychopharmacologia* 1973;29:211–220.

2. Feinberg M, Carroll BJ. Effects of dopamine agonists and antagonists in Tourette's disease. *Arch Gen Psychiatry.* 1979;36:979–985.

3. Caine ED, Ludlow CL, Polinsky RJ, et al. Provocative drug testing in Tourette's syndrome: d- and l-amphetamine and haloperidol. *J Am Acad Child Psychiatry.* 1984;23:147–152.

4. Golden GS. Letter to the editor. *J Am Med Assoc.* 1982;248:1063.

5. Lowe TL, Cohen DJ, Detlor J, et al. Stimulant medications precipitate Tourette's syndrome. *JAMA* 1982;247:1729–1731.

6. Denkla MB, Bemporad JR, MacKay MC. Tics following methylphenindate administration. *JAMA* 1976;235:1349–1351.

7. Shapiro AK, Shapiro E. Do stimulants provoke, cause or exacerbate tics and Tourette syndrome? *Comp Psychiatry.* 1981;22:265–273.

8. Comings DE, Comings BG. Tourette's syndrome and attention deficit disorder with hyperactivity: are they genetically related? *J Am Acad Child Psychiatry.* 1984;23:138–146.

9. Erenberg G, Cruse RP, Rothner AD. Gilles de la Tourette's syndrome: effects of stimulant drugs. *Neurology* 1985;35:1346–1348.

10. Comings DE, Comings BG. A controlled study of Tourette syndrome. I. Attention-deficit disorder, learning disorders, and school problems. *Am J Hum Genet.* 1987;4:701–741.

11. Gadow KD, Sverd J. Stimulants for ADHD in child patients with Tourette's syndrome: the issue of relative risk. *J Dev Behav Pediatr* 1990;11:269–271.

12. Sverd J, Gadow KD, Paolicelli LM. Methylphenidate treatment of attention-deficit hyperactivity disorder in boys with Tourette's syndrome. *J Am Acad Child Adolesc Psychiatry.* 1989;28:574–579.

13. Konkol RJ, Fischer M, Newby RF. Double-blind, placebo-controlled stimulant trial in children with Tourette's syndrome and attention-deficit hyperactivity disorder [Abstract]. *Ann Neurol.* 1990;28:424.

14. Sverd J, Gadow KD, Nolan EE, et al. Methylphenidate in hyperactive boys with comorbid tic disorder: I. Clinic evaluations. In: Chase TN, Friedhoff AJ, Cohen DJ, eds. *Tourette Syndrome: Genetics, Neurobiology, and Treatment.* New York, NY: Raven Press; 1992;58:271–281.

15. Gadow KD, Nolan EE, Sverd J. Methylphenidate in hyperactive boys with comorbid tic disorder: II. Short-term behavioral effects in school settings. *J Am Acad Child Adolesc Psychiatry.* 1992;31:462–471.

16. Sprafkin J, Gadow KD. Four purported cases of methylphenidate-induced tic exacerbation: methodological and clinical doubts. *J Child Adolesc Psychopharm.* 1993;3:231–244.

17. Gadow KD, Sverd J, Sprafkin J, et al. Efficacy of methylphenidate for attention-deficit hyperactivity disorder in children with tic disorder. *Arch Gen Psychiatry.* 1995;52:444–455.

18. Gadow KD, Nolan EE, Sprafkin J, et al. School observations of children with attention deficit hyperactivity disorder and comorbid tic disorder: effects of methylphenidate treatment. *J Dev Behav Pediatr.* 1995;16:167–176.

19. Castellanos FX, Giedd JN, Elia J, et al. Controlled stimulant treatment of ADHD and comorbid Tourette's syndrome: effects of stimulant and dose. *J Am Acad Child Adolesc Psychiatry.* 1997;36:589–596.

20. Nolan EE, Gadow KD. Children with ADHD and tic disorder and their classmates: behavioral normalization with methylphenidate. *J Am Acad Child Adolesc Psychiatry.* 1997;36:597–604.

21. Law SF, Schachar RJ. Do typical clinical doses of methylphenidate cause tics in children treated for attention-deficit hyperactivity disorder? *J Am Acad Child Adolesc Psychiatry.* 1999;38:944–951.

22. Nolan EE, Gadow KD, Sprafkin J. Stimulant medication withdrawal during long-term therapy in children with comorbid attention-deficit hyperactivity disorder and chronic multiple tic disorder. *Pediatrics* 1999;103:730–737.

23. Gadow KD, Sverd J, Sprafkin J, et al. Long-term methylphenidate therapy in children with comorbid ADHD and chronic multiple tic disorder. *Arch Gen Psychiatry.* 1999;56:330–336.

24. Tourette Syndrome Study Group. Treatment of ADHD in children with tics. *Neurology* 2002;58:527–536.

25. Peterson BS, Cohen DJ. The treatment of Tourette's syndrome: multimodal, developmental intervention. *J Clin Psychiatry.* 1998;59:62–72.

26. Riddle MA, Lynch KA, Scahill L, et al. Methylphenidate discontinuation and reinitiation during long-term treatment of children with Tourette's disorder and attention-deficit hyperactivity disorder: a pilot study. *J Child Adolesc Psychopharm.* 1995;5:205–214.

27. Taylor E, Schachar R, Thorley G, et al. Which boys respond to stimulant medication? A controlled trial of methylphenidate in boys with disruptive behaviour. *Psychological Medicine.* 1987;17:121–143.

28. Pliszka SR. Effect of anxiety on cognition, behavior, and stimulant response in ADHD. *J Am Acad Child Adolesc Psychiatry.* 1989;28:882–887.

29. DuPaul GJ, Barkley RA, McMurray MB. Response of children with ADHD to methylphenidate: Interaction with internalizing symptoms. *J Am Acad Child Adolesc Psychiatry.* 1994;33:894–903.

30. Diamond IR, Tannock R, Schachar RJ. Response to methylphenidate in children with ADHD and comorbid anxiety. *J Am Acad Child Adolesc Psychiatry.* 1999;38:402–409.

31. Gadow KD, Nolan EE, Sverd J, et al. Anxiety and depression symptoms and response to methylphenidate in children with attention-deficit hyperactivity disorder and tic disorder. *J Clin Psychopharm.* 2002;22:267–274.

32. Shapiro A, Shapiro E, Young J, et al. *Gilles de la Tourette Syndrome.* New York, NY: Raven Press; 1988.

33. Spencer T, Biederman J, Harding M, et al. Disentangling the overlap between Tourette's disorder and ADHD. *J Child Psychol Psychiatry.* 1998;39:1037–1044.

34. Nolan EE, Sverd J, Gadow KD, et al. Associated psychopathology in children with both ADHD and chronic tic disorder. *J Am Acad Child Adolesc Psychiatry.* 1996;35:1622–1630.

35. Achenbach TM. *Manual for the Child Behavior Checklist/4-18 and 1991 Profile.* Burlington, VT: University of Vermont, Department of Psychiatry, 1991.

36. Achenbach TM. *Manual for the Teacher's Report Form and 1991 Profile.* Burlington, VT: University of Vermont, Department of Psychiatry, 1991.

37. Pierre CB, Nolan EE, Gadow KD, et al. Comparison of internalizing and externalizing symptoms in ADHD

children with and without comorbid tic disorder. *J Dev Behav Pediatr*. 1999;20:170–176.

38. Gadow KD, Nolan EE, Sprafkin J, et al. Tics and psychiatric comorbidity in children and adolescents. *Dev Med Child Neurol*. 2002;44:330–338.

39. Realmuto GM, Main B. Coincidence of Tourette's disorder and infantile autism. *J Autism Dev Disord*. 1982;12:367–372.

40. Barabas G, Matthews WD. Coincident infantile autism and Tourette syndrome: a case report. *J Dev Behav Pediatr*. 1983;4:280–281.

41. Burd L, Fisher WW, Kerbeshian J, et al. Is development of Tourette disorder a marker for improvement in patients with autism and other pervasive developmental disorders? *J Am Acad Child Adolesc Psychiatry*. 1987; 26:162–165.

42. Kano Y, Ohta M, Nagai Y. Two case reports of autistic boys developing Tourette's disorder: indications of improvement? *J Am Acad Child Adolesc Psychiatry*. 1987;26:937–938.

43. Sverd J. Tourette syndrome associated with pervasive developmental disorder: is there an etiological relationship? *J Multihandicapped Person*. 1988;1:281–291.

44. Gadow KD, DeVincent CJ. Clinical significance of tics and ADHD in children with pervasive developmental disorder. *J Child Neurol*. 2005. In press.

45. Bruun RD. The natural history of Tourette's syndrome. In: Cohen DN, Bruun R, Leckman JL, eds. *Tourette Syndrome and Tic Disorders*. New York, NY: John Wiley & Sons; 1988;21–39.

21

Treatment of Co-Morbid Obsessive Compulsive Disorder, Mood, and Anxiety Disorders

Barbara J. Coffey[1] and Rachel L. Shechter[2]

[1]*Department of Psychiatry, New York University School of Medicine, New York, New York;*
[1,2]*Institute for Tourette's and Movement Disorders, New York University Child Study Center, New York, New York*

The objectives of this chapter are to briefly review the prevalence, impact, and treatment of co-morbid obsessive compulsive disorder (OCD), mood, and anxiety disorders in clinically referred youths with Tourette syndrome (TS). Anxiety, mood, and other emotional symptoms have been described in patients with TS for many years. In 1899 in "La Maladies des Tics Convulsif," the first scientific paper on behavioral and emotional aspects of TS, Gilles de la Tourette described "fears, phobias, and arithmomania" in his original report on nine cases (1). In *Case Studies of Hysteria*, Sigmund Freud described facial tics and nervousness in Frau Emmy Von N, who may have had TS, and, in 1907, in "Tics and Their Treatment," (1a) Meige and Feindel described a patient with TS who probably had both OCD, and depression (2).

In recent years, there has been increasing recognition of the clinical and scientific significance of co-morbid emotional disorders in TS, including co-morbid OCD, mood and anxiety disorders (3–16). There appears to be a bidirectional relationship between TS and OCD in most clinically referred patient cohorts (3–5). OC symptoms or OCD have been reported in 20% to 60% of TS patients (6); patients with OCD have about a 7% lifetime risk of TS (7) and 20% risk of tics (8). Family studies indicate that OCD is found at a higher rate in close relatives of individuals with TS than in controls, independent of OCD symptoms in the proband,

which further supports this bidirectional relationship (9–11).

TS and OCD share many common features, including a waxing and waning course, repetitive behaviors and complex movements or rituals, preoccupation with sexual and aggressive themes, and partial voluntary suppression of symptoms with subsequent build up of inner tension. In addition, previous studies have suggested that patients with TS plus OCD have higher levels of disability than those without co-morbid OCD (4,12–15).

Although most studies of co-morbid emotional disorders in TS have focused on OCD, the extant literature suggests that other anxiety and mood disorders may also complicate the course of TS in clinically referred patients (5,14,16–20). This is not surprising, given that OCD is frequently co-morbid with mood and other anxiety disorders (8,14,21–23). However, there have been few rigorous studies of mood and non-OCD anxiety disorders in clinically referred individuals with TS.

Investigators have described elevated rates of trait anxiety, phobias, panic attacks, and generalized anxiety disorder in TS patients (18,24). Although Comings and Comings (24) reported that there was no correlation between the number of tics and phobias in a study of TS and anxiety, fear of crowds and of being alone significantly differentiated TS severity groups (mild, moderate, and severe). In a study of 47 children with ADHD and chronic tics dichotomized by tic severity, Nolan et al. (25) reported that rates of separation anxiety and overanxious disorder were higher in the groups with more severe tics. Pitman et al. (14) studied 16 adult patients with TS, 16 with OCD, and 16 controls, and reported that both the TS and OCD groups had high rates of generalized anxiety disorder compared to controls. In several studies, Robertson et al. (18,26) reported elevated rates of anxiety symptoms (both OCD and non-OCD) in adults with TS in a clinical sample, compared with normal controls. Similarly, Cath et al. (27) reported elevated rates of anxiety symptoms on the Spielberger State-Trait Anxiety Inventory in a clinical sample of adults with TS compared with normal controls (Table 21-1).

PSYCHIATRIC CO-MORBIDITY IN TOURETTE SYNDROME

The prevalence of co-morbid mood and anxiety symptoms and disorders in TS is reported to be rather high in clinical settings, particularly in specialty clinics (18,28,29). This observation could derive from several potential sources, including ascertainment bias that individuals who seek specialty clinical evaluation are likely to be more severely afflicted, and meet criteria for

TABLE 21-1. *Tourette syndrome: co-morbidity with mood/anxiety disorders*

Author	Citation	Findings
Comings et al. 1987	*Am J Hum Gen*, 41; 761–781	Fear of crowds and being alone; differentiated TD severity groups
Comings et al. 1987, 1990	*Am J Hum Gen*, 41; 804–921; 1987; *J Clin Psych* 51; 288–291; 1990	On Diagnostic Interview Scale for mood disorders 23% TS patients versus 2% controls scored in clinical range
Pitman et al. 1987	*Am J Psych* 144; 1166–1171	In 16 adults with TS, 16 with OCD and 16 controls: both TS and OCD groups had higher rates of generalized anxiety disorder and MDD versus controls
Robertson et al. 1993	*Br J Psych* 162; 14–117	Elevated rates of anxiety symptoms (OCD and non-OCD) in clinical sample of adults with TS versus controls
Kerbeshian et al. 1995	*Am J Psych* 152; 1646–1651	Bipolar disorder over-represented in a community sample of adults with TS
Robertson et al. 1997	*Br J Psych* 162; 14–117; *Br J Psych* 171; 283–286	In 22 adults with TS, 19 with MDD and 21 controls, TS and MDD groups scored higher on Beck, Leyton and Spielberger than controls
Berthier et al. 1998	*Biol Psych* 43; 364–370	30/90 (33%) of patients on neurology service met criteria for bipolar disorder
Coffey et al. 2000	*JAACAP* 39(5); 562–568; *JAACAP* 39(5); 556–561	In clinical sample of 190 children with TS, non-OCD anxiety disorders predicted tic severity
		In clinical sample of 156 children with TS, MDD and bipolar disorder were significant predictors of hospitalization and global assessment of functioning <50
Cath et al. 2001	*Psych Res* 101; 171–185	In clinical sample of adults with TS versus controls, elevated rates of depressive symptoms on Montgomery-Asberg Depression Rating Scale

MDD, major depressive disorder; OCD, obsessive compulsive disorder; TS, Tourette syndrome.
Adapted from Coffey BJ, Biederman J, Spencer T, et al. Informativeness of Structured Diagnostic Interviews in the Identification of Tourette's Disorder in Referred Youth. *J Nerv Ment Dis.* 2000;188:584.

TABLE 21-2. *Clinical and demographic characteristics of non-specialized and specialized clinic patients with Tourette syndrome*

Demographic characteristic	Nonspecialized clinic patients (N = 92)		Specialized clinic patients (N = 103)		Overall significance
	Mean	SD	Mean	SD	P
Current age (in years)	10.8	3.23	10.8	3.62	0.89
SES	2.0	1.13	2.2	1.24	0.42
	N	%	N	%	P
Past GAF	47.9	7.50	48.6	7.57	0.54
Current GAF	51.3	7.32	51.9	6.52	0.55
Gender (% Male)	82	90	81	80	0.06

GAF, global assessment of functioning; SES, socioeconomic status.
Adapted from Coffey BJ, Biederman J, Spencer T, et al. Informativeness of Structured Diagnostic Interviews in the Identification of Tourette's Disorder in Referred Youth. *J Nerv Ment Dis.* 2000;188:584.

more than one disorder compared to those who do not seek specialty evaluation. However, a recent study by the authors of this chapter suggests that this may not be the case, and that co-morbid disorders are highly prevalent in youth with TS, even in general child and adolescent psychiatry settings (30).

Subjects were all consecutively referred children and adolescents meeting DSM-III-R diagnostic criteria for TS on structured diagnostic interviews ascertained through a specialized TS clinic (N = 103) and a general pediatric psychopharmacology clinic (N = 92) within the same academic medical center (30a). Although specialized in pediatric psychopharmacology, the latter program was not a tertiary care service because approximately 50% of the referrals had not been evaluated or treated before.

All children in both programs were comprehensively evaluated using the same assessment battery that included the Children's Schedule for Affective Disorders and Schizophrenia for School-Age Children-Epidemiological Version (KSADS-E) (31). Subjects from the TS specialty and the general pediatric psychopharmacology clinic ascertainment sources could not be differentiated with regard to past global assessment of functioning ([GAF]: 48.6 ± 7.6 versus 47.9 ± 7.5, ns) or current (GAF: 51.9 ± 6.5 versus 51.3 ± 7.3, ns) interpersonal functioning, current severity of TS (1.7 ± 0.75 versus 1.5 ± 0.7, ns), mean age of onset of TS (5.5 ± 2.7 versus 6.0 ± 2.8

years, ns), or duration of TS (5.3 ± 3.7 versus 4.3 ± 3.5 years, ns). However, small but statistically significant differences were observed in the rate of current TS (98% versus 83% respectively; $P < 0.005$) and lifetime tic severity (2.2 ± 0.8 versus 1.7 ± 0.73, $P < 0.005$), which were higher in the TS specialty clinic patients (Tables 21-2 and 21-3).

Lifetime rates of psychiatric co-morbidity were overwhelmingly high in youth with TS irrespective of ascertainment source, and rates of individual psychiatric co-morbid disorders were almost identical in the two ascertainment groups. The most prevalent co-morbid disorder in each clinical setting was attention deficit hyperactivity disorder (ADHD) (72% and 84%, ns). However, notable in this study were the high lifetime rates of major mood disorders (57% and 60%, ns) and non-OCD anxiety disorders (40% and 35%, ns), which were overall more prevalent than lifetime rates for OCD (36% and 21%, ns) (Tables 21-4 and 21-5).

Children and adolescents who met criteria for TS on structured diagnostic interviews shared very similar clinical correlates, irrespective of their ascertainment source through specialized or non-specialized TS programs. Overall rates of mood and non-OCD anxiety disorders were high (30).

ANXIETY DISORDERS AND TD

While co-morbidity with OCD has long been recognized as associated with a more severe TS

TABLE 21-3. *Tic characteristics of non-specialized and specialized clinic patients with Tourette syndrome*

Tic characteristic	Nonspecialized clinic patients (N = 92)		Specialized clinic patients (N = 103)		Overall significance
	Mean	SD	Mean	SD	P
TS severity (worst ever) (1 = minimal; 3 = severe)	1.7	0.73	2.2	0.79	0.000
TS severity (current) (1 = minimal; 3 = severe)	1.5	0.70	1.7	0.75	0.031
Duration of TS (in years)	4.3	3.53	5.3	3.69	0.053
Onset of TS (in years)	6.0	2.79	5.5	2.68	0.22
	N	%	N	%	P
Psychiatric hospitalization	13	14	15	14	0.93
Current TS	76	83	101	98	0.000

TS, Tourette syndrome.
Adapted from Coffey BJ, Biederman J, Spencer T, et al. Informativeness of Structured Diagnostic Interviews in the Identification of Tourette's Disorder in Referred Youth. *J Nerv Ment Dis.* 2000;188:585.

TABLE 21-4. *Tourette syndrome co-morbidity: mood disorders*

Diagnosis	Nonspecialized clinic patients (N = 92)		Specialized clinic patients (N = 103)		Overall significance
	N	%	N	%	P
Pure TS (Non-co-morbid)	2	2	5	5	0.31
Major depressive disorder	45	49	56	54	0.49
Any bipolar disorder	20	22	16	16	0.24
Dysthymia	9	10	4	4	0.09
Any mood disorder	55	60	59	57	0.65

TS, Tourette syndrome.
Adapted from Coffey BJ, Biederman J, Spencer T, et al. Informativeness of Structured Diagnostic Interviews in the Identification of Tourette's Disorder in Referred Youth. *J Nerv Ment Dis.* 2000;188:585.

TABLE 21-5. *Tourette syndrome co-morbidity: anxiety disorders*

Diagnosis	Nonspecialized clinic patients (N = 92)		Specialized clinic patients (N = 103)		Overall significance
	N	%	N	%	P
Panic disorder	10	11	15	15	0.45
Agoraphobia	21	23	27	26	0.61
Social phobia	15	16	5	5	0.008
Simple phobia	25	27	30	30	0.73
OCD	19	21	37	36	0.021
Separation anxiety	22	24	39	39	0.028
Multiple anxiety disorders (2+)	32	35	41	40	0.47

OCD, obsessive compulsive disorder.
Adapted from Coffey BJ, Biederman J, Spencer T, et al. Informativeness of Structured Diagnostic Interviews in the Identification of Tourette's Disorder in Referred Youth. *J Nerv Ment Dis.* 2000;188:585.

phenotype (4,32–35), very little is known about the role of non-OCD anxiety disorders in TS patients. However, non-OCD anxiety disorders may be more frequent in TS patients than in the general population, and encompass a wide range of conditions that can also be associated with significant morbidity and dysfunction (14,16,18,24). In order to address the role and impact of non-OCD anxiety in clinically referred youth with TS, the author and her colleagues evaluated the prevalence of anxiety disorders in consecutive referrals to a TS specialty program. In this study of a clinical sample of 190 children with TS, non-OCD anxiety disorders in general, and separation anxiety disorder in particular, were highly associated with tic severity (19). In this study, 190 subjects evaluated in a TS specialty clinic were divided into mild/moderate and severe tic severity groups.

No meaningful differences in age of onset of TS (5.7 ± 2.6 and 5.9 ± 3.0 years), or duration of TS were noted when controlling for age. As expected, the severe TS group had more impairment in psychosocial functioning, as indicated by lower GAF scores (past 44.5 ± 6.4 versus 49.8 ± 7.5, $P < 0.001$; and current 48.3 ± 5.9 versus 53.0 ± 6.9, $P < 0.001$) (Tables 21-6 and 21-7).

Psychiatric co-morbidity was overwhelmingly present irrespective of tic severity status (94.8% for mild/moderate TS and 100% for severe TS). Examination of co-morbidity with anxiety disorders revealed that although OCD was over-represented among the severe TS cases, the difference failed to reach threshold for statistical significance (42% versus 25% for severe and mild/moderate TS, respectively, $P < 0.02$). However, with the exception of social and simple phobia, all other anxiety disorders

TABLE 21-6. *Sample demographic characteristics: mild/moderate versus severe Tourette syndrome in 190 patients*

	Mild/Moderate TS ($N = 134$)		Severe TS ($N = 56$)		Significance
Demographic characteristic	Mean	SD	Mean	SD	P
Current age (in years)	10.2	3.3	12.0	3.4	<0.001
SES	2.03	1.1	2.25	1.33	0.30
	N	%	N	%	P
Gender (% Male)	113	84	49	88	0.57

TS, Tourette syndrome; SES, socioeconomic status.
Adapted from Coffey BJ, Biederman J, Smoller, JW, et al. Anxiety disorders and tic severity in juveniles with Tourette's disorder. *J Am Acad Child Adolesc Psychiatry.* 2000;39:564.

TABLE 21-7. *Clinical characteristics: mild/moderate versus severe Tourette syndrome in 190 patients*

	Mild/Moderate TS ($N = 134$)		Severe TS ($N = 56$)		Significance
Clinical characteristics	Mean	SD	Mean	SD	p
Past GAF	49.8	7.5	44.5	6.4	<0.001
Current GAF	53.0	6.9	48.3	5.9	<0.001
Onset of TS (in years)	5.7	2.6	5.9	3.0	0.75
Duration of TS (in years)	4.3	3.1	6.2	4.4	<0.001
	N	%	N	%	P
Current (past month) symptoms (%)	119	89	55	98	0.03

GAF, global assessment of functioning; TS, Tourette syndrome.
Adapted from Coffey BJ, Biederman J, Smoller, JW, et al. Anxiety disorders and tic severity in juveniles with Tourette's disorder. *J Am Acad Child Adolesc Psychiatry.* 2000;39:564.

TABLE 21-8. *Co-morbidity in Tourette syndrome by severity: mild/moderate versus severe in 190 patients*

Diagnosis	Mild/Moderate TS ($N = 134$)		Severe TS ($N = 56$)		Significance χ^2
	N	%	N	%	P
Any co-morbidity	127	94.8	56	100	0.08
Mood disorders					
Major depressive disorder	66	49.3	33	58.9	0.22
Bipolar disorder	19	14.2	16	28.6	0.02
Dysthymia	9	6.7	4	7.1	0.92
Any mood disorder	75	56.0	36	64.3	0.29
Anxiety disorders					
Panic disorder	12	9.0	13	23.2	0.01
Agoraphobia	25	19.0	22	39.3	0.001
Social phobia	14	10.5	6	10.7	0.97
Simple phobia	34	25.6	21	38.2	0.08
Obsessive compulsive disorder	33	24.8	23	41.8	0.02
Overanxious disorder	36	27.1	25	45.5	0.01
Separation anxiety	32	24.2	28	50.9	0.001
Any anxiety	71	53.0	39	69.6	0.03
Multiple (2+) anxiety disorders	43	32.3	30	53.6	0.01

Adapted from Coffey BJ, Biederman J, Smoller, JW, et al. Anxiety disorders and tic severity in juveniles with Tourette's disorder. *J Am Acad Child Adolesc Psychiatry.* 2000;39:565.

were significantly overrepresented among severe TS subjects including panic disorder (23% versus 9%, $P <0.01$), agoraphobia (39% versus 19%, $P <0.01$), separation anxiety disorder (51% versus 24%, $P <0.001$), and overanxious disorder (46% versus 27%, $P <0.01$). It is noteworthy that separation anxiety disorder most robustly predicted high tic severity, even when controlling for the presence of OCD or other anxiety disorders (OR 2.98, $P <0.001$). In addition, the greater the number of co-morbid anxiety disorders, the higher the tic severity overall (Tables 21-8 and 21-9).

These findings suggest that non-OCD anxiety disorders in general, and separation anxiety disorder in particular, may be predictors of tic severity in referred TS patients (19). Thus, systematic inquiry regarding the spectrum of non-OCD anxiety disorders could be helpful in the identification of TS patients at high risk for severe tics.

Because patients with OCD in this sample had a greater likelihood of non-OCD anxiety disorders, it is possible that OCD could be a modulator of tic severity. Although OCD is frequently co-morbid with other anxiety disorders (21,22,36), these findings suggested that specific associations exist between tic severity and non-OCD anxiety disorders that are not accounted for by the presence of OCD alone.

MOOD DISORDERS AND TOURETTE SYNDROME

Patients with TS have been reported to score higher than normal controls on psychopathology ratings for depression (18). Robertson et al. (18) administered three standardized self-reports of psychopathology (Leyton Obsessional Inventory, Beck Depression Inventory, and Spielberger State-Trait Anxiety Inventory) to 22 adults with TS, 19 with major depression (MD), and 21 normal controls. Results indicated that the groups with TS and MD scored significantly higher than the comparison group on all measures, although scores on the depression scale were lower in the TS than in the MD group (18). Comings et al. (37,38) reported on the Diagnostic Interview Schedule for mood disorders that 23% of the TS patients had a clinically significant

TABLE 21-9. *Demographic and clinical characteristics in Tourette syndrome in 156 patients*

Demographic and clinical characteristic	No hospital (N = 137)		Past hospital (N = 19)		Significance χ^2
	Mean	SD	Mean	SD	P
Current age	10.5	3.0	14.4	3.2	0.001
SES	2.1	1.1	2.5	1.5	NS
Past GAF	51.0	6.1	37.9	6.4	0.000
Current GAF	53.7	5.7	44.7	8.3	0.000
	N	%	N	%	
Gender (% Male)	112	82.4	16	84.2	NS
TS Duration	4.5	3.2	6.9	4.7	0.0058
TS Impairment (worst ever)	—	—	—	—	0.007
Mild	52.0	38.5	2.0	11.1	—
Moderate	52.0	38.5	6.0	33.3	—
Severe	31.0	23.0	10.0	55.6	—

GAF, global assessment of functioning; TS, Tourette syndrome; SES, socioeconomic status.
Adapted from Coffey BJ, Biederman J, Geller D, et al. Distinguishing illness severity from tic severity in children and adolescents with Tourette's disorder. *J Am Acad Child Adolesc Psychiatry.* 2000;39:558.

score compared with 2% of the control group. Pitman et al. (14) studied 16 patients with TS, 16 with OCD, and 16 controls, and reported that both the TS and OCD groups had high rates of unipolar depressive disorders. In a study of personality disorders in TS, Robertson et al. (18,26) reported significantly elevated rates of depressive symptoms on the Beck Depression Rating Scale in adults in a clinical sample, compared to normal controls. Similarly, Cath et al. (27) reported elevated rates of depressive symptoms on the Montgomery-Asberg Depression Rating Scale in a clinical sample of adults with TS, compared to normal controls.

Interestingly, high rates of bipolar disorder have been reported in clinical samples of patients with TS. Kerbeshian et al. (39) reported that bipolar disorder was overrepresented in a community sample of TS patients. Similarly, Berthier and Campos (40) reported high lifetime prevalence for general psychopathology in 90 selected adult TS patients seen on a neurology service and that 30 (33%) met criteria for bipolar disorder (Table 21-1).

Although factors such as social class, duration and complexity of tics have been reported to be associated with TS severity, (12,41) it is not clear whether severely ill TS patients are impaired primarily by their tics or by other non-tic symptoms, such as those that occur in the context of psychiatric co-morbid disorders (17,18,24,37,42).

Moreover, since tic severity is not necessarily synonymous with illness severity, it is feasible that different co-morbidities could be associated with various levels of severity and dysfunction in TS patients. This is particularly the case as recent work by the authors of this chapter and others has documented that in addition to ADHD and OCD, the scope of co-morbidity in TS patients also includes anxiety disorders as well as bipolar and non-bipolar mood disorders, conditions commonly associated with high levels of morbidity and impairment (18,39).

The purpose of this study was to examine factors associated with illness morbidity in youth with TS. Considering that the need for psychiatric hospitalization is a clear measure of poor outcome, we examined whether tic severity, co-morbid disorders or both are associated with psychiatric hospitalization in children with TS.

Subjects were 156 consecutively referred children and adolescents (ages 5 to 20 years) with TS ascertained through an outpatient pediatric psychopharmacology program at a major academic medical center. All subjects were comprehensively evaluated with a clinical interview by a child and adolescent psychiatrist and an assessment battery that included the KSADS-E (31).

Nineteen (12%) of the 156 children and adolescents with TS required psychiatric hospitalization.

TABLE 21-10. *Co-morbidity of hospitalized versus non-hospitalized patients (N = 156) with Tourette syndrome*

Diagnosis	No hospital (N = 137)		Past hospital (N = 19)		Significance
	N	%	N	%	P
Mood disorders					
Major depressive disorder	59	43.4	17	89.5	0.001
Bipolar disorder	13	9.6	11	57.9	0.001
Dysthymia	10	7.4	0	0	NS
Any mood disorder	68	50	18	94.7	0.001
Anxiety disorders					
Panic disorder	14	10.3	7	36.8	0.002
Agoraphobia	30	22.4	6	31.6	NS
Social phobia	15	11.1	4	21.1	NS
Simple phobia	43	31.9	4	21.1	NS
Obsessive compulsive disorder	30	22.1	10	52.6	0.004
Overanxious disorder	36	26.7	11	61.1	0.003
Separation anxiety	36	26.9	9	50	0.044
Multiple (2+) anxiety disorder	47	34.8	10	52.6	NS
Any anxiety disorder	77	56.6	13	68.4	NS

Adapted from Coffey BJ, Biederman J, Geller D, et al. Distinguishing illness severity from tic severity in children and adolescents with Tourette's disorder. *J Am Acad Child Adolesc Psychiatry.* 2000;39:558.

TABLE 21-11. *Illness severity: univariate and multivariate analyses*

	Univariate beta coefficient	SE	Multivariate beta coefficient	SE	Odds ratio	Standard error	z-score	P
MDD	1.94	0.56	2.07	0.68	7.31	4.76	3.05	0.002
BPD	2.07	0.45	1.45	0.49	4.83	2.32	3.27	0.001
TS impairment	0.64	0.28	0.48	0.30	1.74	0.51	1.92	0.055

BPD, bipolar disorder; MDD, major depressive disorder; TS, Tourette syndrome.
Adapted from Coffey BJ, Biederman J, Geller D, et al. Distinguishing illness severity from tic severity in children and adolescents with Tourette's disorder. *J Am Acad Child Adolesc Psychiatry.* 2000;39:559.

Whereas tic severity was marginally significant as a predictor of psychiatric hospitalization (P <0.05), MD (P <0.016) and bipolar disorder (P <0.001) were robust predictors of psychiatric hospitalization, even after adjusting for all other variables. In addition to psychiatric hospitalization, results were also evaluated using GAF score as a binary variable with GAF <50 as the dependent measure in a multiple logistic regression. This analysis confirmed that when GAF score <50 was the outcome variable, the strongest predictor variables remained bipolar disorder (P <0.001), and MD (P <0.001) (20) (Tables 21-10 and 21-11, and Fig. 21-1). In this study of clinically referred youth with TS, our team reported high rates of mood disorders, and a significant association between mood disorders and overall illness morbidity as measured by need for psychiatric hospitalization (20).

The high prevalence rate for bipolar disorder in children with severe tics is both novel and intriguing. Although the diagnosis of childhood mania remains controversial, recent studies document that it can be reliably made when using structured diagnostic interview methodology (43). Interestingly, the rate of co-morbid bipolar disorder observed in this sample of youth with TS is consistent with findings reported in adults with TS (39). In addition, since severe affective dysregulation, often manifested by temper outbursts and aggression, is characteristic of juvenile bipolar disorder (43,44) it is possible that the explosive outbursts ("rage attacks") recently reported in a substantial minority of youth with

Number of Anxiety Disorders and Tic Severity (N=190)

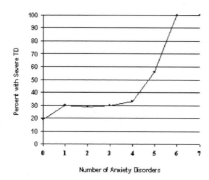

Fig. 21-1. Number of Anxiety Disorders and Tic Severity in 190 Patients. (Adapted with permission from Coffey BJ, Biederman J, Smoller, JW, et al. Anxiety disorders and tic severity in juveniles with Tourette's disorder. *J Am Acad Child Adolesc Psychiatry.* 2000;39:565.)

TS (12) may be a manifestation of undiagnosed bipolar disorder.

TREATMENT CONSIDERATIONS

Overview of Treatment

Because psychiatric co-morbid disorders are so prevalent in clinically referred youth with TS, it is critical to evaluate each individual for the presence of these disorders. TS and co-morbid OCD, mood, and anxiety disorders frequently cluster together; symptoms of each disorder should be evaluated for associated distress and impairment levels. Tics may not always be causing distress or impairment; recent evidence suggests that tics in TS improve as children get older. Thus, tics may simply need monitoring and no treatment (45,46).

If co-morbid conditions are identified as impairing, the next step is parent education regarding the co-morbid mood and anxiety symptoms, and the role these symptoms may be playing in the overall clinical picture. For example, children with significant anxiety symptoms may have an exacerbation of their tics secondary to increased anxiety. The classic situation in which this occurs is the return to school in the fall, at which time many children experience a significant, but most often time limited, increase

in tics related to the transition. Explanation of this phenomenon, and discussion of practical strategies to reduce anxiety is often beneficial.

If multiple co-morbidities are present, the next step is to prioritize the symptoms/diagnostic categories of highest clinical concern. In many cases, the mood and anxiety symptoms will be causing more distress or impairment to the child and/or family than the tics themselves.

The treatment plan should be tailored to the specific diagnostic category or symptoms of most concern. A discussion should take place with the parents and child about the nature of the symptoms/disorder(s) and the available treatments, including evidence for efficacy, of both pharmacologic and non-pharmacologic approaches.

In general, OCD, mood and anxiety disorders should always be treated if they are causing significant impairment or distress to the child. Treatment should be individualized and tailored to the child's specific symptoms and needs, with consideration given to the family's preferences. Developmental issues should be taken into account; for example, for very young children it might be wise to begin with environmental changes, parent guidance, and behavioral strategies rather than medication. In general, a combination of pharmacotherapy with cognitive or behaviorally oriented therapy is helpful.

Tourette Syndrome Plus Obsessive Compulsive Disorder and Other Anxiety Disorders

Medication

For TS plus OCD, in which anxiety symptoms are causing the most distress or impairment, mono-therapy with a selective serotonin reuptake inhibitor (SSRI) is recommended as a first-line approach. SSRI medications with evidence for efficacy in youth for OCD include fluoxetine, fluvoxamine, sertraline, and paroxetine. Clomipramine, a non-SSRI similar in chemical structure to tricyclic antidepressants, is also indicated. Given similar efficacy, the choice of agent will often depend on pharmacokinetic issues such as half-life, potential drug interactions, and side effect profile. Youth are usually started on small doses and titrated up to therapeutic range over several weeks. Adequate duration of a medication trial is approximately 10 to 12 weeks. If there is partial response, the dose can be increased further. If there is no response, switching to another SSRI or clomipramine is indicated. Augmentation strategies with atypical neuroleptics, clonazepam, or buspirone can also be used for partial responders.

The SSRIs are generally well tolerated. Common side effects include gastrointestinal distress, activation, agitation, or akathisia, and headache. There is a small but significant risk of suicidality on SSRIs, so close monitoring is indicated. Side effects can be managed by dosage reduction or switch to another agent in the same class. Clomipramine has a side effect profile similar to that of the tricyclic antidepressants, including weight gain, dry mouth, constipation, and electrocardiogram changes including tachycardia and prolongation of the QTc interval.

Non-Medication Approaches

Cognitive behavioral therapy has been established as an effective treatment for OCD in adults and more recently in youth. The Pediatric OCD Treatment study showed in a multisite randomized controlled trial of 112 youth of sertraline alone, cognitive behavior therapy alone, combined sertraline plus cognitive behavior therapy or placebo, that combination treatment was the most effective treatment overall. However, cognitive behavior therapy alone was effective compared with placebo (48).

Non-OCD Anxiety Disorders

First-line pharmacotherapy for TS and non-OCD anxiety disorders (separation anxiety disorder, generalized anxiety disorder, panic disorder, and social phobia) is also an SSRI, such as fluoxetine, fluvoxamine, and sertraline. There are few randomized controlled studies of these disorders. Clonazepam can be added for short term reduction of non-OCD anxiety or tic flare-ups secondary to anxiety (Table 21-12).

Cognitive-behavioral treatment including relaxation techniques such as breathing exercises and guided imagery for non-OCD anxiety disorders can be helpful.

Tourette Syndrome Plus Mood Disorders

Co-morbid TS and major depressive disorder (MDD) can be treated with an SSRI such as fluoxetine, sertraline, or citalopram. Following review of more than 20 studies, the United States Food and Drug Administration has recently added a black box warning to the use of SSRIs in youth, for evidence suggesting a slightly elevated risk of suicidality (suicidal ideation and behavior) in young patients treated with these agents (47). Approximately 4% of children on medication experienced associated suicidality versus 2% on placebo. In addition, the Food and Drug Administration has published specific guidelines for families and clinicians for youth being treated with the agents (www.parentsmedguide.com). Close monitoring is recommended for the first 4 to 12 weeks of treatment because this appears to represent the period of highest risk. However, because children and adolescents with depression are already at high risk for development of suicidal ideation and behavior, close monitoring of these youth is certainly prudent. As with treatment of OCD, medication should be initiated at a low dose and gradually adjusted upward as tolerated. A reasonable first line approach is fluoxetine, as there is more data available for this agent than other SSRIs; however, its longer half life and greater risk for drug interaction may make its use complicated, and lead to the choice of a shorter acting SSRI with fewer drug interactions.

Co-morbid TS and early onset bipolar disorder can be treated with an atypical neuroleptic such as risperidone, olanzapine, ziprasidone, or aripiprazole. Both the tics and major mood disorder are likely to respond to the atypical neuroleptic (Fig. 21-2). Of the atypical agents, risperidone has been the most widely used. Because the atypical agents are frequently associated with weight gain, sedation, elevated prolactin levels, and extrapyramidal side effects such as akathisia, and Parkinsonism, monitoring of vital signs, height, weight, body mass index, blood lipid profile, and prolactin is indicated at

TABLE 21-12. *Pharmacotherapies for Tourette syndrome and co-morbid disorders in youth*

Co-morbid disorder	Class/Medication	*Starting dose (mg)	*Suggested target daily dose (mg)	Common side effects
Obsessive compulsive disorder	Selective serotonin reuptake inhibitors			
First-line treatment	Fluvoxamine	12.5	75–150	Activation, sedation, gastrointestinal distress. (Potential adverse effect: increased suicidal ideation)
	Fluoxetine	2.5–5	20–60	
	Sertraline	12.5–25	75–150	
	Citalopram	5	20–60	
Non-obsessive compulsive disorder anxiety disorders**	Selective serotonin reuptake inhibitors			
First-line treatment	Fluvoxamine	12.5	75–150	Activation, sedation, gastrointestinal distress. (Potential adverse effect: increased suicidal ideation)
	Fluoxetine	2.5–5	20–40	
	Sertraline	12.5	75–150	
	Benzodiazepine			
Second-line/Adjunctive Short-term treatment	Clonazepam	0.125–0.25	0.5–2.0	Sedation, disinhibition, irritability. dysphoria
Major depressive disorder	Selective serotonin reuptake inhibitors			
First-line treatment	Fluoxetine	2.5–5	20–40	Activation, sedation, gastrointestinal distress. (Potential adverse effect: increased suicidal ideation)
	Sertaline	12.5–25	100–200	
	Citalopram	5	20–40	
Bipolar disorder	Atypical neuroleptics			
First-line treatment	Risperidone	0.125–0.25	1–3	Sedation, extrapyramidal side effects, prolactinemia, weight gain, elevated cholesterol and lipids, blood sugar Extrapyramidal side effects including akathisia
Alternative	Ziprasidone	5–20	20–120	
Alternative	Aripiprazole	1.25–2.5	10–15	

*Starting and suggested target daily doses: lower doses are recommended for prepubertal children, and higher doses for adolescents.

**Non-obsessive compulsive disorder anxiety disorders: social anxiety disorder, generalized anxiety disorder, panic disorder, and social phobia.

baseline and during treatment. Treatment typically begins with low doses, titrated up gradually as tolerated for symptom control. Although no systematic studies have yet been conducted in early onset bipolar disorder and/or TS, these agents may be associated with less appetite increase, and weight gain.

SUMMARY

In summary, OCD, non-OCD anxiety disorders and mood disorders are common co-morbid psychiatric disorders in clinically referred youth with TS. Emotional disorders such as anxiety and depression may be more problematic to the

Tourette's Disorder and Comorbidity: Suggested Treatment Algorithm

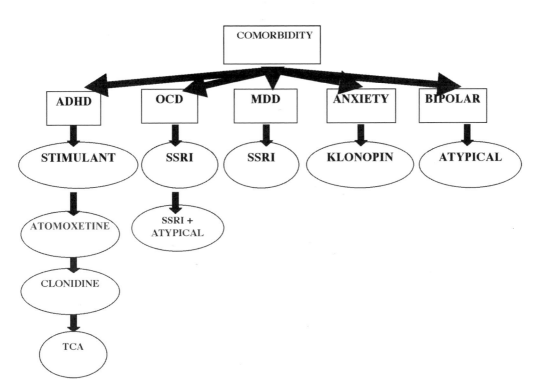

Fig. 21-2. Tourette syndrome and co-morbidity: suggested treatment algorithm.

patient than the tics, with regard to overall illness severity and the potential for adverse outcomes, such as school and social failure. The emotional symptoms and co-morbid mood and anxiety disorders must be comprehensively identified because they will require specific intervention and treatment. Treatment must be tailored to each individual, and should ideally include education, monitoring, and prioritization of symptoms based on distress and impairment. There is growing evidence to support the use of several medications, particularly the selective serotonin reuptake inhibitors, and some cognitive behavioral techniques to treat the psychiatric co-morbid disorders.

ACKNOWLEDGMENTS

This work was supported by Dr. Coffey's career development award MH01415-05 titled Tourette's Disorder in Children: Characterization and Prospective Follow-up of Subtypes.

REFERENCES

1. de la Tourette G. La maladie des tics convulsifs. *La Semaine Medicale*. 1899;19:153–156.
1a. Freud S. Case histories: 2. Frau Emmy von N. In: Breuer J, Freud S. *Studies on Hysteria*. Vienna:1895; chap. II.
2. Coffey B, Miguel E, Savage C, et al. Tourette's disorder and related problems: A review and update. *Harv Rev Psychiatry*. 1994;2:121–132.
3. Frankel M, Cummings JL, Robertson MM, et al. Obsessions and compulsions in Gilles de la Tourette's syndrome. *Neurology* 1986;36:378–382.
4. Comings DE, Comings BG. A controlled study of Tourette syndrome. IV. Obsessions, compulsions, and schizoid behaviors. *Am J Hum Genet.* 1987;41:782–803.
5. Cohen DJ, Leckman JF. Developmental psychopathology and neurobiology of Tourette's syndrome. *J Am Acad Child Adolesc Psychiatry.* 1994;33:2–15.
6. Grad LR, Pelcovits D, Olson M, et al. Obsessive-compulsive symptomatology in children with Tourette's syndrome. *J Am Acad Child Adolesc Psychiatry.* 1987;26:69–73.

7. Rasmussen SA, Eisen JL. Epidemiology and clinical features of obsessive-compulsive disorder. In: Jenike M, Baer L, Minichiello W, eds. *Obsessive Compulsive Disorder: Theory and Management.* 2nd ed. Chicago: Year Book Medical Publishers; 1990;10.

8. Swedo S, Rapoport J, Leonard H, et al. Obsessive compulsive disorder in children and adolescents. *Arch. Gen. Psych.* 1989;46:335.

9. Pauls DL. The genetics of obsessive compulsive disorder and Gilles de la Tourette's syndrome. *Psychiatr Clin North Am.* 1992;15:759–766.

10. Pauls DL, Hurst CR, Kruger SD, et al. Gilles de la Tourette's syndrome and attention deficit disorder with hyperactivity. Evidence against a genetic relationship. *Arch Gen Psychiatry.* 1986;43:1177–1179.

11. Pauls DL, Raymond CL, Stevenson JM, et al. A family study of Gilles de la Tourette syndrome. *Am J Hum Genet.* 1991;48:154–163.

12. Bruun R, Budman C. The course and prognosis of Tourette syndrome. In: Jankovic J, ed. *Tourette Syndrome: Neurologic Clinics.* Philadelphia: WB Saunders; 1997;291–298.

13. Leonard HL, Swedo SE, Rapoport JL, et al. Tourette syndrome and obsessive-compulsive disorder. *Adv Neurol.* 1992;58:83–93.

14. Pitman RK, Green RC, Jenike MA, et al. Clinical comparison of Tourette's disorder and obsessive-compulsive disorder. *Am J Psychiatry.* 1987;144:1166–1171.

15. Coffey B, Miguel E, Biederman J, et al. Tourette's disorder with and without obsessive compulsive disorder: are they different? *J Nerv Mental Dis.* 1998;186:201–215.

16. Coffey B, Frazier J, Chen S. Comorbidity, Tourette syndrome, and anxiety disorders. *Adv Neurol.* 1992; 58:95–104.

17. Comings DE, Comings BG. A controlled study of Tourette syndrome. I. Attention-deficit disorder, learning disorders, and school problems. *Am J Hum Genet.* 1987;41:701–741.

18. Robertson MM, Channon S, Baker J, et al. The psychopathology of Gilles de la Tourette's syndrome: a controlled study. *Br J Psychiatry.* 1993;162:114–117.

19. Coffey BJ, Biederman J, Smoller JW, et al. Anxiety disorders and tic severity in juveniles with Tourette's disorder. *J Am Acad Child Adolesc Psychiatry.* 2000; 39:562–568.

20. Coffey BJ, Biederman J, Geller DA, et al. Distinguishing illness severity from tic severity in children and adolescents with Tourette's disorder. *J Am Acad Child Adolesc Psychiatry.* 2000;39:556–561.

21. Leonard H, Swedo S, Rapoport J. Treatment of childhood obsessive compulsive disorder with clomipramine and desmethylimipramine: a double blind crossover comparison. *Psychopharmacol Bull.* 1988; 24:93–95.

22. Rasmussen SA, Eisen JL. Epidemiology and clinical features of obsessive-compulsive disorder. In: Jenike MA, Baer L, Minichiello W, eds. *Obsessive Compulsive Disorder: Theory and Management.* 2nd ed. Chicago: Year Book Medical Publishers; 1990;10.

23. Swedo S, Leonard H, Rapoport J. Childhood onset obsessive compulsive disorder. In: Jenike MA, Baer L, Minichiello WA, eds. *Obsessive-Compulsive Disorders: Theory and Management.* Boston: Mosby Year Book; 1990;28–38.

24. Comings DE, Comings BG. A controlled study of Tourette syndrome. III. Phobias and panic attacks. *Am J Hum Genet.* 1987;41:761–781.

25. Nolan E, Sverd J, Gadow K, et al. associated psychopathology in children with both ADHD and chronic tic disorder. *J Am Acad Child Adolesc Psychiatry.* 1996;35:1622–1630.

26. Robertson M, Banerjee S, Hiley PJ, et al. Personality disorder and psychopathology in Tourette's syndrome: A controlled study. *Br J Psychiatry.* 1997;171:283–286.

27. Cath D, Spinhoven P, Hoogduin C, et al. Repetitive behaviors in Tourette's syndrome and OCD with and without tics: what are the differences? *Psychiatry Res.* 2001;101:171–185.

28. Stefl ME. Mental health needs associated with Tourette syndrome. *Am J Public Health.* 1984;74: 1310–1313.

29. Singer HS, Rosenberg LA. Development of behavioral and emotional problems in Tourette syndrome. *Pediatr Neurol.* 1989;5:41–44.

30. Coffey B, Biederman J, Spencer T, et al. Informativeness of structured diagnostic interviews in the identification of Tourette's disorder in referred youth. *J Nerv Ment Dis.* 2000;188:583–588.

30a. American Psychiatric Association. *Diagnostic and statistical manual of mental disorders, DSM-IIIR.* Washington, DC: American Psychiatric Press, 1987.

31. Orvaschel H, Puig-Antich J. *Schedule for Affective Disorders and Schizophrenia for School-Age Children: Epidemiologic.* 4th Version. Fort Lauderdale, FL: Nova University, Center for Psychological Study; 1987.

32. de Groot C, Bornstein R, Spetie L, et al. The course of tics. In: Tourette's syndrome: a 5-year follow-up study. *Ann Clin Psychiatry.* 1994;6:227–233.

33. Bornstein RA. Neuropsychological correlates of obsessive characteristics in Tourette syndrome. *J Neuropsychiatry Clin Neurosci.* 1991;3:157–162.

34. Kurlan R, Como PG, Deeley C, et al. A pilot controlled study of fluoxetine for obsessive-compulsive symptoms in children with Tourette's syndrome. *Clin Neuropharmacol.* 1993;16:167–172.

35. Marcus D, Kurlan R. Tics and its disorders. *Neurol Clin* 2001;19:735–758.

36. Steingard R, Dillon-Stout D. Tourette's syndrome and obsessive compulsive disorder: clinical aspects. *Psychiatr Clin North Am.* 1992;15:849–860.

37. Comings BG, Comings DE. A controlled study of Tourette syndrome. V. Depression and mania. *Am J Hum Genet.* 1987;41:804–821.

38. Comings DE, Comings BG. A controlled family history study of Tourette's syndrome, III: affective and other disorders. *J Clin Psychiatry.* 1990;51:288–291.

39. Kerbeshian J, Burd L, Klug M. Comorbid Tourette's disorder and bipolar disorder: an etiologic perspective. *Am J Psychiatry.* 1995;152:1646–1651.

40. Berthier ML, Kulisevsky J, Campos VM. Bipolar disorder in adult patients with Tourette's syndrome: a clinical study. *Biol Psychiatry.* 1998;43:364–370.

41. Shapiro A. Signs, symptoms, and clinical course. In: Shapiro A, Shapiro E, Feinberg T, eds. *Gilles de la Tourette Syndrome.* 1988;169–193.

42. Comings DE, Comings BG. A controlled study of Tourette syndrome. II. Conduct. *Am J Hum Genet.* 1987;41:742–760.

43. Biederman J, Faraone S, Mick E, et al. Attention-deficit hyperactivity disorder and juvenile mania: an

overlooked comorbidity? *J Am Acad Child Adolesc Psychiatry.* 1996;35:997–1008.

44. Wozniak J, Biederman J, Kiely K, et al. Mania-like symptoms suggestive of childhood-onset bipolar disorder in clinically referred children. *J Am Acad Child Adolesc Psychiatry.* 1995;34:867–876.

45. Leckman J, Zhang H, Vitale A, et al. Course of tic severity in Tourette's syndrome: the first two decades. *Pediatrics.* 1998;102:14–19.

46. Coffey B, Biederman J, Geller D, et al. Reexamining tic persistence and tic-associated impairment in Tourette's disorder. Findings from a naturalistic follow-up study. *J Nerv Ment Dis.* 2004;192:776–780.

47. *Physicians' Desk Reference.* 59th ed. Montvale, NJ: Medical Economics Company, Inc; 2005.

48. Pediatric OCD Treatment Study (POTS) Team. Cognitive behavior therapy, sertraline, and their combination for children and adolescents with obsessive compulsive disorder: the Pediatric OCD Treatment Study (POTS) randomized control trial. *JAMA.* 2004; 292:1969–1976.

22

Treatment of Aggression in Tourette Syndrome

Cathy L. Budman

*Departments of Neurology and Psychiatry, North Shore Hospital–Long Island
Jewish Health System, Manhasset, New York*

When present, aggressive symptoms in Tourette syndrome (TS) are a leading cause of morbidity, often associated with severe family distress, impaired interpersonal and/or occupational functioning, psychiatric hospitalizations, and alternative school or residential placements (1–5). Such symptoms encompass both *reactive* and proactive types of aggression including milder temper tantrums, extreme irritability and oppositional-defiant behaviors, explosive outbursts or "rage attacks" as well as bullying or cruelty to animals (1,6–10).

Aggressive symptoms are fairly common in clinical settings where approximately 25% to 70% of TS patients have anger control problems, affective lability, and/or recurrent behavioral dyscontrol (11–16). In a worldwide study of 3,500 outpatients with TS conducted by Freeman et al. (14), 37% reported a history of anger control problems and 25% reported current problems with anger control. A study of 64 outpatients with TS in Japan reported 48% had problems with aggressiveness and impulsivity, 20.3% experienced self-injurious behaviors ranging from head banging to self-mutilation, and 11% suffered domestic violence (17).

Problems with anger control in TS have been reported to occur with significant frequency in community samples as well. For example, among 446 respondents ages 6 to 78 years to a community survey conducted by the Tourette Syndrome Foundation of Canada, 21.4% of children and 15% of adults reported problems with aggression and 30% of children and 19%

of adults described problems with temper control (15). Similarly, a community-based survey of 58 children ages 5 to 15 years in Sweden revealed that 35% were considered by their teachers to suffer from major problems with aggression including repeated verbal assaults, physical aggression or destructive tendencies (18).

RELATIONSHIP WITH PSYCHIATRIC CO-MORBIDITIES

Although the relationship of aggressive symptoms with the underlying tic diathesis of TS has not been fully characterized, some studies suggest that aggressive behavior is not associated with either tic type or severity, but rather with co-morbid psychiatric disorders (1,12,19–22), whereas other studies suggest that aggressive symptoms may correlate with tic severity (23,24), with copro- and echo-phenomenon and a positive family history of tics or TS (25). A clinical study by Stephens and Sandor (20) that examined 33 unmedicated children with TS and aggressive behaviors and compared them with six healthy controls, reported higher rates of co-morbid attention deficit hyperactivity disorder (ADHD) or obsessive compulsive disorder in the aggressive group. In a sample of 113 children with TS between ages 7 to 17 years that compared 48 subjects with explosive outbursts with 65 controls without such symptoms, current co-morbid psychiatric diagnoses of major depression, depression not otherwise specified, bipolar type I, ADHD, oppositional defiant disorder, as well as past history of obsessive compulsive disorder and/or oppositional defiant disorder were all statistically significant predictors of aggressive symptoms (Budman et al. unpublished data, 2003). In this particular study, children with explosive outbursts and TS were also more likely to be receiving mood stabilizers, selective serotonin reuptake inhibitors, or other antidepressants than their control counterparts.

ADHD alone appears to account for a significant proportion of disruptive behaviors in TS patients. In a controlled study of patients from a specialty tic clinic, children with TS-only did not differ from unaffected controls while children with TS and co-morbid ADHD scored significantly higher on both parental and teacher ratings of aggression and delinquent behavior (21,22).

Because most TS clinical studies include subjects with multiple psychiatric co-morbidities that have overlapping symptomatology, it has been difficult to delineate precise causal relationships between particular psychiatric disorders and aggressive symptoms. However, the presentation of aggressive symptoms in a patient with TS should prompt a comprehensive psychiatric and neuropsychological evaluation with thorough review of current psychotropic medications and potential psychosocial stresses.

PHARMACOLOGIC TREATMENT OF AGGRESSION IN TOURETTE SYNDROME

In most cases, effective management of aggression in TS necessitates a combination of both pharmacological and psychosocial interventions. Current research indicates a dichotomy in treatment responsiveness between "impulsive-affective" and "controlled-predatory" subtypes of aggression (26). Impulsive-reactive-affective aggression appears more likely to respond to pharmacologic and psychosocial treatments that target irritability, impulsivity, and arousal whereas controlled, non-reactive, predatory aggressive behaviors are typically addressed with behavioral therapies such as anger management, dialectic behavioral therapy, and relapse prevention programs (27). Because impulsive aggressive symptoms with TS are most commonly

encountered in clinical settings, the following discussion will focus primarily on pharmacological interventions for this specific subtype of aggression.

Although there are few well designed, controlled studies of treatment outcomes for the management of aggressive symptoms in TS, the pharmacologic treatment of impulsive aggression has been evaluated in other psychiatric populations such as in patients with ADHD, conduct disorder, borderline personality disorder, depression, bipolar disorder, intermittent explosive disorder, autism and pervasive developmental disorders, and mental retardation as well as in patients with traumatic head injury or dementia.

A variety of medication classes have been employed to target aggression including: serotonin (5-hydroxytryptophan [5HT]) IA agonists, 5HT2 antagonists, selective serotonin reuptake inhibiters, mixed serotonin/norepinephrine reuptake inhibitors, lithium anticonvulsants, anxiolytics, typical and atypical neuroleptics, $\alpha2$ agonists, β-blockers, opiate antagonists and dopamine agonists (28,29).

The selective serotonin reuptake inhibitors, particularly fluoxetine, fluvoxamine, and sertraline have been most extensively studied for the management of aggressive symptoms (30–32). Citalopram has shown efficacy in an open-label study for the treatment of children and adolescents with impulsive-affective aggression (33). Paroxetine was shown to reduce rage attack frequency and severity in an open-label, uncontrolled study of 45 children and adult with TS and explosive outbursts (34). Trazadone, a weak inhibitor of serotonin reuptake, has been shown in an open-label study to reduce aggressive and impulsive behaviors in hospitalized children with conduct disorder (35).

Mood stabilizers such as carbamazepine, diphenylhydantoin, divalproex sodium, and lithium have demonstrated efficacy in recent placebo-controlled trials of adolescents with explosive outbursts, in children with conduct disorder, and in adult patients with personality disorders and other psychiatric conditions associated with aggressive symptoms (36–41).

Although the conventional neuroleptics have historically been used effectively for reducing aggressive symptoms in a variety of clinical populations, risks of drug-induced tardive dyskinesia, parkinsonism, akathisia, and acute dystonic reactions have lead to their replacement by newer alternatives with relatively fewer adverse side effects. The atypical neuroleptics such as clozapine, risperidone, ziprasidone, and olanzapine have been shown in controlled studies to reduce aggressive behaviors in a variety of conditions (42–50). Among the atypical neuroleptics, risperidone has been widely studied for treatment of aggression in children particularly in subnormal intelligence, pervasive developmental and autistic populations (51–53). Double-blind, placebo-controlled trials have also demonstrated efficacy of risperidone for the treatment of aggressive symptoms in children with conduct disorder (54). Sandor and Stephens (55) reported efficacy of risperidone monotherapy for treatment of aggressive symptoms in children with TS.

The psychostimulants are also helpful for reducing the symptoms of aggression associated with ADHD, such as irritability, anger outbursts, physical assaults, and other conduct problems, particularly in the absence of co-morbid conduct disorder or mental retardation (56). Alpha-adrenergic agonists such as clonidine or guanfacine, either alone or in combination with a psychostimulant have been shown to reduce aggressive behaviors in children with conduct disorder or oppositional defiant disorder (57,58). Beta-agonists such as propranolol, have been reported to be effective for reducing aggressive behaviors in patients with dementia, personality disorders, and traumatic brain injuries (59).

SUMMARY

The largely non-specific and/or multiply-determined etiologies of aggressive symptoms in TS pose significant impediments to effective clinical management. At this time, treatment requires comprehensive neuropsychiatric assessment with a systematic prioritization of the different psychiatric co-morbidities that require intervention. Medication side effects, psychosocial stressors and environmental triggers must also be identified and addressed. The future

elucidation of meaningful clinical and genetic subtypes of TS will have important consequences for the more specific prevention and treatment of aggressive symptoms.

REFERENCES

1. Budman C, Park K, Olson M, Bruun R. Rage attacks in children and adolescents with Tourette syndrome: a pilot study. *J Clin Psychiatry*. 1998;59:576–580.
2. Budman C, Feirman L. The relationship of Tourette's syndrome with its psychiatric comorbidities: is there an overlap? *Psych Annals*. 2000;31:541–548.
3. Coffey B, Biederman J, Geller B, et al. Distinguishing illness severity from tic severity in children and adolescents with Tourette's disorder. *J Amer Acad Child Adolesc Psychiatry*. 2000;39:556–561.
4. Dooley J, Brna P, Gordon K. Parent perceptions of symptoms severity in Tourette's Syndrome. *Arch Dev Child*. 1999;81:440–441.
5. Leckman J, Cohen D, eds. *Tourette's Syndrome: Tics, Obsessions, Compulsions: Developmental Pscyhopathology and Clinical Care*. New York: Wiley; 1999; 155–176.
6. Dodge K. The structure and function of reactive and proactive aggression. In: Pepler D, Rubin K, eds. *The development and treatment of childhood aggression*. Hillsdale, NY: Erlbaum; 1991:201–208.
7. Stefl M. Mental health needs associated with Tourette Syndrome. *Amer J Pub Health*. 1984;74:1310–1313.
8. Nee L, Polinsky R, Eldridge R, et al. Gilles de la Tourette syndrome: clinical and family study of 50 cases. *Ann Neurol*. 1980;7:41–49.
9. Robertson M, Banerjee S, Fox Hiley P, et al. Personality disorder and psychopathology in Tourette's syndrome: a controlled study. *Br J Psychiatry*. 1997;171:283–286.
10. Erenberg G, Cruse R, Rothner A. The natural history of Tourette syndrome: a follow-up study. *Ann Neurol*. 1987;22:383–385.
11. King R, Scahill L. Emotional and behavioral difficulties associated with Tourette syndrome. In: Cohen D, Goetz C, Jankovic J, eds. *Tourette Syndrome*. Philadelphia, PA: Lippincott Williams & Wilkins; 2001:79–88.
12. Budman C, Bruun R, Park K, et al. Explosive outbursts in children with Tourette syndrome. *J Amer Acad Child Adolesc Psychiatry*. 2000;39:1270–1276.
13. Comings D, Comings B. Tourette syndrome: clinical and psychological aspects of 250 cases. *Amer J Hum Genet*. 1985;37:435–450.
14. Freeman R, Rast D, Burd L, et al. An international perspective on Tourette syndrome: selected findings from 3500 cases in 22 countries. *Dev Med Child*. 2000; 42:436–447.
15. Wand R, Matazow A, Shady G, et al. Tourette syndrome: associated symptoms and most disabling features. *Neurosci & Biobehav Rev*. 1993;17:272–275.
16. Santangelo S, Pauls D, Goldstein J. Tourette syndrome: what are the influences of gender and comorbid obsessive compulsive disorder? *J Amer Acad Child Adolesc Psychiatry*. 1994;33:795–804.
17. Kano Y, Ohta M, Nagai Y. Clinical characteristics of Tourette syndrome. *Psychiatry Clinical Neurosci*. 1998; 52:51–57.

18. Kadesjo B, Gillberg C. Tourette's disorder: epidemiology and comorbidity in primary school children. *J Am Acad Child Adolesc Psychiatry*. 2000;39:548–555.

19. Erenberg G, Cruse R, Rothner A. Tourette syndrome. *Cleve Clin Q*. 1986;53:127–131.

20. Stephens R, Sandor P. Aggressive behavior in children with Tourette syndrome and comorbid attention-deficit hyperactivity disorder and obsessive compulsive disorder. *Can J Psychiatry*. 1999;44:1036–1042.

21. Carter A, O'Donnell D, Schultz R, et al. Social and emotional adjustment in children affected with Gilles de al Tourette's syndrome: associations with ADHS and family functioning. *J Child Psychol Psychiatry*. 2000; 41:215–223.

22. Spencer T, Biederman J, Harding M, et al. Disentangling the overlap between Tourette's disorder and ADHD. *J Child Psychol Psychiatry*. 1998;39:1037–1044.

23. DeGroot C, Janus M, Bornstein R. Clinical predictors of psychopathology in children and adolescents with Tourette syndrome. *J Psychiatr Res*. 1995;29:59–70.

24. Nolan E, Sverd J, Gadow K, et al. Associated pathology in children with both ADHD and chronic tic disorder. *J Am Acad Child Adolesc Psychiatry*. 1996;35: 1622–1630.

25. Robertson M, Trimble M, Lees A. The psychopathology of the Gilles de la Tourette syndrome. A phenomenological analysis. *Brit J Psychiatry*. 1988;152: 383–390.

26. Vitielo B, Stoff D. Subtypes of aggression and their relevance to child psychiatry. *J Amer Acad Child Adolesc Psychiatry*. 1997;36:307–315.

27. Malone R, Bennett D, Luebbert J, et al. Aggression classification and treatment response. *Psychopharm Bull*. 1998;34:41–45.

28. Campbell M, Gonzales N, Silva R. The pharmacologic treatment of conduct disorder and rage outbursts. *Psych Clin North Amer*. 1992;15:69–85.

29. Pallanti S, Baldini Ross N, Friedberg J, et al. Psychobiology of impulse-control disorders not otherwise specified (NOS). In: D'haenen H, den Boer J, Willner P, eds. *Biological Psychiatry*. New York: John Wiley & Sons; 2000.

30. Coccaro E, Kavoussi R. Fluoxetine and impulsive aggressive behavior in personality-disordered subjects. *Arch Gen Psychiatry*. 1997;54:1088–1091.

31. Fava M, Rosenbaum J. Anger attacks in depression. *Depress Anxiety*. 1998;8:59–63.

32. Feder R. Treatment of intermittent explosive disorder with sertraline in three patients. *J Clin Psychiatry*. 1999;60:195–196.

33. Amenteros J, Lewis J. Citalopram treatment for impulsive aggression in children and adolescents: An open study. *J Am Acad Child Adolesc Psychiatry*. 2002;159: 266–273.

34. Bruun R, Budman C. Paroxetine treatment of episodic rages associated with Tourette's disorder. *J Clin Psychiatry*. 1998;59:581–584.

35. Zubieta J, Alessi N. Acute and chronic administration of trazodone in the treatment of disruptive behavior disorders in children. *J Clin Psychopharm*. 1992;12: 346–351.

36. Coccaro E, Siever L. Pathophysiology and treatment of aggression. In: David K, Charney D, Coyle J, et al, eds. *Neuropsychopharmacology*. Philadelphia: Lippincott Williams & Wilkins; 2002:1709–1723.

37. Campbell M, Adams P, Small A, et al. Lithium in hospitalized aggressive children with conduct disorder: a double-blind and placebo-controlled study. *J Am Acad Child Adolesc Psychiatry*. 1995;34:445–453.

38. Donovan S, Stewart J, Nunes E, et al. Divalprex treatment for youth with explosive temper and mood lability: a double-blind, placebo-controlled crossover design. *Am J Psychiatry*. 2000;157:818–820.

39. Hollander E, Tracy K, Swann A, et al. Divalproex in the treatment of impulsive aggression: efficacy in cluster B personality disorders. *Neuropsychopharm* 2003;28(6): 1186–1197.

40. Lewin J, Summers D. Successful treatment of episodic dyscontrol with carbamazepine. *Br J Psychiatry*. 1992; 161:262–262.

41. Malone R, Delaney M, Luebbert J, et al. A double-blind placebo-controlled study of lithium in hospitalized aggressive children and adolescents with conduct disorder. *Arch Gen Psychiatry*. 2000;57:649–654.

42. Benedetti F, Sforzini L, Colombo C, et al. Low-dose clozapine in acute and continuation treatment of sever borderline personality disorder. *J Clin Psychiatry*. 1998;59:103–107.

43. Chen N, Bedair H, McKay B, et al. Clozapine in the treatment of aggression in an adolescent with autistic disorder (letter). *J Clin Psychiatry*. 2001;62:479–480.

44. Chengappa K, Vaslie J, Levine J, et al. Clozapine: its impact on aggressive behavior among patients in a state psychiatric hospital. *Schizophren Res*. 2002;53:1–6.

45. Findling R, McNamara N, Branicky L, et al. A double-blind pilot study of risperidone in the treatment of conduct disorder. *J Amer Acad Child Adolesc Psychiatry*. 2000;39:509–516.

46. Krishnamoorthy J, King B. Open-label olanzapine treatment in five preadolescent children. *J Child Adolesc Psychopharma*. 1998;8:107–113.

47. McDougal D, Holmes J, Carlson D, et al. A double-blind placebo-controlled study of risperidone in adults with autistic disorder and other pervasive developmental disorders. *Arch Gen Psychiatry*. 1998;55:633–641.

48. McDougle C, Kem D, Posey D. Case series: use of ziprasidone for maladaptive symptoms in youths with autism. *J Am Acad Child Adolesc Psychiatry*. 2002; 41:921–927.

49. Scheier H. Risperidone for young children with mood disorders and aggressive behavior. *J Child Adolesc Psychopharmacol*. 1998;8:49–59.

50. Synder R, Turgay Aman M, Fisman S. Effects of risperidone on conduct and disruptive behavior disorders in children with subaverage IQs. *J Am Acad Child Adolesc Psychiatry*. 2002;41:1026–1036.

51. Buitelaar J, wan der Gaag R, Cohen-Kettenis P, et al. A randomized controlled trial of risperidone in the treatment of aggression in hospitalized adolescents with subaverage cognitive abilities. *J Clin Psychiatry*. 2001;62:239–248.

52. Aman M, De Smeat G, Derivan A, et al. Double-blind placebo controlled study of risperidone in the treatment of disruptive behaviors in children with subaverage intelligence. *Am J Psychiatry*. 2002;159:1337–1346.

53. McCracken J, McGough H, Shah G, et al. Risperidone in children with autism and serious behavioral problems. *N Eng J Med*. 2002;347:314–321.

54. Findling R, McNamara N, Branicky L, et al. A double-bind pilot study of risperidone for the treatment of

conduct disorder. *J Am Acad Child Adolesc Psychiatry*. 2000;39:509–516.

55. Sandor P, Stephens R. Risperidone treatment of aggressive behavior in children with Tourette's syndrome. *J Clin Psychopharmacol*. 2000;20:710–712.

56. Connor D, Glatt S, Lopez I, et al. Psychopharmacology and aggression. I. A Meta-analysis of stimulant effects on overt/covert aggression-related behavior in ADHD. *J Am Acad Child Adolesc Psychiatry*. 2002;41: 253–261.

57. Connor D, Barkley R, David H. A pilot study of methylphenidate, clonidine, or the combination in ADHD comorbid with aggressive oppositional defiant or conduct disorder. *Clin Pediatr*. 2000;3915–3925.

58. Kemph J, De Vane C, Levin G, et al. Treatment of aggressive children with clonidine: results of an open pilot study. *J Am Acad Child Adolesc Psychiatry*. 1993;32:577–581.

59. Haspel T. Beta-blockers and the treatment of aggression. *Harv Rev Psychiatry*. 1995;23:274–281.

23

Behavioral Treatments for Tic Suppression: Habit Reversal Training

John C. Piacentini and Susanna W. Chang

Department of Psychiatry and Biobehavioral Sciences, University of California–Los Angeles
Los Angeles, California

Although initially developed more than 30 years ago (1), habit reversal training (HRT) has only recently begun to garner widespread acceptance as a viable treatment approach for tic suppression primarily due to positive findings from recent efficacy trials (2) along with an enhanced understanding of what the treatment entails and how it may work. While psychopharmacological approaches remain the most common form of intervention for Tourette syndrome and other chronic tic disorders (CTD), notable side effects, lack of efficacy for some, need for chronic use, and concerns regarding medication use in children serve to limit the utility of medication in many cases (3–6). Recent efforts to more fully establish the efficacy of HRT for tic suppression, including parallel child and adult controlled multi-site treatment trials currently underway by the Tourette Syndrome Association Behavioral Sciences Consortium (TSA BSC), should serve to further enhance treatment options for those tic patients desiring nonmedication treatment or for whom pharmacologic approaches have been hampered by side effects or less than optimal response. This chapter presents a description of HRT and provides a review of available efficacy data for this treatment.

DESCRIPTION OF HABIT REVERSAL TRAINING

HRT is a multicomponent behavioral treatment package originally developed to address a wide variety of repetitive behavior disorders including not only tics, but also trichotillomania, nail biting, thumb sucking, and skin picking (1). Azrin and Nunn described HRT as consisting of five primary intervention components: awareness training, competing response training, contingency management, relaxation training, and generalization training. These components were designed to increase tic awareness, develop an incompatible physical response to tics (i.e., competing response), and/or build and sustain treatment motivation and compliance (7–11).

Awareness training consists of five subcomponents designed to enhance awareness of all tic urges and behaviors as well as specific triggers and environmental factors associated with tic expression. Response description entails having the patient provide a detailed description of the topography of his or her tics (including a detailed description of each tic, the frequency with which each tic occurs, and the presence of any associated premonitory urges, physical sensations, or other triggering factors). Response description is often facilitated by having the patient practice his or her tic in front of a mirror or through use of videotape. During the response detection phase of treatment, the therapist notes to the patient each time the patient performs a previously selected tic, followed by the patient noting these occurrences himself or herself. This procedure is repeated until the patient can reliably identify 80% of tic occurrences. The third component of awareness training involves enhancing awareness of any premonitory urges or sensations associated with tic occurrence using the response detection procedure described previously. Although the presence of a premonitory urge is not mandatory for HRT to be successful, the identification of a premonitory urge prior to tic occurrence can facilitate HRT efficacy by signaling the patient to begin the competing response prior to the onset of tic expression.

During self-monitoring, the fourth awareness training component, patients are asked to record each occurrence of the targeted tic or tics using a wrist counter or paper and pencil. The length of the daily self-monitoring period depends on the frequency of the targeted tic (perhaps ten minutes at a time for a very frequent tic, increasing in length for tics occurring less often). Finally, during situation awareness training, a functional analytic approach is used to identify high risk situations (e.g., places, events, and/or the presence/absence of specific people) where tic are most likely to occur. The identification of situations associated with the highest likelihood of tic expression provides the opportunity for the individual to begin practicing tic management procedures prior to the onset of tic performance. For example, a child who tics most frequently shortly after arriving home at the end of the school day, may elect to practice relaxation training or competing response training immediately upon arriving home instead of waiting for the tics to begin.

The mechanisms underlying the efficacy of the awareness training component of HRT are not well understood, although a number of hypotheses have been put forth. Azrin and Peterson's (1988) speculated that tic reduction was due to increased awareness of tic occurrence. However, this is not supported by the fact that decreases in tic frequency occur even for subjects with limited ability to accurately monitor their tics or who are unable to reliably identify tic occurrence in session (e.g., 12). Others have postulated that self-monitoring may serve to make tic occurrence an aversive event (e.g., via social evaluation or demand characteristics) or that monitoring activities serve as punishers, from an operant conditioning perspective, for tic expression (12–13).

The most distinctive component of habit reversal is the competing response. To be maximally effective, the competing response should be: A) opposite to or incompatible with the tic movement, B) capable of being maintained until the urge to tic has subsided (generally about one minute), C) socially inconspicuous, or at least less conspicuous than the targeted tic, and D) compatible with normal ongoing activity (7). Most commonly, competing response involves isometric tensing of those muscles opposite to the tic movement. In the case of vocal tics, the most commonly used competing response involves slow, rhythmic breathing through the nose. Significant creativity and flexibility may be needed to identify an optimal competing response for some tics. It may not be as important to identify a competing response that is exactly opposite the targeted tic as it is to develop a response that the patient is able to easily and discretely implement. In situations where the tic movement is particularly intense or forceful, a shaping procedure may be used whereby the initial competing response training involves efforts to simply slow down or slightly change expression of the tic (e.g., running one's fingers through their hair to end an arm-jerking tic) (9). As the child gains greater control over the targeted tic, the competing response is shaped to become increasingly more forceful with the ultimate goal of greater tic control. Given that the paroxysmal aspects are typically the most noticeable, distressing, and physically damaging features of tic behaviors, attempts to "slow down" or "de-intensify" targeted tics through the use of shaping procedures may be helpful in some cases.

Competing response training is usually implemented according to a hierarchy of tic symptoms. However, unlike behavioral treatment of obsessive-compulsive disorder where mildest symptoms are targeted first (e.g., 14), in HRT, the most disruptive or frequent tic is often targeted first since the benefits of initial response will often generalize to other, less severe tics. Patients are taught to implement the competing response as soon as they recognize the premonitory urge or sensation. In situations where there is no premonitory urge or for particularly complex tics, the competing response is initiated in response to the initial portion of the tic sequence. Carr (15) provides a list of competing responses for the most commonly seen tics.

The contingency management aspect of HRT is designed to enhance motivation for treatment and maximize compliance with treatment procedures. Social support training refers to the practice of using parents, spouses or other key family members to prompt use of the competing response when appropriate and to provide positive reinforcement for successful use of the procedure (10,16). More structured reward systems are also a useful adjunct for children and adolescents who are less likely than adults to self-refer and, as such, may evidence poorer motivation and compliance. Another motivational procedure is creation of the habit inconvenience review in which the therapist assists the patient in creating a list of all the ways in which his or her tics have been embarrassing, inconvenient, distressing, or impairing. As treatment progresses and the negative aspects of the child's tic disorder dissipate, inconvenience review items that are no longer present are ceremoniously crossed off the list.

The inclusion of relaxation training in HRT is based on the observation that increased stress and/or anxiety often exacerbate tic expression (17). Although a variety of case report and analogue studies (18,19) and one recent controlled trial (20) have not found anxiety management by itself to lead to sustained tic reduction, when included with HRT, relaxation training may have some utility especially for individuals with increased levels of anxiety and/or stress (10). The final HRT component, generalization training, is designed to facilitate the use of those treatment techniques practiced in the clinic and at home in other real world settings. Generalization training typically involves having the patient practice competing response and other treatment techniques in public settings, review of all competing responses covered in treatment, and generation of competing responses for tics not currently present nor targeted in treatment in order to demonstrate generalized knowledge of the principles underlying HRT. The goal of generalization training is to ensure that individuals will be able to generate, on their own, effective intervention strategies for tics that may arise in the future.

DISMANTLING HABIT REVERSAL TRAINING COMPONENTS

Several modifications to the original HRT protocol have been suggested and tested. A number of investigators have considered awareness training and competing response as the only essential components of HRT (21–24), Woods, Miltenberger, and Lumley. Miltenberger, Fuqua, and McKinley (23) found that awareness plus competing response training were as effective for tic reduction as the full Azrin and Nunn procedure. Additionally, this research group established that the competing response must be performed contingently on expression of the targeted tic (22) but it did not have to involve topographically-similar muscles as the targeted tic in all cases (25). Woods, Miltenberger, and Lumley (24) used a multiple baseline design to test four primary HRT components in order of effort (awareness training, self-monitoring, social support and competing response) in four children with motor tics. Although all four youngsters showed a positive treatment response, each child responded to a different combination of interventions. Moreover, compliance tended to decrease as the demands of treatment increased. Collectively, the results of these dismantling studies suggest that the relative contribution of the various HRT components may differ by individual. As a result, use of the full HRT protocol is the preferred approach in most situations (7).

POTENTIAL MECHANISMS OF HABIT REVERSAL TRAINING EFFICACY

Although a growing body of evidence supports the efficacy of HRT for tics, the mechanisms underlying habit reversal remain to be fully elucidated. As noted previously, early hypotheses that HRT efficacy stemmed from heightened tic awareness and strengthening of muscles incompatible with tic expression due to competing response practice, are not consistent with the observed efficacy of topographically-dissimilar competing responses in some cases (25). Others have focused on the aversive nature of the competing response and suggested that it functions as a punisher, in an operant sense, when performed contingently on tic occurrence (22).

More recent conceptualizations of tic maintenance and HRT efficacy have also focused on operant conditioning, albeit from the perspective of negative reinforcement and not punishment paradigms. While strong support exists for a neurobiologic etiology for TS and other CTDs (e.g., 26), evidence also exists supporting the role of environmental factors in the expression and maintenance of tic symptoms (27). Recent behavioral conceptualizations have emphasized the role of premonitory sensory phenomena in an integrative model of tic expression and maintenance (28). Several studies have reported that premonitory urges or sensory phenomena are common antecedents of tic expression (29–33). Most commonly, these premonitions are described as a sense of building tension or a strong urge that are relieved by performance of the associated tic.

Shapiro and Shapiro (34) were among the first to describe the relationship between sensory phenomena and tics as possibly analogous to the relationship between obsessions and compulsions in OCD, although OCD-related compulsions are characteristically triggered by cognitive stimuli and/or physiologic symptoms of anxiety as opposed to sensory phenomena (35). Moreover, while tics have historically been described as involuntary and uncontrollable behaviors, Leckman et al. (36) found that more than 90% of individuals with a tic disorder reported experiencing their tics as controllable or even volitional at times. Premonitory urges and volition both appear to be developmentally related (28). Younger children are less likely to describe their tics as controllable, and premonitory urges are typically absent or much less coherent in children younger than age 10 years (28,37). In addition, simple tics such as eye blinking, are less likely to be controllable than more complex tics.

The fact that tic expression typically leads to relief of the associated premonitory sensation (33), argues that some tics may be negatively reinforced by the contingent dissipation of this noxious state (38). If so, then the efficacy of HRT may be related to disruption of this negative reinforcement cycle since implementation of the competing response serves to preclude performance of the tic and contingent relief of discomfort associated with the premonitory urge. In other words, the use of a competing response to block tic expression and subsequent relief from the associated premonitory urge will ultimately lead to extinction of that premonition as well as the associated tic. Anecdotally, the observation that HRT is often more difficult to implement in very young children and for very simple tics, which are less likely to be triggered by noticeable premonitions, is consistent with the negative reinforcement model. However, this may also reflect the fact that older individuals are typically better able to accurately monitor their tics, especially those that are more complex (e.g., more likely to be accompanied by premonitory sensations).

The negative reinforcement model is also consistent with conceptualization of HRT as a form of exposure plus response prevention, the primary behavioral treatment for obsessive compulsive disorder (39). Recent reports describing successful use of exposure-based interventions for tic suppression provide additional support for this hypothesis (40,41). Additional research is necessary to more thoroughly identify and understand potential mechanisms for HRT efficacy, including enhanced efforts to identify potential neurocognitive factors and biological substrates underlying these processes.

HABIT REVERSAL TRAINING EFFICACY

The efficacy of HRT for tic suppression has been evaluated in dozens of studies, although most of these involved single-case or small case-series designs. However six randomized between-subject studies have been published to date (2,41–45).

Azrin and Peterson (42) used a wait-list controlled design to examine HRT efficacy in fourteen individuals with Tourette syndrome.

Groups were matched for age, medication usage, and tic frequency, and a multimodal assessment strategy, including direct videotape observation of tics, was used to measure outcome. Results indicated an 89% decrease in home-based tic frequency post-HRT improving to 92% decrease at 12 month follow-up. This was in contrast to no change in tic frequency for the comparison group over the three-month wait-list interval. Secondary analyses found HRT to be equally effective for motor and vocal tics with no evidence of symptom substitution. O'Connor et al. (44) found both HRT alone and in combination with cognitive-behavior therapy to be effective for tic reduction in individuals with CTD with cognitive-behavior therapy conferring no additional benefit over that derived from HRT alone. In a second study, O'Connor et al. (45) found HRT superior to wait-list control with 65% of HRT recipients reporting 75% to 100% control over tics post-treatment and 52% reporting this level of control at two year follow-up.

In a study funded by the TSA, Wilhelm et al. (2) randomized a total of 32 adults with CTD to either HRT or a supportive psychotherapy control group (SP). Both treatments consisted of 14 sessions delivered according to detailed treatment manuals. Treatment with HRT was associated with a significant decline in tic severity on the Yale Global Tic Severity Scale (46) (35%; from a mean of $30.5 + 7.13$ at baseline to $19.81 + 7.58$ post-treatment, $P < 0.01$). This mean post-treatment score was significantly lower than the mean for the SP group ($26.88 + 9.19$, $P < 0.05$). HRT was also shown to be durable with individuals in this condition evidencing significantly lower tic severity scores at 10 month follow-up compared to baseline ratings. The Wilhelm et al. study is notable for several design strengths, including the use of a well-characterized and psychiatrically complex sample, a credible psychosocial comparison treatment, and standardized clinical assessment measures. However, study findings need to be evaluated in light of the small sample size and the lack of blind outcome raters.

Verdellen et al. (41) compared HRT to exposure plus response prevention in 43 adults with

TS. Outcome was assessed using a variety of methods including the Yale Global Tic Severity Scale and home and clinic-based tic frequency counts. Both HRT and exposure plus response prevention led statistically significant improvements on all outcome measures. Of interest, there were no significant differences between the two treatments on any of the outcome measures.

Piacentini et al. (47), also funded by TSA, compared standard HRT with an awareness training procedure in 25 children and adolescents (mean age 10.7, 80% male, 48% on stable medications at baseline) with CTD. Youngsters in the awareness training condition were instructed to say the letter "T," either aloud or silently depending on the circumstance, upon each occurrence of the targeted tic or tics. In essence, this condition was analogous to "fixed competing response" HRT with saying "T" serving as the competing response. Both interventions were well accepted and tolerated. Approximately half of the youngsters receiving standard HRT evidenced a clinically significant response as rated by blind clinical interviewers. Although the HRT response rate was approximately twice that found for the awareness training group, this difference was not statistically significant. In addition, response to HRT was durable with treatment gains maintained over a 3-month follow-up period. Similar to Wilhelm et al. (2), the findings from this study must be evaluated in light of the small sample size and limited statistical power to find between group differences. Of interest, neither of the two TSA-funded trials (2,47) found a relationship between response to HRT and baseline medication status suggesting that HRT works equally well as monotherapy or adjunct to medication.

Although highly supportive, the HRT efficacy literature to date can be characterized by a number of design limitations, including relatively small sample sizes, limited characterization of study participants, limited data on children and adolescents, lack of attention to the assessment of treatment integrity and adherence, and limited attention to the identification of potential clinical and neurocognitive mechanisms and predictors of treatment response. In order to address these limitations, the TSA BSC was formed in 2000.

The TSA BSC was charged with the task of developing a research plan for the further development and testing of psychosocial interventions, most notably HRT, for the treatment of CTD. The TSA BSC consists of child and adult Tourette syndrome researchers from Johns Hopkins University, Massachusetts General Hospital/Harvard University; University of California at Los Angeles, University of Wisconsin-Milwaukee, Wilford Hall Medical Center/University of Texas Health Sciences Center at San Antonio, and the Yale Child Study Center. TSA BSC members have collectively been funded by National Institute of Mental Health to conduct two parallel multisite controlled HRT treatment studies for child and adult CTD, respectively. In total, 240 individuals aged 8 to 65 years will be randomized to either HRT or a comparison psychoeducation/supportive therapy condition. HRT will be administered using parallel child and adult treatment manuals developed by this group and incorporating state-of-the-art treatment elements derived from the work of both HAS BSC members and other leading HRT researchers. In addition to providing definitive data about the efficacy and intermediate-term (six month) durability of HRT for CTD, the TSA BSC trials also seek to identify developmental, clinical, psychosocial, and neurocognitive predictors of treatment response. Results from the BSC trials should be available in 2008.

CONCLUSIONS

Numerous smaller-scale studies, including at least six controlled trials, have documented the acceptability, tolerability, efficacy, and durability of HRT for children, adolescents, and adults with CTD. Collectively, this body of research, although tempered by a number of design limitations, supports the use of HRT as a viable first-line or adjunctive (to medication) intervention for tic suppression across the age span. Large-scale randomized controlled trials currently in progress should provide definite evidence regarding HRT efficacy and also provide needed information regarding potential mechanisms of efficacy and predictors of treatment response.

Given that medication is either not a viable option for many individuals with CTD, due to

history or personal choice, or else results in only partial amelioration of tic symptoms, the establishment of HRT as an effective intervention will provide CTD sufferers with a broader range of treatment options and the chance for even better outcomes including enhanced psychosocial functioning. Ultimately, additional controlled trials examining the comparative efficacy of HRT alone and in combination with psychopharmacologic approaches will be necessary to address the question of which treatments (HRT, medication, combined treatment) work best for which individuals under which conditions. In the interim, it is highly reasonable to conclude that based on the existing literature, HRT either alone or in combination with medication should be considered as a viable treatment option for CTD in both children and adolescents.

REFERENCES

1. Azrin NH, Nunn RG. Habit reversal: a method of eliminating nervous habits and tics. *Behav Res Ther*. 1973; 11:619–628.
2. Wilhelm S, Deckersbach T, Coffey BJ, et al. Habit reversal versus supportive psychotherapy for Tourette's disorder: a randomized controlled trial. *Am J Psychiatry*. 2003;160:1175–1177.
3. Carpenter L, Leckman J, Scahill L, et al. Pharmacological and other somatic approaches to treatment. In: Cohen DJ, Leckman JF, Bruun RD, eds. *Tourette Syndrome and Tic Disorders: Clinical Understanding and Treatment*. New York: Wiley; 1988:370–398.
4. Scahill L, Chappell PB, King RA, et al. Pharmacologic treatment of tic disorders. *Psychopharmacology* 2000; 9:99–117.
5. Silva R, Munoz D, Daniel W, et al. Causes of discontinuation in patients with Tourette's disorder: management and alternatives. *J Clin Psychiatry*. 1996;57: 129–135.
6. The Tourette Syndrome Study Group. Short versus longer term pimozide therapy in Tourette's syndrome: a preliminary study. *Neurology* 1999;52:874–877.
7. Peterson A, Woods D, Piacentini J. Psychosocial management of tics and intentional repetitive behaviors. In: Woods D, Piacentini J, Walkup J, eds. *Management of Tourette's Syndrome*. New York: Guilford. In press.
8. Peterson AL, Campise RL, Azrin NH. Behavioral and pharmacological treatments for tic and habit disorders: A review. *J Dev Behav Pediat*. 1994;15:430–441.
9. Piacentini J, Chang S. Behavioral treatments for Tourette syndrome: state of the art. In: Cohen DJ, Jankovic J, Goetz C, eds. *Advances in Neurology: Tourette Syndrome* Vol. 85. Philadelphia: Lippincott Williams & Wilkins; 2001:319–332.
10. Piacentini J, Chang S. Habit Reversal Training for Tic Disorders in Children and Adolescents, Behavior Modification. 2005;29:1–21.
11. Woods DW, Miltenberger RG. *Tic Disorders, Trichotillomania, and Other Repetitive Behavior Disorders:*

Behavioral Approaches to Analysis and Treatment. Norwell, MA: Kluwer Academic Publishers; 2001.

12. Wright K, Miltenberger R. Awareness training in the treatment of head and facial tics. *J Behav Ther Exp Psychiatry.* 1987;18:269–274.

13. Azrin NH, Peterson AL. Behavior therapy for Tourette's syndrome and tic disorders. In: Cohen DJ, Leckman JF, Bruun RD, eds. *Tourette Syndrome and Tic Disorders: Clinical Understanding and Treatment.* New York: Wiley; 1988:237–255.

14. Piacentini J, Langley A. Cognitive-behavior therapy for children with obsessive compulsive disorder. *J Clin Psychol.* 2004;60:1181–1194.

15. Carr JE. Competing responses for the treatment of Tourette syndrome and tic disorders. *Behav Res Ther.* 1995;33:455–456.

16. Miltenberger RG, Fuqua RW, Woods DW. Applying behavior analysis to clinical problems: review and analysis of habit reversal. *J Appl Behav Anal.* 1998; 31:447–469.

17. Cohen DJ, Friedhoff AJ, Leckman JF, et al. Tourette syndrome: extending basic research to clinical care. In: Chase TN, Friedhoff AJ, Cohen DJ, eds. *Advances in Neurology: vol 58. Tourette syndrome: Genetics, Neurobiology and Treatment.* New York: Raven Press, 1992; 341–362.

18. Peterson AL, Azrin NH. An evaluation of behavioral treatments for Tourette syndrome. *Behav Res Ther.* 1992;30:167–174.

19. Turpin G. The behavioural management of tic disorders: a critical review. *Adv Behavior Res Ther.* 1983;5: 203–245.

20. Bergin A, Waranch H, Brown J, et al. Relaxation therapy in Tourette syndrome: a pilot study. *Pediatr Neurol.* 1998;18:136–141.

21. Azrin NH, Peterson AL. Reduction of an eye tic by controlled blinking. *Behav Ther.* 1989;20:467–473.

22. Miltenberger R, Fuqua R. A comparison of contingent vs. non-contingent competing response practice in the treatment of nervous habits. *J Behav Ther Exp Psychiatry.* 1985;16:39–50.

23. Miltenberger R, Fuqua R, McKinley T. Habit reversal with muscle tics: replication and component analysis. *Behav Ther.* 1985;16:39–50.

24. Woods D, Miltenberger R, Lumley V. Sequential application of major habit-reversal components to treat motor tics in children. *J Appl Behav Anal.* 1996;29: 483–493.

25. Sharenow E, Fuqua R, Miltenberger R. The treatment of muscle tics with dissimilar competing response practice. *J Appl Behav Anal.* 1989;22:35–42.

26. McCracken J. Tic Disorders. In: Kaplan H, Sadock B, eds. *Comprehensive Textbook of Psychiatry.* 7th ed. Philadelphia: Lippincott Williams & Wilkins; 2000:2711–2719.

27. Woods D, et al. Behavioral treatment of problems associated with TS (this volume).

28. Woods D, Piacentini J, Himle M, et al. Premonitory urge for tics scale (PUTS): initial psychometric results and examination of the premonitory urge phenomenon in youth with tic disorders. *J Dev Behavior Pediat.* 2005;26:1–7.

29. Banaschewski T, Woerner W, Rothenberger A. Premonitory sensory phenomena and suppressibility of tics in Tourette syndrome: developmental aspects in children and adolescents. *Dev Med Child Neurol.* 2003;45: 700–703.

30. Bruun RD. The natural history of Tourette's syndrome. In: Cohen DJ, Leckman JF, Bruun RD, eds. *Tourette Syndrome and Tic Disorders: Clinical Understanding and Treatment.* New York: Wiley; 1988:21–39.

31. Leckman JF, Walker DE, Cohen DJ. Premonitory urges in Tourette's syndrome. *Am J Psychiatry.* 1993;150: 98–102.

32. Miguel EC, Rosario-Campos MC, Prado HS, et al. Sensory phenomena in obsessive-compulsive disorder and Tourette's disorder. *J Clin Psychiatry.* 2000;61:150–156.

33. Scahill L, Leckman J, Marek K. Sensory phenomena in Tourette's syndrome. In: Weiner WJ, Lang AE, eds. *Advances in Neurology: Behavioral Neurology of Movement Disorders.* vol. 65. New York: Raven Press; 1995:273–280.

34. Shapiro A, Shapiro E. Evaluation of the reported association of obsessive-compulsive symptoms or disorder with Tourette's disorder. *Comprehensive Psychiatry*, 1992;33:152–165.

35. Miguel EC, Coffey BJ, Baer L, et al. Phenomenology of intentional repetitive behaviors in obsessive-compulsive disorder and Tourette's syndrome. *J Clin Psychiatry.* 1995;56:246–255.

36. Leckman J, Walker D, Cohen D. Premonitory urges in Tourette's syndrome. *Am J Psychiatry.* 1993;150:98–102.

37. Leckman JF, Cohen DJ, eds. *Tourette's syndrome—Tics, Obsessions, Compulsions: Developmental Psychopathology and Clinical Care.* New York: John Wiley and Sons; 1999.

38. Evers RAF, van de Wetering BJM. A treatment model for motor tics based on specific tension-reduction technique. *J Behav Ther Exp Psychiatry.* 1194;25:255–260.

39. Hoogduin K, Verdellen C, Cath D. Exposure and response prevention in the treatment of Gilles de la Tourette's syndrome: four case studies. *Clinical Psychology and Psychotherapy* 1997;4:125–135.

40. Woods DW, Hook SS, Spellman DF, et al. Case study: exposure and response prevention for an adolescent with Tourette's syndrome and OCD. *J Am Acad Child Adol Psychiatry.* 2000;39:904–907.

41. Verdellen CW, Keijsers GP, Cath DC. Exposure with response prevention versus habit reversal in Tourette's syndrome: a controlled study. *Behav Res Ther.* 2004; 42:501–511.

42. Azrin NH, Peterson AL. Treatment of Tourette syndrome by habit reversal: a waiting-list control group comparison. *Behav Ther.* 1990;21:305–318.

43. Azrin NH, Nunn RG, Frantz SE. Habit reversal vs. negative practice treatment of nervous tics. *Behav Ther.* 1980;11:169–178.

44. O'Connor K, Gareau D, Borgeat F. A comparison of a behavioural and a cognitive-behavioural approach to the management of chronic tic disorders. *Clinical Psychology and Psychotherapy.* 1997;4:105–117.

45. O'Connor KP, Brault M, Robillard S, et al. Evaluation of a cognitive-behavioral program for the management of chronic tic and habit disorders. *Behav Res Ther.* 2001;39:667–681.

46. Leckman J, Riddle MA, Hardin MT, et al. The Yale Global Tic Severity Scale (YGTSS): Initial testing of a clinical-rated scale of tic severity. *J Am Acad Child Adol Psychiatry.* 1989;28:566–573.

47. Piacentini J, et al. Comparison of habit reversal and awareness training for chronic tic disorder in children and adolescents. Manuscript in prep.

24

Behavior Therapy: Other Interventions for Tic Disorders

Douglas W. Woods, Michael B. Himle, and Christine A. Conelea

Department of Psychology, University of Wisconsin-Milwaukee, Milwaukee, Wisconsin

Throughout the past several decades, a variety of behavior therapies have been used to treat the symptoms of tic disorders. These interventions have been met with varying levels of acceptance in the professional community, perhaps because they are based on antiquated theories, have shown inconsistent results in efficacy studies, and have not been subjected to the level of empirical scrutiny necessary to justify their widespread use in tic disorder patients. More recently, however, behavior therapists have attempted to understand interactions between the neurobiological underpinnings of tic disorders and environmental variables that affect tic expression. Understanding the functional relationships between tic expression and environmental variables has led to increased understanding of the nature of tic disorders and renewed interest in function-based behavior therapies for tics. This chapter outlines several behavior therapies that have been used in the past and the empirical support for each. Recent research examining the impact of the environment on tic expression is then reviewed. Finally, a function-based behavior therapy approach to the management of tics is discussed.

BEHAVIOR THERAPY: OTHER INTERVENTIONS FOR TIC DISORDERS

For more than 40 years, behavior therapists have considered behavior therapy procedures to be viable interventions for tic disorders. The procedures have demonstrated varying levels of success, however, and efficacy studies have often employed designs that lack sufficient experimental control. This chapter reviews the various behavioral treatment approaches that have been proposed, discusses the empirical basis for claims of efficacy, and presents trends in the application of behavioral technology in the understanding and treatment of tics.

Before reviewing the history of behavior therapy for Tourette syndrome (TS), a brief discussion about the appropriateness of behavioral approaches to tic management is required. Some have questioned the utility of nonpharmacologic interventions for a neurological disorder (1). Although the basis for claims cautioning against the use of such procedures for TS is not clear, the authors of this chapter suspect that they derive from various misconceptions. First, a number of professionals believe that behavior therapists use environmental variables to affect change in tics, thereby suggesting that behavior therapists believe tic are caused by an identifiable learning history. Conversely, behavioral psychologists understand that variables that cause a disorder are often separate from the variables that maintain the disorder. What behavioral psychologists do contend is that the environment interacts with the biological organism (including its neurological deficiencies). By adopting this view, one can appreciate that A) the impact the environment can exert on an organism is limited by the biology of the subject, and B) the organism (including its biology and corresponding biological manifestations) is shaped by the environment. This latter realization relates directly to the second misconception, namely, behavior therapists believe they are *curing* TS via nonpharmacologic means. Again, this is not the case. Behavior therapists view behavior therapy as involving specific environmental modifications and the training of behaviors that may allow the individual to effectively cope with or manage the tics. A final potential area for argument against the use of behavior therapy for TS involves the history of psychotherapy in TS interventions. Unfortunately, the early history of TS treatment involved the use of various psychotherapeutic techniques based on theories with little empirical support (e.g., psychoanalysis) (2). Although behavior therapy developed uniquely from other psychotherapies with its reliance on efficacy testing and a basis in empirically sound operant learning principles, it may be the case that behavior therapy is unwittingly lumped into a broad class of activities called *psychotherapy* and subsequently discounted out of hand. Nevertheless, the data supporting the efficacy of behavioral interventions for tics associated with TS is now large enough to suggest that such interventions are worthy of further investigation and clinical consideration (3–7).

The primary behavioral treatment for TS has been a procedure called *habit reversal* (8). However, several other behavior therapy procedures have been documented. The empirical support for these other procedures are fewer in number and have often been tested using questionable empirical methods. This chapter reviews these procedures and discuss other areas in which behavior therapy and more broadly, behavioral sciences, have made progress in understanding and treating the interactions between the environment and organism to influence tic expression.

Description of Other Behavior Therapy Procedures and Evidence for Efficacy

Relaxation Training

Relaxation training teaches an individual to become more aware of tic (and pre-tic) sensations

and tension and to engage in one of two types of relaxation: A) active, targeted relaxation of muscles involved in the tic (9), or B) general, progressive muscle relaxation training (10). The rationale behind relaxation training is intuitively strong. First, relaxation training is thought to teach the patient to relax specific muscles involved in the tic, thereby directly competing with the muscle contraction that produces the tic. Second, because anxiety and stress are thought to increase tic symptoms (11), relaxation training is believed to indirectly reduce tics by decreasing anxiety. Furthermore, reports outlining the influence of environmental variables on tics have suggested that tics are lessened when an individual is relaxed (12), providing support for relaxation training as a potential treatment modality for TS.

Interestingly, relaxation training is rarely employed as a monotherapy for TS. Rather, it is typically included as one of multiple components in a behavioral treatment package (13,14). A few reports on the efficacy of treatments that include relaxation training have been promising; however, the relative contribution of the relaxation training component and the degree to which treatment gains are maintained outside of the treatment setting remains unknown. Thomas et al. (15), for example, combined relaxation training with self-monitoring in the treatment of a patient with TS and reported a 90% reduction in tic frequency. However, the respective contribution of each of the two procedures was unclear and treatment gains were only measured within the context of the treatment setting, thereby restricting conclusions regarding generalization. Similar results have been reported with other treatment combinations (16). In a component analysis study, Peterson and Azrin (4) evaluated relaxation training (along with self-monitoring and habit reversal) in six adults with TS in a randomized, counterbalanced reversal design. They found that relaxation training was the least effective of the three treatment components. However, it was the most effective component for one participant.

To date, only one randomized, controlled study has evaluated the efficacy of relaxation training as a monotherapy for TS. Bergin et al. (17)

compared relaxation training to a minimal therapy control group for 23 randomized (stratified according to TS severity and presence of ADHD) TS patients. In this study, those who received the relaxation training did not differ in TS severity following 6 weeks of treatment when compared to the control group, providing initial evidence that relaxation training alone may not be a viable treatment modality for TS. Indeed, other studies have reported that treatment gains from relaxation training are typically transient (18) and restricted to the treatment setting (19,20). Although relaxation training continues to be included in many behavioral treatment packages or as a treatment adjunct, current research has failed to show that relaxation training alone has a significant contribution in the behavioral treatment of TS.

Biofeedback

Biofeedback involves the use of physiological recording equipment to provide feedback on a specific domain of physiological functioning. Typically for tic disorders, the feedback domain is muscle tension (17,21,22), although body temperature (23) and electroencephalogram signals (24) have also been used.

Biofeedback procedures are often embedded within a treatment package, thereby making it difficult to determine the independent efficacy of the procedure. For example, Culbertson (23) used a finger-tip temperature biofeedback procedure within a four-step hypnotherapy model that also included progressive relaxation training, Spiegel's eye-roll procedure, and imagery. Patient reports suggested improvement, but there was no independent confirmation. Similar improvements have been found with other procedural combinations (22,24).

Despite the promise of these early reports, the specific utility of biofeedback for tic disorders remains uncertain for two primary reasons. First, most of the designs used to evaluate the procedure have been uncontrolled case studies (21–24). In the one exception (17), biofeedback was a small part of a much larger treatment package, thus complicating efforts to make a definitive statement about the individual utility

of biofeedback. This latter issue of incorporating biofeedback with other treatment components has made the isolated effect of biofeedback unclear. Typically the biofeedback component has been combined with some other self-management strategy such as explicit instructions to relax, or even more explicit relaxation training. Only one study to date appears to have evaluated the efficacy of biofeedback alone (21). In an open trial of nine individuals with tics, O'Connor et al. (21) showed that providing electromyographic muscle tension biofeedback reduced tics in six of the subjects by 40%. In summary, due to the lack of controlled studies that examine the individual impact of biofeedback procedures alone, the efficacy of such procedures as a treatment for tics remains unclear.

Massed Negative Practice

Massed negative practice (MNP) has also been used to treat tics. When using MNP, a therapist instructs a patient to "practice" his/her tics continuously for some period of time, several times each day. The rationale for MNP is based on a Hullian learning theory, which views tics as maladaptive habits (i.e., a tic) that are strengthened by repetition and can be replaced by the strengthening of more adaptive habits (i.e., not having tics). According to the model, as a patient engages in repeated (i.e., "massed") practice of the tic, a conditioned inhibition or conditioned fatigue builds up until a critical level is reached, and the individual is required to rest (i.e., engage in the more adaptive habit, essentially not having tics). These periods of incompatible rest are thought to be strengthened until they eventually replace the tics.

Early empirical support for the Hullian theory of tic maintenance was based on a few case studies. Walton (25) reported the successful treatment of a child with tics using MNP and medication. In a second case report, Walton (26) used MNP and medication to treat multiple motor and vocal tics in a young child. According to the report, massed practice resulted in "considerable amelioration" of the child's tics and treatment gains were maintained at a five month follow-up. Despite their numerous methodological limitations, these case reports were considered to support the Hullian account of tics and MNP commenced as a potentially viable treatment for individuals with TS.

Overall, the results of efficacy studies evaluating MNP as a treatment for TS are mixed. Nicassio et al. (27) used daily, 10-minute MNP practice sessions to treat two individuals with motor tics. They reported significant tic reduction in one, but not both participants. Interestingly, the patient suffering from a single motor tic benefited from the treatment and the patient with multiple tics did not. Topenhoff (28) reported the successful treatment of an adolescent with TS using massed practice, but the intervention also involved social contingency management, confounding the effects of massed practice. A variety of other case studies have reported successful (29) and unsuccessful (30,31) treatment of tics with MNP. In other cases, MNP has been discontinued because tics increased following treatment with MNP (31). To date, only one controlled trial has evaluated the efficacy of MNP. Azrin et al. (32) compared MNP with habit reversal training (HRT) by randomly assigning 22 participants to one of the two treatments. They found that MNP decreased tics by approximately 33% whereas HRT decreased tics almost completely. The lack of an inactive control group and the use of self-report as the primary dependent variable, however, limits conclusions from the study. Overall, evaluations of MNP as a treatment for TS provide an insufficient base upon which to draw conclusions regarding the treatment's efficacy.

Self-Monitoring

Self-monitoring is frequently employed as a method of data collection in studies on TS (33). Less often, self-monitoring is used as a monotherapy for TS. Thomas et al. (15) treated a patient with multiple motor and vocal tics using self-monitoring alone. They reported that although one of the patient's vocal tics decreased significantly, the patient's other vocal and motor tics did not improve until other treatment modalities were added. Billings (34) utilized a multiple baseline design to evaluate the effectiveness of self-monitoring in reducing an adolescent's motor and phonic tics. Billings (34) found that self-monitoring resulted in a reduction in both the frequency and intensity of the patient's tics. In addition, Billings (34) found that during self-monitoring, immediate recording was more effective than delayed recording for some tics during self-monitoring. The only study to compare self-monitoring to other treatment modalities was conducted by Peterson and Azrin (4). Utilizing a counterbalanced design, self-monitoring was compared to relaxation training and HRT. Self-monitoring was shown to be more efficacious than relaxation training, but less efficacious than HRT.

The exact mechanisms by which self-monitoring may be effective in some cases are unknown. It is plausible that teaching a patient to be more aware of tics and the context in which they occur will allow the person to compensate for tics by engaging in natural, non-tic behavior (i.e., a natural competing response, suppression, etc.). However, research has not yet ruled out the potential role of placebo, social demand, inconvenience, and several other plausible explanations. Randomized, controlled studies are needed before conclusions regarding the efficacy of self-monitoring, and the related mechanisms of change, can be drawn.

Contingency Management

Research examining the effectiveness of reinforcement and punishment procedures for tics have shown that tics can be influenced (at least temporarily) by consequences delivered contingently upon the tic (33,35). Specific interventions include reinforcement procedures, such as token economies, and punishment procedures such as time out. For example, Lahey et al. (36) reported the successful use of time-out procedures to reduce the frequency of an obscene vocal tic in a child with TS. Varni et al. (37) successfully treated a child with TS and hyperactivity using self-monitoring, reinforcement, and time-out. Treatment gains not only generalized to untreated tics, but were maintained at 8-week follow-up. Still, as with most research on other behavioral interventions for TS, the wait-list and placebo controlled outcome studies have not been conducted, and thus the efficacy of the procedures remains unclear.

The literature base on behavioral interventions other than HRT is large but insufficient. There is preliminary evidence that a number of different interventions may be effective for reducing tics associated with TS, however, the exact mechanisms of change remain unclear. Most recently, behavioral research has begun to investigate the effects of environmental variables on tic expression and suppression. The research group of the authors of this chapter recently developed an individualized approach to environmental assessment and modification as a potentially useful approach to tic reduction. The following discussion reviews this approach to environmental assessment and modification and advances in behavioral research aimed at understanding tic expression and suppression.

ADVANCES IN BEHAVIORAL RESEARCH ON TIC EXPRESSION/REDUCTION

Recent research concerning environment-tic interactions has demonstrated the systematic impact of environmental events on tic expression. Broad survey studies of persons with TS show that various environmental events lead to exacerbation or reduction of tics (12). For example, Silva et al. (12) surveyed 14 persons with TS and found that 79% of them reported tic exacerbation when exposed to anxiety producing situations and 42% reported tic exacerbation when in social gatherings.

Other research investigating the control of various antecedent environmental events include a study by Malatesta (38), who demonstrated that tics were more frequent when a child was in the presence of his critical father, and a study by Woods et al. (39), which experimentally showed that vocal tics, but not motor tics, were under the control of tic-related conversation.

Recent research has begun to focus on the consequences of tics and their impact on tic expression. Some research has shown that chronic tics can, under some circumstances, be maintained by contingent attention. For example, Watson and Sterling (35) showed that a child's coughing tic occurred primarily at the dinner table, and was most frequent when a parent provided attention following the tic. When the parents were instructed to stop attending to the tic, it was eliminated. Other studies (40) have also reported cases in which tics were maintained by social reinforcement.

Research has also begun to systematically investigate the impact of environmental consequences on the suppression of tics. Woods and Himle (41) experimentally demonstrated that delivering tangible reinforcers for 10-second tic-free periods temporarily reduced tics 76% from baseline levels. This was in comparison with a 10% reduction observed when children were simply asked to suppress their tics with no environmental consequences for tic free periods. Subsequent research in this area suggests that the findings are robust and that the use of environmental variables to induce brief tic suppression does not subsequently produce a rebound in tic frequency or severity (42). An additional finding from this latter study showed a significant correlation ($r = -0.89$, $P < 0.01$) between degree of tic suppression and attentional problems as measured by the parent report of the Child Behavior Checklist. This supports research (43) that suggests tic suppression may involve attentional processes, and suggests that combined therapies (attention deficit hyperactivity disorder medication plus behavior therapy) may be beneficial for children with TS and comorbid attention deficit hyperactivity disorder.

FUNCTIONAL ASSESSMENT AND MODIFICATION OF ENVIRONMENT

The aforementioned research has empirically demonstrated the functional relationships between tics and environmental variables. Although these studies have led to a greater understanding of the impact of environment on tics, relatively little work has been conducted to systematically modify the environment for therapeutic benefit in an individualized fashion.

The process by which one systematically determines functional relations between tics and their environmental antecedents and consequences is known as functional assessment. The goal of the functional assessment as applied to TS is to generate hypotheses regarding the functional impact of various environmental events on tics and then systematically modify the environment to alter their occurrence.

Functional assessment procedures have been successfully used to guide treatment planning and implementation across a number of different repetitive behavior problems (44). Still, it has only rarely been applied to tic disorders. One example of the application of functional assessment to tic disorders can be found in the previously described study by Watson and Sterling (35). These researchers showed that a child's parents were actually reinforcing (i.e., strengthening) the tic. As such, treatment involved ignoring the tic, which produced an elimination of the behavior. Although this case was just one example, it points to the broader approach of function-based treatments.

A number of antecedent and consequence variables should be considered when conducting a functional assessment. For example, the tics may be more common at school, at home immediately after school, when anxious, while watching television, during meals, while doing homework, etc. Likewise, the tics may produce a number of environmental outcomes such as parents or peers confronting the child about tics, someone laughing at or teasing the child, asking the child to leave the area, or getting out of completing a task. These outcomes may worsen tics.

Antecedents and consequences that appear to worsen tic frequency should be targeted for change. In cases where it is possible to change specific environmental antecedents and consequences, it should be done. For example, if anxiety is a specific tic-exacerbating stimulus, then relaxation training should occur. Likewise, if parental reminders to stop ticcing or peer teasing seems to worsen tics, then ignoring tics and a school-wide intervention to stop the teasing would be recommended as they may directly impact tic frequency and may have the added benefit of improving the child's overall mental health. However, sometimes it may not be possible to modify the environment (e.g., it may be difficult

to stop riding in cars). In such cases, it may be useful to teach and have the child practice specific tic management skills (e.g., competing responses for tics). The targeted practice of such procedures in high-risk situations should facilitate the transfer of treatment effects to these situations.

Clearly, these function-based procedures are just beginning to be applied to the treatment of TS, and data supporting their use is limited. Nevertheless, there is intuitive appeal in their application, and similar procedures have been widely applied in the treatment of a number of other behavior problems (45,46). Before widespread use is recommended, however, systematic evaluations of functional assessment and derived treatments for tics should be conducted, standards for implementation should be defined, and the efficacy of environmental manipulations must be demonstrated.

SUMMARY

This chapter reviewed other behavioral interventions for TS and discussed their efficacy. Clearly, the majority of behavioral interventions (habit reversal excluded) have not been systematically evaluated enough to be deemed empirically supported monotherapies for TS. In addition to reviewing these interventions, recent advances in behavioral research on TS and a function-based model of treatment development and implementation were presented. Both of these areas are in their infancy, but point to exciting new directions in the application of behavioral sciences to the understanding of TS.

REFERENCES

1. Burd L, Kerbeshian J. Treatment-generated problems associated with behavior modification in Tourette disorder. *Dev Med Child Neurol.* 1987;29:831,832.
2. Kushner HI. *A Cursing Brain? The Histories of Tourette Syndrome.* Cambridge MA: Harvard University Press; 1999.
3. Azrin NH, Peterson AL. Habit reversal for the treatment of Tourette syndrome. *Behav Res Ther.* 1988;26:347–351.
4. Peterson AL, Azrin NH. An evaluation of behavioral treatments for Tourette syndrome. *Behav Res Ther.* 1992; 30:167–174.
5. O'Connor KP, Brault M, Robillard S, et al. Evaluation of a cognitive-behavioral program for the management of chronic tic and habit disorders. *Behav Res Ther.* 2001; 39:667–681.

6. Wilhelm A, Deckersbach T, Coffey BJ, et al. Habit reversal versus supportive psychotherapy for Tourette's disorder: a randomized controlled trial. *Am J Psychiat.* 2003;160:1175,1176.

7. Woods DW, Twohig MP, Flessner C, et al. Treatment of vocal tics in children with Tourette syndrome: investigating the efficacy of habit reversal. *J Appl Behav Anal.* 2003;36:109–112.

8. Azrin NH, Nunn RG. Habit reversal: a method of eliminating nervous habits and tics. *Behav Res Ther.* 1973; 11:619–628.

9. Evers RAF, van de Wetering BJM. A treatment model for motor tics based on specific tension-reduction technique. *J Behav Ther Exp Psychiat.* 1994;25:255–260.

10. Bernstein DS, Borkovec TD. *Progressive Relaxation Training.* Champaign, IL: Research Press; 1973.

11. Moldofsky H. A psychophysiological study of multiple tics. *Arch Gen Psychiatry.* 1971;25:79–87.

12. Silva RR, Munoz DM, Barickman J, et al. Environmental factors and related fluctuations of symptoms in children and adolescents with Tourette's disorder. *J Child Psychol Psychiatry.* 995;36:305–312.

13. Azrin NH, Nunn RG. *Habit Control in a Day.* New York: Simon & Shuster; 1977.

14. Michultka DM, Blanchard EB, Rosenblum EL. Stress management and Gilles de la Tourette's syndrome. *Biofeedback Self-Regul.* 1989;14:115–123.

15. Thomas EJ, Abrams KS, Johnson JB. Self-monitoring and reciprocal inhibition in the modification of multiple tics of Gilles de la Tourette syndrome. *J Behav Ther Exp Psychiatry.* 1971;2:159–171.

16. Savicki V, Carlin, AS. Behavioral treatment of Gilles de la Tourette syndrome. *Int J Child Psychother.* 1972; 1:97–109.

17. Bergin A, Waranch HR, Brown J, et al. Relaxation therapy in Tourette syndrome: a pilot study. *Pediatr Neurol.* 1998;18:136–142.

18. St. James-Roberts N, Powell GE. A case-study comparing the effects of relaxation and massed practice upon tic frequency. *Behav Res Ther.* 1979;17:401–403.

19. Canavan AGM, Powell GE. The efficacy of several treatments of Gilles de la Tourette's syndrome as assessed in a single case. *Behav Ther Res.* 1981;19:549–556.

20. Crawley B, Powell G. A comparison of the effects of massed practice and relaxation upon the frequency of a facial tic. *Behav Psychother.* 1986;14:249–257.

21. O'Connor K, Gareau D, Borgeat F. Muscle control in chronic tic disorders. *Biofeedback Self-Regul.* 1995;20: 111–122.

22. Stanwood JK, Lanyon RI, Wright MH. Treatment of severe hemifacial spasm with biofeedback: a case study. *Behav Modif.* 1984;8:567–580.

23. Culbertson FM. A four-step hypnotherapy model for Gilles de la Tourette's syndrome. *Am J Clin Hypn.* 1989;31:252–256.

24. Tansey MA. A simple and a complex tic (Gilles de la Tourette's syndrome): their response to EEG sensorimotor rhythm biofeedback training. *Int J Psychophysiol.* 1986;4:91–97.

25. Walton D. Experimental psychology and the treatment of a ticqueur. *J Child Psychol Psychiat.* 1961;2:148–155.

26. Walton D. Massed practice and simultaneous reduction in drive level. Further evidence of the efficacy of this approach to the treatment of tics. In: HJ Eysenck, ed. *Experiments in Behavior Therapy.* London: Pergamon, 1964;398–400.

27. Nicassio FJ, Liberman RP, Patterson RL, et al. The treatment of tics by negative practice. *J Behav Ther Exp Psychiat.* 1972;3:281–287.

28. Topenhoff M. Massed practice, relaxation and assertion training in the treatment of Gilles de la Tourette's syndrome. *J Behav Ther Exp Psychiat.* 1973;4:71–73.

29. Storms L. Massed negative practice as a behavioral treatment for Gilles de la Tourette's syndrome. *Am J Psychother.* 1985;39:277–281.

30. Feldman RB, Werry JS. An unsuccessful attempt to treat a tiqueur by massed practice. *Behav Res Ther.* 1966;4:111–117.

31. Hollandsworth JG Jr, Bausinger L. Unsuccessful use of massed practice in the treatment of Gilles de la Tourette's syndrome. *Psychol Rep.* 1978;43:671–677.

32. Azrin NH, Nunn RG, Frantz SE. Habit reversal vs. negative practice treatment of nervous tics. *Behav Ther.* 1980;11:169–178.

33. Carr JE, Taylor CC, Wallander RJ, et al. A functional-analytic approach to the diagnosis of a transient tic disorder. *J Behav Ther Exp Psychiat.* 1996;27:291–297.

34. Billings A. Self-monitoring in the treatment of tics: a single-subject analysis. *J Behav Ther Exp Psychiat.* 1978;9:339–342.

35. Watson TS, Sterling HE. Brief functional analysis and treatment of a vocal tic. *J Appl Behav Anal.* 1998; 31:471–474.

36. Lahey BB, McNees MP, McNees MC. Control of an obscene "verbal tic" through timeout in an elementary classroom. *J Appl Behav Anal.* 1973;6:101–104.

37. Varni JW, Boyd EF, Cataldo MF. Self-monitoring, external reinforcement, and timeout procedures in the control of high rate tic behaviors in a hyperactive child. *J Behav Ther Exp Psychiat.* 1978;9:353–358.

38. Malatesta VJ. Behavioral case formulation: an experimental assessment study of transient tic disorder. *J Psychopathol Behav Assess.* 1990;12:219–232.

39. Woods DW, Watson TS, Wolfe E, et al. Analyzing the influence of tic-related conversation on vocal and motor tics in children with Tourette's syndrome. *J Appl Behav Anal.* 2001;34:353–356.

40. Schulman M. Control of tics by maternal reinforcement. *J Behav Ther Exp Psychiat.* 1974;5:95–96.

41. Woods DW, Himle MB. Creating tic suppression: comparing the effects of verbal instruction to differential reinforcement. *J Appl Behav Anal.* 2004:37:417–420.

42. Himle, MB, Woods DW. An experimental evaluation of tic suppression and the tic rebound effect. *Behav Res Ther.* 2005. In press.

43. Peterson BS, Skudlarski P, Anderson AW, et al. A functional magnetic resonance imaging study of tic suppression in Tourette syndrome. *Arc Gen Psychiat.* 1998; 55:326–333.

44. Ringdahl JE, Wacker DP, Berg WK, et al. Repetitive behavior disorders in persons with developmental disabilities. In: Woods DW, Miltenberger RG, eds. *Tic disorders, Trichotillomania, and Other Repetitive Behavior Disorders. Behavioral Approaches to Analysis and Treatment.* Boston: Kluwer Academic Press. 2001;297–314.

45. Kratochwill TR, McGivern JE. Clinical diagnosis, behavioral assessment, and functional analysis: Examining the connection between assessment and intervention. *Sch Psychol Rev.* 1996;25:342–355.

46. Hanley GP, Iwata BA, McCord BE. Functional analysis of problem behavior: a review. *J Appl Behav Anal.* 2003;36:147–185.

25

Behavioral Neurosurgery

Donald A. Malone Jr. and Mayur M. Pandya

Department of Psychiatry, Cleveland Clinic Foundation, Cleveland, Ohio

Tourette syndrome (TS) is a neuropsychiatric condition characterized by waxing and waning motor and vocal tics. Georges Gilles de la Tourette emphasized the triad of multiple tics, coprolalia, and echolalia (1). In addition to the neurologic aspects of the syndrome, the common comorbidity of psychiatric manifestations may be just as debilitating. These conditions may include obsessive compulsive disorder (OCD), attention-deficit disorder, hyperactivity, and mood disorders among others (2). Although pharmacologic and behavioral therapies remain the mainstay of treatment (3), various neurosurgical interventions have been sought to better control the vast array of neuropsychiatric symptoms.

A relatively new neurosurgical technique known as deep brain stimulation (DBS) has had promising results (4). Successfully introduced for the treatment of movement disorders (5), such as Parkinson disease, this procedure has been experimentally used in a number of patients with OCD (6,7). The success of DBS in patients with OCD, combined with the similarities and often coexistence with TS, makes the use of DBS in patients with TS more intriguing.

TOURETTE SYNDROME

TS is a tic disorder characterized by multiple motor and one or more vocal tics beginning before the age of 18 years (8). The frequency, severity, and location typically change over time. It occurs in around 1% of youngsters between the ages of 5 and 16 years with a male predominance (9). Motor tics typically precede vocal tics. The most common initial motor and vocal tics are eye blinking and throat clearing, respectively. Other common tics include licking, spitting, coprolalia, echolalia, grunting, coughing, touching, and hitting. Tics are generally aggravated by anxiety, stress, fatigue, and excitement, while they are often suppressed by sleep, alcohol, fever, and relaxation (10).

Many psychiatric and behavioral disturbances are associated with TS, including OCD, attention deficit hyperactivity disorder, self-injury, phobias, antisocial personality, and aggressiveness. Behavioral symptoms of TS are subject to the same waxing and waning as motor and vocal symptoms and may even persist beyond the disappearance of the tics. It is reported that 30% to 90% of TS patients manifest obsessive-compulsive behavior in addition to their tics and vocalizations (11). The significance of recognizing the coexistence of OCD and TS and its implications to treatment are yet to be fully defined. However, enough evidence exists to suggest a common link and the possibility of a tic-related OCD phenotype (12). The importance of appropriately treating this special OCD subset is demonstrated by the observation that those individuals with both disorders may represent a more severe form than either disorder alone. These individuals have higher rates of mood and anxiety disorders, disruptive behavior, and substance abuse than those subjects with TS or OCD alone (13).

OCD occurs in 2% to 3% of the population (14). Often it begins in childhood or adolescence and takes on a chronic course. The disability resulting from this illness can be devastating (15). The World Health Organization has determined OCD to be the tenth leading cause of disability worldwide (16). History of OCD in a first-degree family carries up to a three times greater risk than the general population though family history is certainly not a prerequisite. Patients with OCD are often reluctant to present for treatment. They can see their symptoms as bizarre and untreatable. Fear of embarrassment or humiliation can provide impediments. Therefore, there is often a substantial time delay between the onset of symptoms and receiving professional help.

When comparing TS and OCD, many common features are observed, including intrusive, involuntary, ego-alien behavior as well as bizarre sexual, aggressive, and viscero-eliminative themes (11). Tics are similar to compulsive behaviors in that they are "voluntarily" suppressible, but eventually are performed to relieve an uncomfortable sensation or tension. Localizing information through neuroimaging studies reveal association to the basal ganglia and related structures in both disorders. Furthermore, the involvement of dopaminergic neurotransmitter system has also been hypothesized for both disorders. However, the most impressive observations for a link have been inheritance and genetic relationship studies. A number of reports (17–19) have discovered a higher frequency of OCD in biologic families of patients with TS and tic disorders, suggesting a common genetic abnormality with variable phenotypic expression. Due to this commonality, further investigation of their similarities and the implications for treatment strategies is appropriate.

BASAL GANGLIA: CORTICO-STRIATO-THALAMO-CORTICAL CIRCUIT

Hypothetical models of the role of basal ganglia in TS are due to the observation of the development of tic disorders in patients with basal ganglia lesions such as in cases of encephalitis and carbon monoxide poisoning (20–22). Likewise, development of OCD has also been documented with basal ganglia lesions (23). The basal ganglia consist of the striatum (caudate nucleus,

putamen, and nucleus accumbens), subthalamic nucleus, globus pallidus (pars interna and externa), and substantia nigra (pars compacta and pars reticulata). The globus pallidus pars interna and substantia nigra pars reticulata (receiving inhibitory projections from the striatum) are the primary output nuclei sending inhibitory connections to the thalamus and brainstem. Dysfunction of this cortico-striato-thalamo-cortical circuit has been proposed as the basis for TS and OCD (24–27). Although the exact mechanism is yet unknown, investigations have targeted an increased dopaminergic release and/or sensitivity.

In a review of 172 documented structural computerized tomography brain scans of patients with TS (10), only 18 were found to be abnormal, with most having no etiologic significance. Another review of volumetric studies (28), however, found significant discrepancies between TS children and adults in various brain regions, including lenticular nuclei, corpus collosum, and prefrontal cortex, suggesting possible activity-dependent neuronal plasticity as symptoms change later in life. Functional neuroimaging studies of TS patients have demonstrated significant activation of a number of neural systems. Positron emission tomography and single photon emitted computed tomography studies have revealed decreased metabolism and blood flow in the basal ganglia in TS adults relative to healthy controls (29,30). Another investigation revealed abnormal activity in anterior cingulate, premotor, and dorsolateral prefrontal cortex, as well as activation in the dopaminergic-rich midbrain tegmentum, suggesting abnormal modulation of the striatal circuits by excess dopamine (31). Some subtle volumetric abnormalities in the striatum of OCD patients have been noted, though these findings are not present in all studies (32,33). Functional studies have been more consistent. These studies have found fairly consistent increases in activity within the orbitofrontal cortex, anterior cingulate, and the caudate nucleus (34). When functional neuroimaging is combined with provocation of OCD symptoms, increases in the activity of these brain regions can also be seen (35). Combined, these findings suggest that there is overactivity to this neural circuit in patients with OCD.

TREATMENT STRATEGIES

The traditional scope of treatment strategies in patients with TS consists of behavioral therapy and/or pharmacologic management. A few refractory cases have experimentally undergone neurosurgical intervention. This chapter briefly discusses the current mainstays of treatment and investigates the use of neurosurgical techniques in the treatment of TS.

Behavioral

Numerous behavioral techniques have been documented in the literature. Due to pharmacologic side effects and noncompliance, behavioral techniques have long been a mainstay of treatment. These techniques are commonly used in conjunction with pharmacologic treatment or following an unsuccessful or partially successful medication trial. Techniques employed include massed (negative) practice, operant conditioning, anxiety management techniques, awareness training, and habit-reversal training. Unfortunately, the efficacy of these techniques has been difficult to determine due to studies of small sample size, poor sample characterization, lack of control groups, short follow-up, and multi-technique treatment packages (36). Nevertheless, promising results have been seen with certain techniques, especially habit-reversal training (37). Habit-reversal training consists of eight primary components focusing on awareness and competing responses to tic occurrence.

Pharmacologic

Dopamine has long been implicated in the pathogenesis of TS. This has been speculated clinically due to the effectiveness of dopamine receptor antagonists, such as haloperidol, trifluoperazine, and pimozide, in the suppression of tics; while the administration of dopaminergic stimulants tends to elicit or exacerbate TS symptomatology. A number of cellular analysis studies have confirmed some type of dopaminergic dysfunction in patients with TS. These range from elevated intrasynaptic dopamine release to abnormal modulation of basal ganglia circuits by hypersensitive striatal neurons to dopamine receptor binding (27,38,39). Other studies, however, have not reproduced these findings (40,41). Newer "atypical" antipsychotics, such as risperidone, and alpha-2-adrenergic agonist, clonidine, have also been shown to be efficacious in tic control in TS (42).

Neurosurgical

Neurosurgical interventions for human psychiatric disorders date back to the early 20th century. One of the most notable surgeons was the American neurosurgeon Walter Freeman. Due to the lack of medications available for mental illness and the overcrowding of psychiatric institutions, Freeman began to apply his relatively untested procedure, the prefrontal lobotomy, in which he transorbitally inserted an ice pick into the frontal cortex. From 1936 to the mid-1950s, these neurosurgical procedures were widely performed in the United States (43). Although therapeutic benefit in a variety of psychiatric disorders (including OCD) was reported, the large area of brain affected by the procedure resulted in significant cognitive and behavioral sequelae. The controversy of these procedures, combined with the discovery of pharmacologic therapy, eventually shut the door on the popularity of behavioral psychosurgery for the next few decades. However, with the advancement of neurosurgical precision and technique, the possibility of more focused behavioral neurosurgery has emerged.

Stereotactic procedures utilized in OCD have included subcaudate tractotomy, cingulotomy, limbic leucotomy, and capsulotomy. Subcaudate tractotomy targets the white matter region beneath the head of the caudate in order to interrupt white matter tracts between orbital cortex and subcortical structures (an area believed to be responsible for OCD symptomatology). Cingulotomy typically involves bilateral lesioning of the anterior cingulate gyrus, which was noted to be involved with highly integrated motor behavior upon stimulation (44). Limbic leucotomy is a multi-target procedure combining subcaudate tractotomy and cingulotomy. Lastly, capsulotomy targets the anterior limb of the internal capsule with the purpose of interrupting presumed fronto-thalamic connections. Evaluating the effectiveness of these procedures in OCD is difficult. Recent literature only documents the procedure in very treatment-refractory illnesses while earlier patient populations may have responded to either medication or behavior therapy, if they had been available. An ongoing study by Rasmussen and Greenberg (45) is evaluating the effectiveness of gamma knife anterior capsulotomy in truly treatment-refractory OCD. By placing two 4-mm lesions bilaterally, they have found a 62% response at 3-year follow-up. An initial study with only a single bilateral lesion noted minimal improvement. It was only with the addition of the second lesion more ventrally located in the capsule that response was seen.

A few cases of TS that have been refractory to conventional methods of treatment have undergone surgical lesioning in an attempt to control debilitating symptoms (46). Neurosurgical treatment of TS remains experimental, as only anecdotal experiences with these operations have been reported. The introduction of stereotactic targeting has greatly improved target accuracy, reducing major side effects. The advantages of stereotactic surgery include a reduction of trauma and operative risk, anatomical control, reduced risk of parenchymal hemorrhage, and reduced risk of sepsis (47). The thalamus has been a target of intervention in neurosurgical treatments of TS due to basic studies of its association in various types of movement disorders (48). Cases of successful thalamic lesioning in TS have been reported (49). The thalamus is made up of four parts—the epithalamus, ventral thalamus, hypothalamus, and dorsal thalamus—divided into 50 to 60 nuclei. The midline and intralaminar nuclei within the dorsal thalamus have been speculated to have functional importance with motor control within the basal ganglia (50). The center median-parafascicular complex, specifically, has been found to have large projections to and from the basal ganglia (51). As discussed in the following text,

this has been the area of focus with DBS in patients with TS.

In 1962, the first leucotomy and first thalamectomy for TS were carried out by Baker (52) and Cooper (53), respectively. Cooper (53) targeted the ventrolateral nucleus of the thalamus. Hassler and Dieckman (54) in 1970 performed bilateral thalamotomies, targeting the intralaminar and medial nuclei, resulting in tic reductions between 70% and 100%. Criticisms or questions regarding most early neurosurgical procedures in TS, however, involve rationale and accuracy of target localization, as well as reliable diagnosis and tic measurements (46).

Review of the literature reveals 21 reports of 69 individuals undergoing neurosurgical procedures for TS (46,55,56). Twenty-three cases had no mention of or reported side effects. Side effects in the other cases included transient confusion and speech loss, gait problems, cognitive deficits, cerebellar signs, dysarthria, dystonia, "severe neurologic deficits," hemiparesis, hemiballism, and spastic hemiplegia, and quadriplegia. As discussed later in text, the "reversible" nature of DBS may significantly reduce the risks of these permanent side effects.

Deep Brain Stimulation

The use of DBS for the treatment of OCD is in a very early stage of evaluation. Only very treatment-refractory cases are currently being considered in closely monitored research protocols. Guidelines for conducting this research have been published by a multi-center collaborative group to help ensure ethical research, which will provide information useful to the ongoing assessment of this procedure (57). Nuttin et al. (58) have published an initial series of six patients who received bilateral DBS to the anterior limb of the internal capsule. Results note response rates similar to those in the best studies of anterior capsular lesioning. Overall the procedure is well tolerated. Some complications have included relatively short battery life, abrupt symptom worsening upon cessation of stimulation, hypomanic or manic conversion, and the significant time and effort involved in optimizing stimulation parameters. In addition to these cases, a multi-center collaborative group has reported on an additional 14 patients who have received a similar procedure (59). Approximately 50% of these patients have noted significant response with corresponding improvements in functionality. It is important to re-emphasize, however, that these results are highly preliminary and further study is required before this procedure becomes a potential standard of care for treatment-refractory OCD.

There are currently five reports of DBS in patients with TS (60–62). In four cases Visser-Vandewalle et al. (60) targeted the midline and intralaminar thalamic nuclei based on previous lesioning techniques by Hassler and Dieckman and the hypothesis that these nuclei may play a role in the gating of the output of the basal ganglia to the thalamocortical system (52). Each patient experienced significant reductions in their tics, as well as complete disappearance of their obsessive-compulsive behaviors. Follow-ups were 5 years for case one, 1 year for case two, and 8 months for case three. Tic reductions were 90%, 72%, and 82%, respectively, at each follow-up. Case four (61) involved the implantation of two additional electrodes in the globus pallidus interna, which was found to have a slightly better effect than the thalamic DBS. The fifth, and most recent, case (62) also involved stimulation of the intralaminar thalamic nuclei. Preoperatively, the patient displayed more than 50 motor tics per minute. Postimplantation, the patient reported only a few tics per week.

Although long-term follow-up is needed to validate the success of DBS in patients with TS, initial success provides hope. Stimulation-dependent side effects reported include dizziness, decreased energy, and changes in sexual function. Only patients with severe, debilitating, and treatment-refractory illness should be considered; while those with severe personality disorders and substance abuse problems should be excluded. And as with all surgical interventions, the potential benefits must be weighed against the risks of surgery. In summary, the use of neurosurgical procedures for the treatment of OCD and TS is encouraging but remains experimental. It should only be performed in careful research settings with extensive cooperation between neurosurgery, neurology, neuropsychiatry, psychiatry, and bioethics. If preliminary findings hold, DBS may provide a safe, well tolerated, and potentially reversible procedure for the treatment of the most debilitated and refractory patients.

REFERENCES

1. Lajonchere C, Nortz M, Finger S. Gilles de la Tourette and the discovery of Tourette syndrome. Includes a translation of his 1884 article. *Arch Neurol.* 1996;53: 567–574.
2. Kurlan R, Como PG, Miller B, et al. The behavioral spectrum of tic disorders: a community-based study. *Neurology* 2002;59:414–420.
3. Sadock B, Sadock V. *Kaplan and Sadock's Comprehensive Textbook of Psychiatry.* Philadelphia: Lippincott Williams & Wilkins; 7th edition. 2000:2717–2719.
4. Greenberg B. Update on deep brain stimulation. *J ECT.* 2002;18:193–196.
5. Tronnier VM, Fogel W, Krause M, et al. High frequency stimulation of the basal ganglia for the treatment of movement disorders: current status and clinical results. *Minim Invasive Neurosurg.* 2002;45:91–96.
6. Nuttin B, Cosyns P, Demeulemeester H. Electrical stimulation in anterior limbs of internal capsules in patients with obsessive-compulsive disorder. *Lancet* 1999;354:1526.
7. Gabriels L, Cosyns P, Nuttin B. Deep brain stimulation for treatment-refractory obsessive-compulsive disorder: psychopathological and neuropsychological outcome in three cases. *Acta Psychiatr Scand.* 2003;107:275–282.
8. American Psychiatric Association. *Diagnostic and Statistical Manual of Mental Disorders. Fourth ed. Text revision (DSM-IV-TR).* Washington DC: American Psychiatric Association, 2000.
9. Robertson MM. Diagnosing Tourette syndrome: is it a common disorder? *J Psychosom Res.* 2003;55:3–6.
10. Robertson MM. The Gilles de la Tourette Syndrome: the current status. *Br J Psychiatry.* 1989;154:147–169.
11. Cummings JL, Frankel M. Gilles de la Tourette syndrome and the neurological basis of obsessions and compulsions. *Biol Psychiatry.* 1985;20:1117–1126.
12. Miguel EC, do Rosario-Campos MC, Shavitt RG. The tic-related obsessive-compulsive disorder phenotype and treatment implications. *Adv Neurol.* 2001;85: 43–55.
13. Coffey BJ, Miguel EC, Biederman J, et al. Tourette's disorder with and without obsessive-compulsive disorder in adults: are they different? *J Nerv Ment Dis.* 1998;186:201–206.
14. Narrow WE, Rae DS, Robins LN, et al. Revised prevalence estimates of mental disorders in the United States: using a clinical significance criterion to reconcile 2 surveys' estimates. *Arch Gen Psychiatry.* 2002;59: 115–123.
15. Rasmussen SA, Eisen JL. The epidemiology and clinical features of obsessive compulsive disorder. *Psychiatr Clin North Am.* 1992;15:743–758.

16. Murray CJ, Lopez AD. Global mortality, disability, and the contribution of risk factors: global burden of disease study. *Lancet* 1997;349:1436–1442.

17. Pauls DL, Alsobrook JP 2nd, Goodman W, et al. A family study of obsessive-compulsive disorder. *Am J Psychiatry*. 1995;152:76–84.

18. Pauls DL, Leckman JF. The inheritance of Gilles de la Tourette's syndrome and associated behaviors. *N Engl J Med*. 1986;315:993–997.

19. Pauls DL, Towbin KE, Leckman JF, et al. Gilles de la Tourette's syndrome and obsessive-compulsive disorder: evidence supporting a genetic relationship. *Arch Gen Psychiatry*. 1986;43:1180–1182.

20. Northam RS, Singer HS. Postencephalitic acquired Tourette-like syndrome in a child. *Neurology* 1991; 41:592–593.

21. Dale RC, Church AJ, Heyman I. Striatal encephalitis after varicella zoster infection complicated by Tourettism. *Mov Disord*. 2003;18:1554–1556.

22. Pulst SM, Walshe TM, Romero JA. Carbon monoxide poisoning with features of Gilles de la Tourette's syndrome. *Arch Neurol*. 1983;40:443–444.

23. Laplane D, Levasseur M, Pillon B, et al. Obsessive-compulsive and other behavioral changes with bilateral basal ganglia lesions. *Brain* 1989;112:699–725.

24. Stahl SM. Basal ganglia neuropharmacology and obsessive-compulsive disorder: the obsessive-compulsive disorder hypothesis of basal ganglia dysfunction. *Psychopharmacol Bull*. 1988;24:370–374.

25. Insel TR, Winslow JT. Neurobiology of obsessive-compulsive disorder. *Psychiatr Clin North Am*. 1992;15:813–824.

26. Berardelli A, Curra A, Fabbrini G, et al. Pathophysiology of tics and Tourette syndrome. *J Neurol*. 2003;250: 781–787.

27. Mink JW. Basal ganglia dysfunction in Tourette's syndrome: a new hypothesis. *Pediatr Neurol*. 2001;25: 190–198.

28. Gerard E, Peterson BS. Developmental processes and brain imaging studies in Tourette syndrome. *J Psychosom Res*. 2003;55:13–22.

29. Riddle MA, Rasmusson AM, Woods SW, et al. SPECT imaging of cerebral blood flow in Tourette syndrome. *Adv Neurol*. 1992;58:207–211.

30. Moriarty J, Costa DC, Schmitz B, et al. Brain perfusion abnormalities in Gilles de la Tourette's syndrome. *Br J Psychiatry*. 1995;167:249–254.

31. Stern E, Silbersweig DA, Chee K, et al. A functional neuroanatomy of tics in Tourette syndrome. *Arch Gen Psychiatry*. 2000;57:741–748.

32. Jenike MA, Breiter HC, Baer L, et al. Cerebral structural abnormalities in obsessive-compulsive disorder: a quantitative morphometric magnetic resonance imaging study. *Arch Gen Psychiatry*. 1996;53:625–632.

33. Aylward EH, Harris GJ, Hoehn-Saric R, et al. Normal caudate nucleus in obsessive-compulsive disorder assessed by quantitative neuroimaging. *Arch Gen Psychiatry*. 1996;53:577–584.

34. Baxter LR, Schwartz JM, Mazziotta JC, et al. Cerebral glucose metabolic rates in non-depressed obsessive-compulsives. *Am J Psychiatry*. 1988;145:1560–1563.

35. Breiter HC, Rauch SL, Kwong KK, et al. Functional magnetic resonance imaging of symptom provocation in obsessive-compulsive disorder. *Arch Gen Psychiatry*. 1996;49:595–606.

36. Piacentini J, Chang S. Behavioral treatments for Tourette syndrome and tic disorders: state of the art. *Adv Neurol*. 2001;85:319–31.

37. Azrin NH, Nunn RG. Habit-reversal: a method of eliminating nervous habits and tics. *Behav Res Ther*. 1973;11:619–628.

38. Singer HS, Butler IJ, Tune LE, et al. Dopaminergic dysfunction in Tourette syndrome. *Ann Neurol*. 1982; 12:361–366.

39. Singer HS, Szymanski S, Giuliano J, et al. Elevated intrasynaptic dopamine release in Tourette's syndrome. *Am J Psychiatry*. 2002;159:1329–1336.

40. Turjanski N, Sawle GV, Playford ED, et al. PET studies of the presynaptic and postsynaptic dopaminergic system in Tourette's syndrome. *J Neurol Neurosurg Psychiatry*. 1994;57:688–692.

41. Meyer P, Bohnen NI, Minoshima S, et al. Striatal presynaptic monoaminergic vesicles are not increased in Tourette's syndrome. *Neurology* 1999;53:371–374.

42. Gaffney GR, Perry PJ, Lund BC, et al. Risperidone versus clonidine in the treatment of children and adolescents with Tourette's syndrome. *J Am Acad Child Adolesc Psychiatry*. 2002;41:330–336.

43. Kopell BH, Rezai AR. Psychiatric neurosurgery: a historical perspective. *Neurosurg Clin N Am*. 2003;14:181–197.

44. Talairach J, Bancaud J, Geier S, et al. The cingulate gyrus and human behaviour. *Electroencephalogr Clin Neurophysiol*. 1973;34:45–52.

45. Greenberg BD, Price LH, Rauch SC, et al. Neurosurgery for intractable obsessive-compulsive disorder and depression: critical issues. *Neurosurg Clin N Am*. 2003;14:199–212.

46. Temel Y, Visser-Vanderwalle V. Surgery in Tourette syndrome. *Mov Disord*. 2004;91:3–14.

47. Cappabianca P, Spaziante R, Carrabs G, et al. Surgical sterotactic treatment for Gilles de la Tourette's syndrome. *Acta Neurol (Napoli)*. 1987;9:273–280.

48. Ohye C. Use of selective thalamotomy for various kinds of movement disorder, based on basic studies. *Stereotact Funct Neurosurg*. 2000;75:54–65.

49. Babel TB, Warnke PC, Ostertag CB. Immediate and long term outcome after infrathalamic and thalamic lesioning for intractable Tourette's syndrome. *J Neurol Neurosurg Psychiatry*. 2001;70:666–671.

50. Herrero MT, Barcia C, Navarro JM. Functional anatomy of thalamus and basal ganglia. *Childs Nerv Syst*. 2002;18:386–404.

51. Kimura M, Minamimoto T, Matsumoto N, et al. Monitoring and switching of cortico-basal ganglia loop functions by the thalamo-striatal system. *Neurosci Res*. 2004;48:355–360.

52. Baker EFW. Gilles de la Tourette syndrome treated by bimedial leucotomy. *Can Med Assoc J*. 1962;86: 746–747.

53. Cooper IS. Dystonia reversal by operation in the basal ganglia. *Arch Neurol*. 1962;7:64–74.

54. Hassler R, Dieckmann G. Stereotaxic treatment of tics and inarticulate cries or coprolalia considered as motor obsessional phenomena in Gilles de la Tourette's disease. *Rev Neurol*. (Paris). 1970;123(2):89–100.

55. de Divitiis E, D'Errico A, Cerillo A. Stereotactic surgery in Gilles de la Tourette syndrome. *Acta Neurochirurgica*. 1977;73:

56. Kulisevsky J, Berthier ML, Avila A. Longitudinal evolution of prefrontal leucotomy in Tourette's syndrome. *Mov Disord*. 1995;10:345–348.

57. OCD-DBS Collaborative Group. Deep brain stimulation for psychiatric disorders. *Neurosurgery.* 2002;51:519.

58. Nuttin BJ, Gabriels LA, Cosyns PR, et al. Long-term electrical capsular stimulation in patients with obsessive-compulsive disorder. *Neurosurgery.* 2003;52:1263–1274.

59. Rezai AR, Friehs G, Nuttin B, et al. Deep brain stimulation for the treatment of obsessive-compulsive disorder: preliminary results from a multicenter prospective trial. Presented at: Annual Meeting of the American Association of Neurological Surgeons; April 29, 2003; San Diego, CA.

60. Visser-Vandewalle V, Temel Y, Boon P, et al. Chronic bilateral thalamic stimulation: a new therapeutic approach in intractable Tourette syndrome. *J Neurosurg.* 2003;99:1094–1100.

61. Visser-Vandewalle V, Temel Y, Cath D. Deep brain stimulation in patients with intractable Tourette syndrome: two targets? Poster abstract at: Fourth International Scientific Symposium on Tourette Syndrome; June 2004; Cleveland, OH.

62. Maddux B, Riley D, Whitney C, et al. Chronic deep brain stimulation for medically intractable Tourette Syndrome: a case report of the first successful North American clinical experience. Poster abstract at: Fourth International Scientific Symposium on Tourette Syndrome; June 2004; Cleveland, OH.

26

Future and Alternative Therapies in Tourette Syndrome

Roger Kurlan

Department of Neurology, University of Rochester, Rochester, New York

The ultimate therapy of Tourette syndrome (TS) will involve prevention of the condition and complete elimination of all symptoms for any individual developing the disorder. Such prevention and cure are not currently in sight because they await the elucidation of the detailed molecular pathogenesis of TS, which is far from complete. In the past few years there has been dramatic and exciting progress in the understanding of the etiology of other neurologic movement disorders that have similarities to TS. This chapter reviews some of this information since it may provide a window into the types of neurobiologic abnormalities and therapeutic targets that might emerge as the molecular mechanisms of TS are uncovered.

This discussion of potential neurobiologic mechanism-based future therapies in TS will be followed by a review of "alternative" or "complementary" therapies, a very different approach that is generally not based on scientific data or testing, but remains of great interest to individuals with TS and their families.

FUTURE THERAPIES

Molecular Genetics of Other Movement Disorders

Dystonia is an involuntary movement characterized by sustained tightening of muscles and twisting of the trunk or limbs. Individuals with TS sometimes exhibit so-called "dystonic" tics (1), a form of motor tics that resembles dystonia in that there is tonic tightening of body areas (e.g., abdomen, shoulders, buttocks) or sustained twisting of a body region (e.g., neck, arm, foot/ankle). Disturbances of dopamine neurotransmission and a motor control physiologic disturbance of surround inhibition have been implicated in both tics (2,3) and dystonia (4,5). To date, mutations at a total of 14 different genetic loci (termed *DYT1* through *DYT14*) have been identified to cause different hereditary dystonia syndromes (6). For two of these with some similarities to TS, the abnormal gene product has been characterized, thereby providing new etiologic insights.

Genetic linkage studies, like those currently in progress for TS, led in 1997 to the successful identification of the DYT1 gene on chromosome 9 as the disease locus for most cases of early-onset, early-limb involvement autosomal dominant dystonia (7). Shortly thereafter, it was found that the DYT1 gene coded for a protein termed torsinA, a member of the newly discovered AAA+ superfamily of adenosine triphosphatases that function as molecular chaperones in a variety of intracellular activities, including protein folding, degrading misfolded proteins and trafficking membranes and newly assembled organelles (8,9). TorsinA appears to be widely distributed throughout the central nervous system but torsinA messenger RNA expression in the dopaminergic neurons of the substantia nigra pars compacta is particularly robust (10,11). Recent information suggests that mutant torsinA might affect presynaptic release of striatal dopamine resulting in increased dopamine turnover (12). Because it has been localized to the intracellular sites of aggregations of misfolded proteins, co-localized with ubiquitin, mutant torsinA might disrupt neuronal homeostasis and neurotransmission by failing to properly manage malformed protein structures (13). Evidence suggests that this process may be particularly disturbed in the setting of oxidative stress, which is known to accompany dopamine metabolism in the striatum (14).

Recent molecular data suggest that DYT1 dystonia may not be a model for a hyperkinetic movement disorder like TS, but rather is more accurately viewed as a hypokinetic, parkinsons-like condition with progressive immobility over time. TorsinA has been shown to form aggregates along with two proteins implicated in the pathogenesis of forms of inherited parkinsonism, α-synuclein and parkin (15,16). All 3 proteins have been localized to vesicles within presynaptic neuronal terminals and all have been associated with perturbations in dopamine homeostasis (4,15–18).

Hereditary myoclonus-dystonia (DYT11) may be a better model for TS. It is an autosomal dominant condition characterized by dystonia and rapid muscle jerks of myoclonus (described as "jerky dystonia"). The gene for this condition has been mapped to 7q21 (19) and it codes for epsilon-sarcoglycan, a protein with unclear function in the brain (20). Preliminary evidence points to a general role in structurally supporting the intracellular cytoskeleton and perhaps a more specific role in maintaining the architecture of postsynaptic gamma-butyric acid (GABA) receptors (21). Disturbed GABAergic inhibition in certain brain areas could result in the involuntary movements of dystonia and myoclonus.

Myoclonus-dystonia is a condition with interesting parallels to TS. In addition to the movement disorder, like TS, myoclonus-dystonia is associated with obsessive compulsive disorder (22). Like TS (23), there is evidence of maternal imprinting of the myoclonus-dystonia gene. There is significantly reduced penetrance if the disease allele is passed on by the mother (21). Of interest to TS, a condition with childhood onset, parental imprinting has been described for many genes, particularly those involved in early embryonic development (21).

Genetic loci and gene products have been identified in other neurologic movement disorders with more tenuous links to TS. Most of these conditions begin in adulthood and are neurodegenerative, causing progressive neurologic decline and death. This course is very different from TS, where symptoms wax and wane over time and typically lessen or disappear in adulthood so that the long-term prognosis is excellent. These natural history characteristics of TS are undoubtedly important clues into the types of developmental processes that will be found to be disturbed in the disorder.

Thus, recent advances in understanding other conditions with similarities to TS might provide examples of the types of molecular genetic mechanisms and therapeutic targets that could be involved in TS. These include disturbances of protein folding and degradation as seen in DYT1 dystonia and structural abnormalities of neurotransmitter receptors as may be occurring in myoclonus-dystonia. Based on its natural course, the systems affected in TS are likely involved in brain development, are disturbed in a fashion that does not cause progressive illness and have the capacity to normalize over time.

ALTERNATIVE THERAPIES

The knowledge of the detailed pathophysiology of TS is fragmentary and has not progressed to the levels described above for the hereditary dystonias. Intensive research efforts to identify disease genes in TS have been largely futile so far. In the absence of mechanistic information, our treatments for TS have largely evolved from empirical observations. In fact, the observation from the 1960s that neuroleptic dopamine receptor antagonist drugs suppress tics remains the strongest support for the prevailing notion of dopamine receptor supersensitivity underlying TS, resulting in a kind of circular mechanism-based pharmacotherapy. Nevertheless, solid scientific data from randomized, double-blind, placebo-controlled trials have documented the efficacy of classical neuroleptic antipsychotics, atypical antipsychotics, and alpha agonists in reducing tics. Similar proof exists for the efficacy of selective serotonin-reuptake inhibitors for associated obsessive compulsive disorder and stimulants, atomoxetine and alpha agonists for co-morbid attention deficit hyperactivity disorder (ADHD) (as discussed in other chapters of this volume).

Despite the availability of proven medications for TS and its most common behavioral co-morbidities, drugs that have successfully passed the rigorous testing for efficacy and safety demanded by the United States Food and Drug Administration (FDA), the use of alternative therapies remains of great interest to the community of individuals with TS. Although there has been little data collected, this interest probably stems from a variety of sources: the absence of neurobiologic understanding of the detailed pathogenesis of TS so that current treatments are not clearly rational and mechanism-based, the potentially bothersome side effects of current medications and a lay press that tends to focus on side effects and ignore therapeutic successes, a belief that alternative remedies are safer than prescription drugs, a lack of confidence that physicians are knowledgeable about alternative treatments, an attempt to lower medication costs, and a desire to take therapeutic control since most alternative treatments are readily available without a physician's prescription.

Because no alternative therapy proposed for TS has been subjected to standard scientific testing in a controlled clinical trial, this chapter will focus on general principles of alternative treatments, particularly herbal alternative medicines, as they may relate to TS (24,25).

Scope of the Issue

Treatments not part of the conventional medical system for managing health and disease were initially called *alternative*, probably reflecting a dissatisfaction with regular medicine and a kind of rebellion against the traditional biomedical community. Later, other terms, such as *complementary* or *non-traditional* treatments were added to reflect the view that standard and alternative therapies were not mutually exclusive and might be used together to treat or prevent illness. A number of academic medical centers have now established departments or centers of complementary medicine and National Institutes of Health has established the National Center for Complementary and Alternative Medicine to provide education and to fund research for this approach.

Alternative therapies include a variety of forms, including mind-body interventions (e.g., biofeedback, meditation, hypnosis), the use of electrical currents or magnetic fields, acupuncture and other Asian healing methods, manual treatments (e.g., acupressure, massage, spinal manipulation), biologic treatments (e.g., chelation), dietary approaches, and herbal medicines (24). A 1998 survey found that 40% of adult respondents in the United States had used alternative therapy during the previous year (26). Dietary supplements accounted for $6.5 billion in sales in the United States in the mid 1990s (27).

Studies have consistently shown that patients typically fail to report their use of alternative medicines to physicians even when specifically requested on health questionnaires (28). Thus, patients should be specifically asked about such treatments to obtain accurate information about the full scope of their medicinal regimen.

Do Alternative Therapies Improve Neurobehavioral Symptoms?

Of the alternative therapies, herbal medicines have been the mainstay of healing approaches throughout the world. Among the medical conditions most commonly reported by patients seeking herbal medicines, three are neurobehavioral, namely insomnia, anxiety, and depression (24).

Consumers should be aware that most herbal remedies in the United States are considered dietary supplements and thus are not regulated as medicines and are not required to meet the standards for drugs set forth in the Federal Food, Drug, and Cosmetic Act (25). They are marketed without prior approval of their efficacy or safety by the FDA. Manufacturers are permitted to claim that their herbal product affects the structure or function of the body but there must be no claim of effectiveness for treatment of a specific disease (25). Because the herbal industry is not required to demonstrate efficacy, only a tiny fraction of herbal medicines have been tested rigorously in appropriate clinical trials. Furthermore, there is little data available on direct comparisons between herbal and conventional medicines.

For the common neurobehavioral symptoms, randomized controlled trials have produced conflicting results for the efficacy of St. John's wort for depression (29) but suggest some benefit of kava for the treatment of anxiety (30). In the case of kava, however, potential therapeutic benefit may be outweighed by an unpredictable risk of serious hepatic toxicity (25). Trials of valerian root for the treatment of insomnia have provided inconclusive results (25,31).

It is reasonable to consider that herbal medicines might have benefit for some neurobehavioral symptoms. Roughly 25% to 50% of current pharmaceuticals were procured from plants (32). A number of herbal products have demonstrated actions within the brain. St. John's wort, for example, shows evidence of inhibition of serotonin reuptake (33) and some actions on GABA-A and GABA-B receptors (29).

A variety of alternative treatments have been recommended for TS, such as dietary restrictions, vitamins A, B, C, and E; niacin; magnesium; and calcium supplements. Gingko biloba has been proposed for the treatment of ADHD and there has been recent interest in St. John's wort for obsessive compulsive disorder (34). As mentioned earlier, however, no clinical trial has been performed to support the efficacy of any alternative therapy for TS or its associated behavioral disorders. Natural history features of TS demand the performance of scientifically controlled trials to establish efficacy of any therapy. First, the natural waxing and waning of tics means that exacerbations are inevitably followed by remissions. Thus, any intervention made at the time of peak symptoms will appear to improve the illness but, in the absence of randomized, placebo-controlled and double-blind treatment, the effect will be indistinguishable from the spontaneous improvement that will almost always follow. Similar trial designs are

needed to distinguish long-term efficacy of an intervention for tics from the natural tendency of the condition to improve over time. Finally, clinical trials of conventional tic-suppressing medications have documented that a substantial response to placebo occurs in TS, necessitating inclusion of placebo control to test the efficacy of any possible treatment.

It is recommended that clinicians should not prescribe or recommend herbal medicines in the absence of evidence of efficacy derived from rigorous study (25). In a recent editorial, former Surgeon General, Dr. C. Everett Koop, wrote that the potential role of alternative treatments in meeting current and future health care needs "can only be played if that industry and its proponents are prepared to meet real scientific and regulatory tests of safety and effectiveness" (35). The multicenter research collaboration, the Tourette Syndrome Study Group, currently headed by the author of this chapter, has great interest in conducting randomized controlled clinical trials of alternative therapies that show promise in treating TS.

Are Alternative Therapies Safe?

Aside from data about efficacy, recommendations regarding any form of treatment for TS must be based on information about safety. The oath of "do no harm" must guide therapy. Contrary to popular belief, alternative medicines are not necessarily safe and may be associated with potentially life threatening side effects and interactions with prescription drugs. Adverse effects on the heart, liver, kidney, and brain (e.g., seizures) can occur with a variety of herbal remedies (25). There is growing appreciation of potentially dangerous interactions between herbs and conventional drugs (25,36). As examples, Gingko biloba combined with aspirin or warfarin can result in bleeding reactions (25). Relevant to TS, St. John's wort can influence plasma levels of other drugs, including selective serotonin reuptake inhibitors and tricyclic antidepressants (25). It appears that any medication that is a substrate for cytochrome P450 3A4 or the P-glycoprotein transmembrane pump may pose interaction risks when combined with

St. John's wort (36). The issue of potential drug interactions is highlighted by a recent United States survey that found one in six adults taking prescription drugs reported concomitant use of at least one alternative product during the prior week (37). Consumers should be aware that proof of safety is not required prior to the marketing of herbal medicines in the United States. Under current regulations, if a safety concern arises, the burden of proof lies not with the manufacturer, but with the FDA, which must prove that the product is unsafe (25).

Aside from direct adverse effects and adverse drug interactions, the use of alternative medications may cause problems by delaying appropriate medical evaluation, diagnosis, and treatment. This is a cost of missed opportunity. It is now well-established, for example, that delay in the diagnosis and treatment of ADHD is associated with poorer long-term outcomes (38,39). Another potential problem of alternative treatments are their costs, which can cause significant financial burdens to the individuals purchasing them. In the case of TS, in the absence of evidence of efficacy, such monies might be better spent on established medications or potentially more helpful interventions, such as counseling or tutoring.

systems implicated in the disorder, and the functional consequences stabilize or resolve over time once synaptogenesis is completed. Clarification of the molecular mechanisms of TS will undoubtedly present new therapeutic targets and is the key to the development of preventive and curative therapies, whether by pharmacologic, genetic or other approaches.

Lack of knowledge about the molecular pathogenesis of TS is not adequate justification to use non-conventional alternative therapies. Any recommended treatment should have scientifically valid evidence of efficacy and safety. Such evidence is currently lacking for any alternative product in the treatment of TS. Alternative treatments can be expensive and are not necessarily benign since they can cause potentially dangerous side effects and drug interactions. Promising alternative therapies for TS should be rigorously evaluated in randomized controlled trials. A multicenter collaborative research group and potential sources of funding are now in place to accomplish this. Not only for safety reasons but also to provide clues to possibly effective products, clinicians should directly question TS patients about their use of and experience with alternative therapies.

CONCLUSIONS

The failure to localize disease genes and elucidate its molecular pathogenesis has greatly hampered progress toward better treating TS. The recent uncovering of the molecular genetic mechanisms in related hereditary movement disorders might shed light on the types of disease processes that could underlie TS. DYT1 dystonia points to mishandling of misfolded intracellular proteins. If relevant, perhaps in TS the mishandled proteins are those synthesized only during brain development so that later in life the pathogenic processes cease and the functional consequences stabilize or resolve. An underlying architectural instability of neurotransmitter receptors is suggested by hereditary myoclonus-dystonia. If relevant, perhaps in TS there is a structural disturbance of dopamine or norepinephrine receptors, neurotransmitter

REFERENCES

1. Jankovic J, Stone L. Dystonic tics in patients with Tourette's syndrome. *Mov Disord.* 1991;6:248–252.
2. Singer HS, Butler IJ, Tune LE, et al. Dopaminergic dysfunction in Tourette's syndrome. *Ann Neurol.* 1982;12:361–366.
3. Mink JW. Basal ganglia dysfunction in Tourette syndrome: a new hypothesis. *Pediatr Neurol.* 2001;25: 190–198.
4. Augood SJ, Hollingsworth Z, Albers DS, et al. Dopamine transmission in DYT1 dystonia. *Adv Neurol.* 2004;94:53–60.
5. Hallett M. Dystonia: abnormal movements result from loss of inhibition. *Adv Neurol.* 2004;94:1–9.
6. Bressman SB. Dystonia genotypes, phenotypes and classification. *Adv Neurol.* 2004;94:101–107.
7. Ozelius LJ, Hewett JA, Page C, et al. The early-onset-torsion dystonia gene (DYT1) encodes an ATP-binding protein. *Nat Genet.* 1997;17:40–48.
8. Neuwald AF, Aravind L, Spouge JL, et al. AAA+: a class of chaperone-like ATPases associated with the assembly, operation and disassembly of protein complexes. *Genome Res.* 1999;9:27–43.
9. Vale RD. AAA proteins: lords of the ring. *CJ Cell Biol.* 2000;150:F13–F19.

10. Augood SJ, Penney JB, Friberg I, et al. Expression of the early-onset torsion dystonia gene (DYT1) in human brain. *Ann Neurol.* 1998;43:669–673.

11. Augood SJ, Martin DM, Ozelius LJ, et al. Distribution of the mRNAs encoding torsinA and torsinB in the adult human brain. *Ann Neurol.* 1999;46:761–769.

12. Augood SJ, Hollingsworth Z, Albers DS, et al. Dopamine transmission in DYT1 dystonia: A biochemical and autoradiolographical study. *Neurology* 2002;59: 445–448.

13. Bragg DC, Slater DJ, Breakefield XO. TorsinA and early-onset torsion dystonia. *Adv Neurol.* 2004;94:87–93.

14. Hewett JA, Ziefer P, Bergeron D, et al. TorsinA in PC12 cells: localization in the endoplasmic reticulum and responses to stress. *J Neurosci Res.* 2003;72:158–168.

15. Sharma N, Hewett JA, Ozelius LJ, et al. TorsinA has a tight intermolecular association with alpha synuclein in Lewy bodies: a fluorescence resonance energy transfer study. *Am J Pathol.* 2001;159:339–344.

16. Augood SJ, Keller-McGandy CE, Siriani A, et al. Distribution and ultrastructural localization of torsinA immunoreactivity in the human brain. *Brain Res.* 2003; 12–21.

17. Kahle PJ, Neurmann M, Ozmen L, et al. Subcellular localization of wild-type and Parkinson's disease-associated mutant alpha-synuclein in human and transgenic mouse brain. *J Neurosci.* 2000;20:6365–6373.

18. Maroteaux L, Campanelli JT, Scheller RH. Synuclein: a neuron-specific prtein localized to the nucleus and presynaptic nerve terminal. *J Neurosci.* 1998;8:2804–2815.

19. Nygaard TG, Raymond D, Chen C, et al. Localization of a gene for myoclonus-dystonia to chromosome 7q21-q31. *Ann Neurol.* 1999;46:794–798.

20. Zimprich A, Grabowski M, Asmus F, et al. Mutations in the gene encoding epsilon-sarcoglycan cause myoclonus-dystonia syndrome. *Nat Genet.* 2001;29:66–69.

21. Asmus F, Gasser T. Inherited myoclonus-dystonia. *Adv Neurol.* 2004;94:113–119.

22. Saunders-Pullman R, Ozelius LJ, Bressman SB. Inherited myoclonus-dystonia. *Adv Neurol.* 2002;89:185–191.

23. Lichter DG, Jackson LA, Schachter M. Clinical evidence of genomic imprinting in Tourette's syndrome. *Neurology* 1995;45:924–928.

24. LaFrance WC, Lauterbach EC, Coffey CE, et al. The use of herbal alternative medicines in neuropsychiatry. *J Neuropsychiatry Clin Neurosci.* 2000;12:177–192.

25. DeSmet PAGM. Herbal remedies. *N Engl J Med.* 2002; 347:2046–2056.

26. Austin JA. Why patients use alternative medicine: results of a national survey. *JAMA* 1998;279:1548–1553.

27. Brody JE. In vitamin mania, millions take a gamble on health. *New York Times.* October 26,199:7 Sect. 1.

28. Hensrud DD, Engle DD, Scheitel SM. Underreporting the use of dietary supplements and nonprescription medications among patients undergoing a periodic health examination. *Mayo Clinic Proc.* 1999;74: 443–447.

29. Meltzer-Brody SE. St. John's wort: clinical status in psychiatry. *CNS Spectrums.* 2001;6:835–840.

30. Pittler MH, Ernst E. Kava extract for treating anxiety. *Cochrane Database Syst Rev.* 2002;2:CD003383.

31. Krystal AD, Ressler I. The use of valerian in neuropsychiatry. *CNS Spectrums.* 2001;6:841–847.

32. Frug-Berman A. Clinical trials of herbs. *Primary Care.* 1997;24:889–903.

33. Neary JT, Bu Y. Hypericum LI 160 inhibits uptake of serotonin and norepinephrine in astrocytes. *Brain Res.* 1999;816:358–363.

34. Taylor LVH, Kobak KA. An open-label trial of St. John's wort (Hypericum perforatum) in obsessive-compulsive disorder. *J Clin Psychiatry.* 2000;61:575–578.

35. Koop CE. The future of medicine. *Science* 2002; 295:233.

36. Cott JM. Herb-drug interactions: focus on pharmacokinetics. *CNS Spectrums.* 2001;6:827–832.

37. Kaufman DW, Kelley JP, Rosenberg L, et al. Recent patterns of medication use in the ambulatory adult population of the United States: the Slone survey. *JAMA* 2002;287:337–344.

38. Diagnosis and treatment of attention deficit hyperactivity disorder (ADHD). *NIH Consensus Statement.* 1998; 16:1–37.

39. Manuzza S, Gittelman Klein R, Bonagura N, et al. Hyperactive boys almost grown up. V. Replication of psychiatric status. *Arch Gen Psychiatry.* 1991;48: 77–83.

Subject Index